Minor Emergencies:

Splinters to Fractures

MINOR EMERGENCIES:

SPLINTERS TO FRACTURES

Philip Buttaravoli, M.D., FACEP
Medical Director of the Emergency Department
Palm Beach Gardens Medical Center
Palm Beach, Florida

Thomas Stair, M.D., FACEP
Attending Emergency Physician
Department of Emergency Medicine
Brigham and Women's Hospital
Lecturer
Harvard Medical School
Boston, Massachusetts

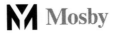 Mosby

An Imprint of Elsevier Science
St. Louis   London   Philadelphia   Sydney   Toronto

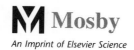

An Imprint of Elsevier Science

Editor: Elizabeth Fathman
Project Manager: Carol Sullivan Weis
Production Editor: Rachel E. McMullen
Designer: Judi Lang

NOTICE

Pharmacology is an ever-changing field. Standard safety precautions must be followed, but as new research and clinical experience broaden our knowledge, changes in treatment and drug therapy may become necessary or appropriate. Readers are advised to check the most current product information provided by the manufacturer of each drug to be administered to verify the recommended dose, the method and duration of administration, and contraindications. It is the responsibility of the treating physician, relying on experience and knowledge of the patient, to determine dosages and the best treatment for each individual patient. Neither the Publisher nor the editor assume any liability for any injury and/or damage to persons or property arising from this publication.

Mosby, Inc.
An Imprint of Elsevier Science
11830 Westline Industrial Drive
St. Louis, Missouri 63146

Printed in the United States of America

ISBN 0-323-00756-2

02   03   TG/FF   9   8   7   6   5

To my wife Susan, my son Frank, my father Frank,
and especially my mother Dorothy, who
removed all my childhood splinters.

PB

To Lucy

TS

Foreword

The first edition of *Common Simple Emergencies* was published in 1985. This new edition, *Minor Emergencies: Splinters to Fractures,* has been a long time coming but worth the wait. In the 15 years since the first edition was published, my good friends and colleagues, Drs. Buttaravoli and Stair, have gained that much more practical clinical and academic experience, which they have professionally infused into this new book. More information and tips are drawn from this experience, and the text is referenced with current and similarly practical journal articles. Although much is written in the numerous dense textbooks on emergency medicine, neither the texts nor the curricula in medical schools or training programs provide the quick and practical approach to those everyday encounters that the reader will find in this book.

Directed primarily at the practicing emergency physician, *Minor Emergencies: Splinters to Fractures* provides a wealth of practical and extremely useful information for a broad audience. It should prove a convenient reference for paramedics, medical students, nurses, physician assistants, and nurse practitioners, as well as house officers from all specialties. Many practicing physicians and housestaff do not come across the problems addressed in the book often enough to be familiar with them but do confront these issues frequently enough to need a quick guiding hand in dealing with them. It is also a useful addition to the library of the local urgent care or remote, isolated rural clinic. Even the diagrams and photographs are simple yet useful. This book tells you what to do and how to do it in a clear, concise, and enjoyable manner. Perhaps as importantly, the reader learns what not to do in a given circumstance.

From the recognition of hysterical coma to the repair of an earlobe from which an earring has been plucked, this book is brimming with interesting and practical tips. Not a shift will go by that you won't find something of use to see, do, or teach from this handy reference. Despite the proliferation of textbooks, continuing education courses, home study aids, and computer based resources, there is clearly a place for this book—in your pocket.

Robert J. Rothstein, M.D.

Preface

Much has happened in emergency medicine over the past 15 years. Since the first publication of this book under the title *Common Simple Emergencies,* Dr. Stair and I have accumulated over 45 years of combined experience in the practice of emergency medicine, his being more academic experience and mine more of a community hospital practice. We have tried to incorporate the advances in emergency medicine, including the latest research, in this present publication to produce an advanced, comprehensive, yet very practical and useful book for managing minor emergencies.

New topics have been added and original topics have been updated and expanded. Due to the more comprehensive review of this material, bold print has been added to highlight the key elements and thereby allow you to quickly review and treat a specific problem.

As much as things have changed over the past 15 years, some things never change. Patients continue to seek care from us for their minor emergencies, and they are still remarkably grateful when their problems are managed with compassion and respect, as well as clinical confidence and accuracy.

My hope is that this book will help more of these patients by being a useful resource for their respective caregivers.

Philip Buttaravoli

Preface to *Common Simple Emergencies*

Patients seeking medical care for minor emergencies are often experiencing as much anguish and/or pain as those experiencing truly life- or limb-threatening emergencies. These patients trust that the physicians who treat them will be as caring, confident, and thorough in their duties as they would be when presented with a major medical problem.

On the other hand, it is quite possible to find today's young physicians either totally perplexed or falsely confident when confronted with a simple clinical problem that they just haven't seen before. The risk, then, is that they will lose rapport with the patient, be unable to provide any useful service to the patient, or at worst, harm the patient.

It was with these problems in mind that in 1977 I began a lecture series for medical students at Georgetown University. *Common Simple Emergencies* grew out of that series.

Like the lectures, this book provides a review of the management of simple, acute, clinical problems and should assist the physician in dealing properly with these ubiquitous yet sometimes difficult situations.

I have found that, after providing patients with competent and sensitive care for the most minor and routine problems, I have been rewarded with gratitude no less intense that if I had performed major surgery.

Philip Buttaravoli

This book is written for the health care professional just beginning work in an emergency department or clinic, to provide some guidance with the majority of patient problems, which somehow are not covered in schools or textbooks. Even experienced practitioners, however, who have already learned many of these approaches from the oral traditions of medicine or who have evolved their own methods, may benefit from comparing their approaches with those in this book.

The approaches to common simple emergencies described herein are sometimes unorthodox but are the best we have come up with so far and do reflect our own current clinical practices. Whenever possible, our recommendations are based on our own or others' clinical research. Where formal studies were unavailable, as was often the case, we fell back on our clinical experience. We have avoided, as far as possible, promulgating unexamined medical traditions or repeating "the way we've always done it."

Much more basic and clinical research remains to be done on the management of common simple emergencies, and we welcome contributions from our readers concerning topics, approaches, insights, clinical trials, quantification, and analysis.

Thomas Stair

Acknowledgments

We would like to give special thanks for the professional input of Randolph G. Cleveland, M.D.; Linda Pao, M.D.; Douglas Leder, D.O.; John Li, M.D.; Michael Cassatly, D.M.D.; Rogelio A. Choy, M.D.; Mitchell S. Flaxman, M.D.; Stuart J. Schwartz, M.D.; Jerry Swyers, M.D.; Frank Cook, M.D.; Charles Eaton, M.D.; Brian Hass, M.D.; Alan Sara, M.D.; and Scott Fayne, M.D.

We would also like to express our sincere appreciation for both Liz Fathman's and Kathy Falk's trust, support, and perseverance, as well as the efficient and expert help from Robin Sutter, Christine Carroll Schwepker, Carol Sullivan Weis, Rachel E. McMullen, and Craig Hoffman.

A final thanks goes to Susan Mattern Buttaravoli for her eagle eye proofreading.

Contents

Contents

part 1

Neurologic and Psychiatric Emergencies

Bell's Palsy (Idiopathic Facial Paralysis)

Presentation

The patient with this condition is often frightened by his facial disfigurement. He complains of sudden onset of "numbness," a feeling of fullness or swelling, periauricular pain, or some other change in sensation on one side of the face; a crooked smile, mouth "drawing," or some other asymmetric weakness of facial muscles; an irritated, dry, or tearing eye; drooling out of the corner of the mouth; or changes in hearing or taste. Symptoms develop over several hours or days. Often there will have been a viral illness 1 to 3 weeks before or there may have been another trigger, such as stress, fever, dental extraction, or cold exposure. On initial observation of the patient, it is immediately apparent that he is alert and oriented, with a partial or complete unilateral facial paralysis that includes one side of the forehead (Figure 1-1).

What To Do:

✔ Perform a thorough neurologic examination of the cranial and upper cervical nerves and limb strength, noting which nerves are involved and whether unilaterally or bilaterally. **Ask the patient to wrinkle his forehead, close his eyes forcefully, smile, puff his cheeks, and whistle, observing closely for facial asymmetry.** Central or cerebral lesions result in relative sparing of the forehead. **Check tearing, ability to close the eye and protect the cornea,** corneal desication, hearing, and, when practical, taste. Examine the ear canal and pinna for herpetic vesicles and the tympanic membrane for signs of otitis media or cholesteatoma.

✔ Patients with facial paralysis accompanied by acute otitis media, chronic suppurative middle ear disease, otorrhea, or otitis externa require otolaryngologic consultation. Facial weakness progressing to paralysis over weeks to months, progressive twitching, or facial spasm suggests a neoplasm affecting the facial nerve. When facial paralysis is associated with pulsatile tinnitus and hearing loss, suspect a glomus tumor or cerebellar pontine angle tumor. **Diplopia, dysphagia, hoarseness, facial pain, or hypesthe-**

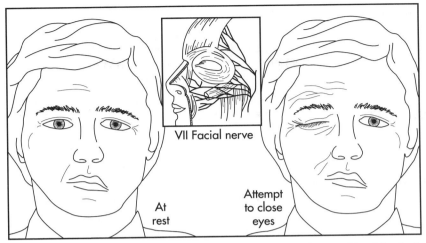

VII Facial nerve

At rest

Attempt to close eyes

Figure 1-1 Partial or complete unilateral facial paralysis that includes one side of the forehead.

sia suggests involvement of cranial nerves other than the seventh and calls for neurologic consultation.

✔ If there is a history of head trauma, obtain a CT scan of the head (including the skull base) to rule out a temporal bone fracture.

✔ **Because the most widely accepted cause at present is a neuropathy induced by herpes simplex virus, when a patient presents within 7 to 10 days of the onset of acute paresis or paralysis and there is no other suspected etiology, prescribe a 10-day course of either acyclovir (Zovirax) 200 to 400 mg 5 times a day or valacyclovir (Valtrex) 1000 mg bid. In addition, if there are no contraindications to steroid use** (i.e., hypertension, diabetes, peptic ulcer disease, tuberculosis, AIDS, or immunosuppression), **begin therapy with prednisone 60 mg qd, tapering after 5 days to 10 mg qd for another 5 days.**

✔ If the cornea is dry or injured as a result of the patient's inability to produce tears and blink, protect it by patching. If patching is not necessary, **recommend that the patient wear eyeglasses, apply methylcellulose artificial tears regularly during the day, and use a protective bland ointment or tape the eyelid shut at night.**

✔ Send a serum specimen for acute-phase Lyme disease titers, if available, because this is another treatable disorder that can present as a facial neuropathy. **In areas where Lyme disease is endemic, a 10-day course of tetracycline or doxycycline may be indicated.**

✔ If the cause appears to be herpes zoster-varicella or shingles of the facial nerve (e.g., grouped vesicles on the tongue), acyclovir or famciclovir should still be effective. If the geniculate ganglion is involved (i.e., Ramsay Hunt syndrome, with vesicles in the ear, decreased hearing, encephalitis, meningitis, etc.), the patient may require hospitalization for IV treatment.

✔ **Inform the patient that symptoms may progress for 7 to 10 days, reassure him that 70% to 80% of cases of Bell's palsy recover completely within a few weeks, and provide for definite follow up and reevaluation.**

✔ Provide appropriate specialty referral when there is a mass in the head or neck or a history of any malignancy.

What Not To Do:

✘ Do not overlook alternate causes of facial palsy that require different treatment, such as cerebrovascular accidents and cerebellopontine angle tumors (which usually produce weakness in limbs or defects of adjacent cranial nerves), multiple sclerosis (which usually is not painful, spares taste, and often produces intranuclear ophthalmoplegia), and polio (which presents as fever, headache, neck stiffness, and palsies).

✘ Do not order a CT scan unless there is a history of trauma or the symptoms are atypical and include such findings as vertigo, central neurologic signs, or severe headache.

✘ Do not make the diagnosis of Bell's palsy in patients who report gradual onset of facial paralysis over several weeks or facial paralysis that has persisted for 3 months or more. These patients require further evaluation by a neurologist or otolaryngologist.

 DISCUSSION

Idiopathic nerve paralysis is a common malady, affecting 1 in 5000 people every year, especially diabetic or pregnant patients and those between the ages of 15 and 45. Up to 10% of patients have a recurrence on the same or other side of the face. Although Bell's palsy was described classically as a pure facial nerve lesion and physicians have tried to identify the exact level at which the nerve is compressed, the most common presenting complaints are related to trigeminal nerve involvement. The mechanism is probably a spotty demyelination of several nerves at several sites caused by reactivated herpes simplex virus. Genetic, metabolic, autoimmune, vascular, and nerve entrapment etiologies have been proposed without definitive proof.

SUGGESTED READINGS

Adour KK, Ruboyianes JM, Von Doersten PG, et al: Bell's palsy treatment with acyclovir and prednisone compared with prednisone alone: a double-blind, randomized, controlled trial, *Ann Otol Rhinol Laryngol* 105:371-378, 1996.

Austin JR, Peskind SP, Austin SG, et al: Idiopathic facial nerve paralysis: a randomized double-blind controlled study of placebo versus prednisone, *Laryngoscope* 103:1326-1333, 1993.

Baringer JR: Herpes simplex virus and Bell's palsy (editorial), *Ann Intern Med* 124:63-65, 1996.

Murakmi S, Mizobuchi M, Nakashiro Y, et al: Bell's palsy and herpes simplex virus: identification of viral DNA in endoneural fluid and muscle, *Ann Intern Med* 124:27-30, 1996.

Stankiewicz JA: A review of the published data on steroids and idiopathic facial paralysis, *Otolaryngol Head Neck Surg* 97:481-486, 1987.

2

Dystonic Drug Reaction

Presentation

The patient arrives at the emergency department (ED) or clinic with peculiar posturing or difficulty speaking and is usually quite upset and worried about having a stroke. Often there is no history offered. The patient may not be able to speak, may not be aware she took any phenothiazines or butyrophenones (e.g., Haldol has been used to cut heroin), may not admit she takes psychotropic medication, or may not make the connection between her symptoms and drug use (e.g., one dose of Compazine given to treat vomiting). Acute dystonias usually present with one or more of the following symptoms:

Buccolingual—protruding or pulling sensation of the tongue

Torticollic—twisted neck or facial muscle spasm

Oculogyric—roving or deviated gaze

Tortipelvic—abdominal rigidity and pain

Opisthotonic—spasm of the entire body

These acute dystonias can resemble partial seizures, the posturing of psychosis, or the spasms of tetanus, strychnine poisoning, or electrolyte imbalances. More chronic neurologic side effects of phenothiazines, including the restlessness of akathisia, tardive dyskinesias, and parkinsonism, do not usually respond as dramatically to drug treatment as do the acute dystonias (Figure 2-1).

What To Do:

✔ **Administer 2 mg of benztropine (Cogentin) or 50 mg of diphenhydramine (Benadryl) IV, and watch for improvement of the dystonia over the next 5 minutes.** This step is both therapeutic and diagnostic. Benztropine produces fewer side effects (mostly drowsiness) and may be slightly more effective, but diphenhydramine is more likely to be on hand in the ED or physician's office.

✔ **Instruct the patient to discontinue use of the offending drug, and arrange for follow-up if medications must be adjusted. If the culprit is long acting, prescribe benztropine 2 mg or diphenhydramine 25 mg PO q6h for 24 hours to prevent a relapse.**

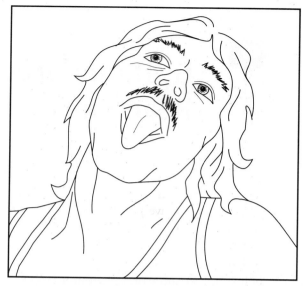

Figure 2-1 Patient with dystonic drug reaction.

What Not To Do:

✗ Do not persist with treatment in the face of a questionable response or no response, but get on with the work up in an attempt to find another cause for the dystonia (e.g., tetanus, seizures, hypomagnesemia, hypocalcemia, alkalosis, muscle disease).

✗ Do not use IV diazepam first because it relaxes spasms resulting from other causes and thus leaves the diagnosis unclear.

 DISCUSSION

The extrapyramidal motor system depends on excitatory cholinergic and inhibitory dopaminergic neurotransmitters, the latter being susceptible to blockage by phenothiazine and butyrophenone medications. Anticholinergic medications restore the excitatory-inhibitory balance. One IV dose of benztropine or diphenhydramine is relatively innocuous, rapidly diagnostic, and probably justified as an initial step in the treatment of any patient with a dystonic reaction.

SUGGESTED READINGS

Lee AS: Treatment of drug-induced dystonic reactions, *JACEP* 8:453-457, 1979.

3

Hyperventilation

Presentation

The patient is anxious and complains of shortness of breath and an inability to fill the lungs adequately (Figure 3-1). The patient also may have palpitations, chest or abdominal pain, tingling or numbness around the mouth and fingers, and possibly even flexor spasm of the hands and feet. His respiratory volume is increased, which may be apparent as increased respiratory rate, increased tidal volume, or frequent sighing. The remainder of the physical examination is normal. The patient's history may reveal an obvious precipitating emotional cause (such as having been caught stealing or being in the midst of a family quarrel).

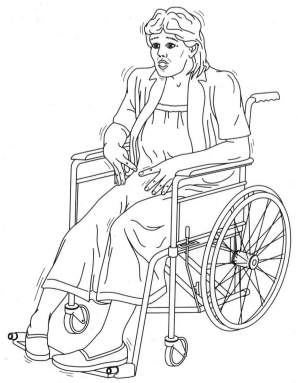

Figure 3-1 The patient experiences anxiety and shortness of breath and is unable to fill the lungs.

What To Do:

✔ Perform a brief physical examination, checking especially that the patient's mental status is good; there is no unusual breath odor; there are good, equal excursion and breath sounds in both sides of the chest; and there is no swelling, pain, or inflammation of the legs.

✔ **Measure pulse oximetry, which should be between 98% and 100%.**

✔ Explain to the patient the cycle in which rapid, deep breathing can cause physical symptoms upsetting enough to cause further rapid, deep breathing. Repeat a cadence ("in . . . out . . . in . . .") to help him voluntarily slow his breathing, or have him voluntarily hold his breath for a while.

✔ **If the patient cannot reduce his ventilatory rate and volume, provide a paper bag or length of tubing through which he can breathe (Figure 3-2), keeping the pulse oximetry monitor on to avoid hypoxia.** This will allow him to continue moving a large quantity of air but will provide air rich in carbon dioxide (CO_2), allowing the blood partial CO_2 (P_{CO2}) to rise toward normal. (Carbogen gas [5% CO_2] also may be used, if available.) **Administration of 50 to 100 mg of hydroxyzine (Vistaril) IM often helps to calm the patient.**

✔ **If these symptoms cannot be reversed and respiratory effort cannot be reduced in this manner within 15 to 20 minutes, double check the diagnosis by obtaining arterial blood gas measurements and looking for a metabolic acidosis or hypoxia indicative of underlying disease.**

✔ Reexamine the patient after hyperventilation is controlled.

✔ Ensure that the patient understands the hyperventilation syndrome and knows some strategies for breaking the cycle next time. (It may be valuable to have the patient reproduce the symptoms voluntarily.) Arrange for follow-up as needed.

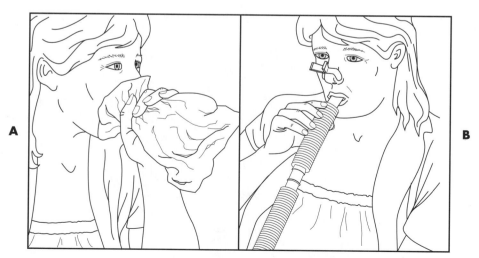

Figure 3-2 Instruct the patient to breathe through a paper bag **(A)** or length of tubing **(B)** to increase the percentage of inspired CO_2.

What Not To Do:

✗ Do not overlook the true medical emergencies, including pneumothorax, pneumonia, pulmonary embolus, diabetic ketoacidosis, salicylate overdose, sepsis, uremia, asthma, substance abuse, myocardial infarction, and stroke, that also may present with hyperventilation.

✗ Do not allow a patient with a low oxygen-saturation level determined by pulse oximetry (<96%) to breathe through a paper bag.

 ## DISCUSSION

The acute respiratory alkalosis of hyperventilation causes transient imbalances of calcium, potassium, and perhaps other ions, with the net effect of increasing the irritability and spontaneous depolarization of excitable muscles and nerves. First-time victims of the hyperventilation syndrome are the most likely to visit the emergency department or doctor's office, and this is an excellent time to educate them about its pathophysiology and the prevention of recurrence. Repeat visitors may be overly excitable or may have emotional problems and need counseling.

During recovery after hyperventilation, the transition from hypocapnia to normocapnia is associated with hypoventilation. Be aware that patients may experience significant hypoxemia after hyperventilation. Some investigators believe that there is no benefit in having a patient rebreathe his own exhaled air and that any benefit provided is the result of the reassurance of "instructional manipulation" and the patient's belief in the treatment rather than the elevated fractional concentration of CO_2 in inspired gas (F_{ICO2}).

SUGGESTED READINGS

Callaham M: Hypoxic hazards of traditional paper bag rebreathing in hyperventilating patients, *Ann Emerg Med* 18:622-628, 1989.

Chin K, Ohi M, Kita H, et al: Hypoxic ventilatory response and breathlessness following hypocapnic and isocapnic hyperventilation, *Chest* 112:154-163, 1997.

Demeter SL, Cordasco EM: Hyperventilation syndrome and asthma, *Am J Med* 81:989-994, 1986.

Saisch SGN, Wessely S, Gardner WN: Patients with acute hyperventilation presenting to an inner-city emergency department, *Chest* 110:952-957, 1996.

4

Hysterical Coma or Seizure

Presentation

The patient is unresponsive and brought to the emergency department on a stretcher. There is usually a history of recent emotional upset—an unexpected death in the family, school or employment difficulties, or the breakup of a close relationship. Hysterical coma and pseudoseizures rarely occur in social isolation. The patient may be lying still on the stretcher or demonstrating bizarre posturing or even asynchronous or thrashing, seizure-like movements. Head turning from side to side and pelvic thrusting are typical of psychogenic seizures. The patient's general color and vital signs are normal, without any evidence of airway obstruction. Commonly the patient will be fluttering her eyelids or will resist having her eyes opened. Tearfulness during the event argues against true epileptic seizure. There should not be fecal or urinary incontinence or lateral tongue biting. A striking finding is that the patient may hold her breath when the examiner breaks an ammonia capsule over the patient's mouth and nose. (Real coma victims usually move the head or do nothing.) A classic finding is that when the patient's apparently flaccid arm is released over her face, it does not fall on the face but drops off to the side. The patient may show remarkably little response to painful stimuli, but there should be no true focal neurologic findings and the remainder of the physical examination should be normal.

What To Do:

✔ Obtain any old medical records.

✔ **Perform a complete physical examination. Patients under stress of illness or injury sometimes react with hysterical coma.**

✔ **Do not allow any visitors, and place the patient in a quiet observation area, minimizing any stimulation until she "awakens." Check vital signs every 30 minutes.**

✔ **When there is significant emotional stress involved, administer a mild tranquilizing agent, such as hydroxyzine pamoate (Vistaril) 50 to 100 mg IM.**

✔ Consider obtaining a drug screen and investigating for possible sexual abuse. In women, consider ordering a pregnancy test.

✔ If a generalized seizure is questionable, verify with a lactate or blood gas level, which shows metabolic acidosis.

✔ When the patient becomes more responsive, reexamine her, obtain a more complete history, and offer follow-up care, including psychologic support if appropriate.

✔ **If the patient is not awake, alert, and oriented after about 90 minutes, begin a more comprehensive medical work up. Illnesses to consider include electrolyte disorders, hypoglycemia, hyperglycemia, renal failure, occult neoplasm, dysrhythmias, systemic infection, toxins, and neurologic disorders.**

What Not To Do:

✗ Do not get angry with the patient and torture her with painful stimuli in an attempt to "wake" her.

✗ Do not administer anticonvulsants when pseudoseizures are suspected.

✗ Do not perform expensive work ups routinely.

✗ Do not ignore or release the patient who has not fully recovered. Instead, she must be fully evaluated for an underlying medical problem, which may require hospital admission.

 DISCUSSION

True hysterical coma is an unconscious act that the patient cannot control. Antagonizing the patient often prolongs the condition, whereas ignoring her seems to take the spotlight off of her peculiar behavior, allowing her to recover. Some psychomotor or complex partial seizures are difficult to diagnose because of dazed confusion or fugue-like activity and might be labeled hysterical. If the diagnosis is not obviously hysteria, the patient might require an EEG administered during sleep and deserves a referral to a neurologist. Psychiatric disorders as potential causes of syncope or coma should be sought in young patients who faint frequently, patients in whom syncope does not cause injury, and patients who have many symptoms (e.g., nausea, lightheadedness, numbness, fear, dread).

SUGGESTED READINGS

Dula DJ, DeNaples L: Emergency department presentation of patients with conversion disorder, *Acad Emerg Med* 2:120-123, 1995.

5

Migraine Headache

Presentation

The patient complains of a steady, severe pain in the left or right side of his head, usually with photophobia and nausea but without vomiting. Sometimes the headache follows ophthalmic or neurologic symptoms that resolved as the headache developed. Scintillating castellated scotomata in the visual field corresponding to the side of the subsequent headache are the classic aura, but transient weakness, vertigo, or ataxia is more likely to bring a patient to the emergency department (ED). Unlike other headaches, migraines are especially likely to wake the patient in the morning. There may be a family or personal history of similar headaches as well.

What To Do:

✔ **Migraine headaches (and similar recurrent headache syndromes, with or without nausea and vomiting) are usually treated successfully with IV prochlorperazine (Compazine) 10 mg or metoclopramide (Reglan) 10 mg, with or without a liter of saline to counteract vasodilatation and orthostasis.**

✔ If the migraine is of recent onset, the patient has not already taken ergotamines, and starting an IV line may be difficult, begin treatment with sumatriptan (Imitrex) 6 mg SC or dihydroergotamine (DHE 45) 1 mg IM. These drugs are more expensive than prochlorperazine and metoclopramide and can have adverse cardiovascular effects. If dihydroergotamine is administered IV, pretreatment with an antiemetic, such as prochlorperazine, is necessary.

✔ **If the pain has been present most of the day and has precipitated a secondary muscle headache, evinced by scalp tenderness, add ketorolac (Toradol) 60 mg IM or ibuprofen (Motrin) 800 mg PO for nonsteroidal antiinflammatory effect.**

✔ If the pain persists and narcotic analgesics should be avoided, administer intranasal 4% lidocaine (Xylocaine). Use a 1-ml syringe. Have the patient lie supine with his head hyperextended 45 degrees and rotated 30 degrees toward the side of the headache, and drip 0.5 ml of the lidocaine solution into the ipsilateral nostril over 30 seconds. If the headache is bilateral, repeat on the other side. If after 2 minutes the headache persists, instill a second dose. Another relatively benign and inexpensive alternative to narcotics is IV infusion of magnesium sulfate 1 g in a 10% solution over 5 minutes. Most patients will have complete resolution of pain, photophobia, and nausea within 15 minutes.

✔ If the pain remains severe, add narcotic analgesics (e.g., meperidine 50 to 100 mg IM or IV) and have the patient lie down in a dark, quiet room. It can be cruel to attempt to obtain a complete history and physical examination (and is unrealistic to expect the patient to cooperate) before some relief of pain has been achieved.

✔ After 20 minutes, when the patient is feeling a little better, undertake the history and physical examination. **If there are persistent changes in mental status or on neurologic examination, a stiff neck, or fever, proceed with CT examination, lumbar puncture (LP), or both to rule out intracranial hemorrhage or infection as the cause of the "migraine."**

✔ **Other danger signals that should trigger a more intensive diagnostic work up include sudden onset of a new, severe headache ("the worst ever"); a progressive course; onset with exertion or during sexual intercourse; onset during or after middle age; and presence of a systemic malignant disease or infection or compromised immune system.**

✔ If the presentation is indeed consistent with a migraine, allow the patient to sleep in the ED, undisturbed except for a brief neurologic examination each hour. Typically the patient will awaken after 1 to 3 hours, with the headache completely resolved or much improved and no neurologic residua.

✔ For future attacks, if there are no cardiovascular risks, prescribe a self-injector preloaded with 6 mg of sumatriptan. If the patient prefers to take medication orally, try tablets of ergotamine 2 mg and caffeine 100 mg (Cafergot), two at the first sign of the aura, then one every half hour up to a total daily dosage of six tablets. If nausea and vomiting prevent oral medication, Cafergot is also available in rectal suppositories at the same dosage, but one or two suppositories are usually sufficient to relieve a headache. Sumatriptan can also be administered as a nasal spray. Use the lowest effective dose, either one or two 5 mg sprays or one 20 mg spray. The dose may be repeated once after 2 hours, not to exceed a total daily dose of 40 mg.

✔ Instruct the patient to return to the ED if there is any change in or worsening of the usual migraine pattern, and make arrangements for medical follow-up. First-time migraine attacks warrant a thorough elective neurologic evaluation to establish the diagnosis.

What Not To Do:

✘ Do not prescribe medications containing ergotamine, caffeine, or barbiturates for continual prophylaxis. They will not be effective used this way, and withdrawal from these drugs may produce headaches.

✘ Do not omit follow-up, especially for first attacks.

✘ Do not overlook possible meningitis, subarachnoid hemorrhage, glaucoma, or stroke, conditions that may deteriorate rapidly if undiagnosed.

13

💡 DISCUSSION

Even more characteristic of migraine than the aura is the unilateral pain. ("Migraine" is a corruption of "hemicranium.") The pathophysiology is probably unilateral cerebral vasospasm (producing the neurologic symptoms of the aura) followed by vasodilatation (producing the headache). Neurologic symptoms may persist into the headache phase, but the longer they persist, the less likely it is that they are caused by the migraine. Cluster headaches, probably also of vascular origin, are characterized by lacrimation, rhinorrhea, and clustering in time, but the treatment of an attack is usually the same as that for migraines.

Acute migraine headaches are self-limited and respond well to placebos, so many therapies are effective. Medications for acute migraine pass in and out of style, and the aforementioned represent popular regimens at the time of writing. Ergotamines, phenothiazines, and serotonin inhibitors may all work by cerebral vasoconstriction. Be cautious in the use of ergot or serotonin agonists to treat any patient who has angina, focal weakness, or sensory deficits. It is possible to precipitate ischemia of the brain or heart in such patients by using preparations that act by causing vasoconstriction. One recommendation is that sumatriptan not be administered to postmenopausal women, men older than 40 years, and patients with vascular risk factors, such as hypertension, hypercholesterolemia, obesity, diabetes, smoking, or a strong family history of vascular disease. Sumatriptan also should not be used within 24 hours after administration of an ergotamine-containing medication.

Patients with aneurysms or arteriovenous malformations can present clinically as migraine patients. If there is something different about the severity or nature of this headache, consider the possibility of a subarachnoid hemorrhage. Headaches that are always on the same side and in the same location are very suspicious for an underlying structural lesion (e.g., aneurysm, arteriovenous malformation).

Many patients seeking narcotics have learned that faking a migraine headache is even easier than faking a ureteral stone, but they usually do not follow the typical course of falling asleep after being given a shot and waking up a few hours later with pain relief. It is a good policy to limit narcotics for treatment of migraine headaches to one or two shots and avoid prescribing oral narcotics in the ED or doctor's office.

SUGGESTED READINGS

Cameron JD, Lane PL, Speechley M: Intravenous chlorpromazine vs intravenous metoclopramide in acute migraine headache, *Acad Emerg Med* 2:597-602, 1995.

Coppola M, Yealy DM, Leibold RA: Randomized, placebo-controlled evaluation of prochlorperazine versus metoclopramide for emergency department treatment of migraine headache, *Ann Emerg Med* 26:541-546, 1995.

Klapper JA, Stanton J: Current emergency treatment of severe migraine headaches, *Headache* 33:560-562, 1993.

Maizels M, Scott B, Cohen W, et al: Intranasal lidocaine for treatment of migraine, *JAMA* 276:319-321, 1996.

Mauskop A, Altura BT, Cracco RQ, et al: Intravenous magnesium sulfate rapidly alleviates headaches of various types, *Headache* 36:154-156, 1996.

Salomone JA, Thomas RW, Althoff JR, et al: An evaluation of the role of the ED in the management of migraine headaches, *Am J Emerg Med* 12:134-137, 1994.

6

Minor Head Trauma (Concussion)

Presentation

A patient is brought to the emergency department or clinic after suffering a blow to the head. There may or may not be a laceration, scalp hematoma, headache, transient sleepiness, or nausea, but there is no loss of consciousness, amnesia involving the injury or preceding events, seizure, neurologic change, or disorientation. The patient or family may express concern about a "mild concussion," the possibility of a skull fracture, or a rapidly developing scalp hematoma or "goose egg."

What To Do:

✔ Corroborate and record the history as given by witnesses. Ascertain why the patient was injured (Was there a seizure or sudden weakness?), and rule out particularly dangerous types of head trauma. (A blow inflicted with a brick or hammer is likely to produce a depressed skull fracture.)

✔ Perform and record a physical examination of the head, looking for signs of a skull fracture, such as hemotympanum or bony depression, and examine the neck for spasm, bony tenderness, limited range of motion, and other signs of associated injury.

✔ **Perform and record a neurologic examination, paying special attention to mental status, cranial nerves, strength, and deep tendon reflexes to all four limbs.**

✔ If the history or physical examination suggests a clinically significant intracranial injury, obtain a noncontrast CT scan of the head. **Criteria for obtaining a CT scan include documented loss of consciousness, amnesia, severe headache, persistent nausea and vomiting, cerebrospinal fluid leaking from the nose or ear, blood behind the tympanic membrane or over the mastoid (Battle's sign), confusion, stupor, coma, or any focal neurologic sign. The threshold for ordering a CT scan is lower if the patient is elderly (over 60 years of age), is taking anticoagulant medications, or has a known or suspected bleeding diathesis.**

✔ **If the history or physical examination suggests a clinically significant depressed skull fracture, obtain skull x-ray films. Criteria for obtaining skull x-ray films**

include a blow inflicted with a heavy object, suspected skull penetration, and palpable depression. If a depressed skull fracture is discovered, obtain a CT scan and arrange for neurosurgical consultation.

✔ **If there is no clinical indication for a CT scan or skull films, explain to the patient and concerned family and friends why x-ray images are not being ordered.** Many patients expect x-ray examinations but will gladly forego them once they understand that they are of little value. Also, provide reassurance as to the benign nature of a scalp hematoma despite the sometimes frightening appearance.

✔ Explain to the patient and a responsible family member or friend that the more important possible sequelae of head trauma are not always diagnosed by reading x-ray films but rather by noting certain signs and symptoms that occur later. Ensure that they understand and are given written instructions to seek immediate emergency care if any abnormal behavior, increasing drowsiness or difficulty in rousing the patient, headache, neck stiffness, vomiting, visual problems, weakness, or seizures are noted.

✔ Recommend that the appropriate length of time to abstain from sports participation after concussion ranges from 20 minutes for individuals manifesting only confusion without amnesia to 1 month for those experiencing loss of consciousness.

What Not To Do:

✗ Do not skimp on the neurologic examination or its documentation.
✗ Do not be reassured by normal skull films, which do not rule out intracranial bleeding or edema.

DISCUSSION

Because of the risks of late neurologic sequelae (e.g., subdural hematoma, seizure disorder, meningitis, postconcussional syndrome), good follow-up is essential after any head trauma, but the majority of patients without findings on initial examination do well. It is probably unwise to describe to the patient all of the subtle possible long-term effects of head trauma because many may be induced by suggestion. Concentrate on explaining the danger signs that patients should watch for over the next few days.

There is no universally accepted rule for determining whether CT head scanning is necessary. The criteria for ordering a CT scan suggested earlier represent a conservative but not scientifically proved approach. Patients with minor head injuries who meet the criteria for a CT scan but have a normal scan and neurologic examination may be safely discharged and sent home.

A large scalp hematoma may have a soft central area that mimics a depression in the skull when palpated directly but allows palpation of the underlying skull when pushed to one side. Cold packs may be recommended to reduce the swelling, and the patient may be reassured that the hematoma will resolve over days to weeks.

SUGGESTED READINGS

Borczuk P: Predictors of intracranial injury in patients with mild head trauma, *Ann Emerg Med* 25:731-736, 1995.

Davis RL, Hughes M, Gubler D, et al: The use of cranial CT scans in the triage of pediatric patients with mild head injury, *Pediatrics* 95:345-349, 1995.

Holmes JF, Baier ME, Derlet RW, et al: Failure of the Miller criteria to predict significant intracranial injury in patients with a Glasgow coma scale score of 14 after minor head trauma injury, *Acad Emerg Med* 4:788-792, 1997.

Madden C, Witzke DB, Sanders AB, et al: High yield selection criteria for cranial computed tomography after acute trauma, *Acad Emerg Med* 2:248-253, 1995.

Miller EC, Derlet RW, Kinser D: Minor head trauma: is computed tomography always necessary? *Ann Emerg Med* 27:290-294, 1996.

Miller EC, Holmes JF, Derlet RW, et al: Utilizing clinical factors to reduce head CT scan ordering for minor head trauma patients, *J Emerg Med* 15:453-457, 1997.

Mitchell KA, Fallat ME, Raque GH, et al: Evaluation of minor head injury in children, *J Ped Surg* 29:851-854, 1994.

Schunk JE, Rogerson JD, Woodward GA: The utility of head computed tomographic scanning in pediatric patients with normal neurologic examinations in the emergency department, *Pediatr Emerg Care* 12:160-165, 1996.

Shackford SR, Wald SL, Ross SE, et al: The clinical utility of computed tomographic scanning and neurologic examination in the management of patients with minor head injuries, *J Trauma* 33:385-394, 1992.

Staffeld L, Levitt A, Simon, et al: Identification of ethanol-intoxicated patients with minor head trauma requiring computed tomography scans, *Acad Emerg Med* 1:227-234, 1993.

Stiell IG, Wells GA, Vandemheen K, et al: Variation in ED use of computed tomography for patients with minor head injury, *Ann Emerg Med* 30:14-22, 1997.

7

Seizures
(Convulsions, Fits)

Presentation

The patient experiencing seizures may be found in the street, the hospital, or the emergency department (ED). The patient may complain of an "aura," feel she is "about to have a seizure," experience a brief petit mal "absence," exhibit the repetitive stereotypical behavior of continuous partial seizures, display the whole-body tonic stiffness or clonic jerking of grand mal seizures, or simply be found in the gradual recovery of the postictal phase. Patients experiencing grand mal seizures can injure themselves, most often by biting the tongue laterally, and generalized seizures prolonged for more than a couple of minutes can lead to hypoxia, acidosis, and even brain damage.

What To Do:

✔ If the patient is having a grand mal seizure, stand by her for a few minutes, until her thrashing subsides, to guard against injury or airway obstruction. Usually, only suctioning or turning the patient on her side is required, but breathing will be uncoordinated until the tonic–clonic phase is over.

✔ Watch the pattern of the seizure for clues to the etiology. (Did clonus start in one place and "march" out to the rest of the body? Did the eyes deviate one way throughout the seizure? Did the whole body participate?)

✔ **If the seizure lasts more than 2 minutes or recurs before the patient regains consciousness,** it has overwhelmed the brain's natural buffers, and drugs may be required to stop the seizure. **This is defined as** *status epilepticus* **and is best treated with diazepam (Valium) 5 to 10 mg IV, followed by gradual loading with IV phenytoin (Dilantin), 1 g given at less than 50 mg per minute.**

✔ Check the patient's blood glucose level (especially if she is wearing a "diabetes" MedicAlert bracelet or medallion) by performing a quick finger stick, and administer IV glucose if the level is below normal.

✔ If the patient arrives in the postictal phase, examine her thoroughly for injuries and record a complete neurologic examination (the results of which are apt to be bizarre). Repeat the neurologic examination periodically. **If the patient is indeed recovering,**

you may be able to obviate much of the diagnostic work up by waiting until she is lucid enough to give a history.

✔ If the patient arrives awake and oriented after an alleged seizure, corroborate the history through witness accounts or the presence of injuries, such as a scalp laceration or a bitten tongue. Doubt a grand mal seizure if there is no prolonged postictal recovery period.

✔ **If the patient has a history of seizure disorder** or is taking anticonvulsant medications, check her records, speak to her physician, find out whether an etiology has been determined, **look for reasons for this relapse (e.g., infection, ethanol poisoning, lack of sleep), and draw blood to determine levels of anticonvulsants.**

✔ **If the seizure is clearly related to alcohol withdrawal, ascertain why the patient reduced her consumption. She may be broke, be suffering from pancreatitis or gastritis that requires further evaluation and treatment,** or have decided to "dry out" completely. If she is demonstrating signs of delirium tremens, such as tremors, tachycardia, and hallucinations, her withdrawal should be medically supervised and treated with benzodiazepines (e.g., Librium, Valium, Ativan). Many emergency department physicians presumptively treat alcohol withdrawal symptoms with an IV infusion containing glucose, 100 mg of thiamine, 2 g of magnesium, and multivitamins.

✔ **If the seizure is a new event, make arrangements for a work up, including an EEG. About half of all patients with a new onset of seizure require hospitalization, and most of these patients can be identified by abnormalities evident on physical examination, head CT scans, or blood counts.** Other tests (lumbar puncture and serum electrolyte, glucose, and calcium measurements) may also identify new seizure victims who require admission.

✔ If the work up will be conducted on an outpatient basis, the patient should be given a loading dose of phenytoin (Dilantin) 17 to 20 mg/kg over 30 minutes IV or over 6 hours PO to protect her from further seizures. (With oral loading, 1 g of phenytoin capsules is divided into 3 doses [400 mg, 300 mg, 300 mg,] and administered at 2-hour intervals.) If there is any question, check a serum phenytoin level before administering this loading dose. Patients should be on cardiac monitoring during IV loading, which should be slowed if conduction blocks or dysrhythmias develop. **A neurologist should be consulted before phenytoin treatment is initiated for new-onset seizures. Many neurologists believe it is in the patient's best interest to withhold long-term anticonvulsant therapy until a second seizure occurs.** Fosphenytoin (Cerebyx) is a prodrug; its active metabolite is phenytoin. It is considerably more expensive than phenytoin, but it has the advantage of IM administration, which can be important in cases in which IV access cannot be easily obtained.

What Not To Do:

✘ Do not stick anything in the mouth of a seizing patient. The ubiquitous padded throat sticks may be nice for a patient to hold and bite on at the first sign of a seizure, but they do nothing to protect the airway and are ineffective when the jaw is clenched.

19

✘ Do not rush to give IV diazepam to a seizing patient. Most seizures stop within a few minutes. It is diagnostically useful to see how the seizure resolves on its own; also, the patient will awaken sooner if she has not been medicated. Reserve diazepam treatment for genuine status epilepticus.

✘ Be careful not to assume an alcoholic etiology. Ethanol abusers sustain more head trauma and seizure disorders than the population at large.

✘ Do not treat alcohol withdrawal seizures with phenobarbital or phenytoin. Both are ineffective (and unnecessary because the problem is self-limiting) and can themselves produce withdrawal seizures.

✘ Do not rule out alcohol withdrawal seizures on the basis of a toxic serum ethanol level. The patient may actually be withdrawing from an even higher baseline.

✘ Do not be fooled by pseudoseizures. Even patients with genuine epilepsy occasionally fake seizures for various reasons, and an exceptional performer can be convincing. Amateurs may be roused with ammonia or smelling salts, and few can simulate the fluctuating neurologic abnormalities of the postictal state. Probably no one can voluntarily produce the pronounced metabolic acidosis or serum lactate elevation of a grand mal seizure (see Chapter 4).

✘ Do not release a patient who has persistent neurologic abnormalities before a head CT scan or specialty consultation is obtained.

✘ Do not allow a patient who experienced a seizure to drive home.

DISCUSSION

Grand mal seizures are frightening and inspire observers to "do something," but usually it is necessary only to stand by and prevent the patient from injuring herself.

The age of the patient makes some difference as to the probable underlying etiology of a first seizure and therefore makes some difference in disposition. Up to 3 years of age, rapid rise in temperature can cause a generalized febrile seizure that does not lead to epilepsy and is best treated by control of fever. Brief febrile seizures may not require an LP to evaluate the cause of the fever, but these children should be managed in consultation with the primary care physician to ensure early follow-up. In the 12- to 20-year-old patient, the seizure is probably "idiopathic," although other causes are certainly possible. In the 40-year-old patient experiencing a first seizure, neoplasm, posttraumatic epilepsy, and withdrawal must be excluded. In the 65-year-old patient experiencing a first seizure, cerebrovascular insufficiency must also be considered. With such a patient, the possibility of an impending stroke in addition to the other possible causes should be kept in mind during treatment and work up.

For these reasons, a patient experiencing a first seizure who is 30 years of age or older must undergo a CT scan, preferably while in the ED. A noncontrast study can be obtained initially. If there are abnormalities present or if there are still suspicions of a focal abnormality, a contrast study can be obtained at the same time or later, whichever is most convenient.

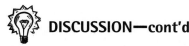 **DISCUSSION—cont'd**

Also, patients should be discharged for outpatient care only if there is full recovery of neurologic function, should possibly be given a full loading dose of phenytoin, and should make clear arrangements for follow-up or return to the ED if another seizure occurs. An EEG can usually be done electively, except in cases of status epilepticus. A toxic screen may be needed to detect the many drug overdoses that can present as seizures, including overdoses of drugs such as amphetamines, cocaine, isoniazid, lidocaine, lithium, phencyclidine, phenytoin, and tricyclic antidepressants.

SUGGESTED READINGS

Eisner RF, Turnbull TL, Howes DS, et al: Efficacy of a "standard" seizure workup in the emergency department, *Ann Emerg Med* 15:33-39, 1986.

Henneman PL, DeRoos F, Lewis RJ: Determining the need for admission in patients with new-onset seizures, *Ann Emerg Med* 24:1108-1114, 1994.

8

Tension (Muscle Contraction) Headache

Presentation

The patient complains of a mild-to-moderate, dull, steady pain, described as a pressing, tightening, squeezing, or constricting band, located bilaterally anywhere from the eyes to the occiput, perhaps including the neck or shoulders. Most commonly the headache develops near the end of the day or after some particular stressful event. There is usually no nausea or vomiting, although there may be anorexia, and these headaches may be associated with lightheadedness and feeling tired. The pain may improve with rest or administration of aspirin, acetaminophen, or other medications. The physical examination is unremarkable except for cranial or posterior cervical muscle spasm or tenderness and difficulty relaxing.

What To Do:

✔ **Obtain a complete general history (including environmental factors and foods that precede the headaches) and perform a physical examination (including a neurologic and funduscopic examination).**

✔ If the patient complains of sudden onset of the "worst headache of my life," a thunderclap headache that reaches maximal intensity within 1 minute, or a headache accompanied by any change in mental status, weakness, seizures, stiff neck, or persistent neurologic abnormalities, suspect a cerebrovascular cause, especially a subarachnoid hemorrhage, intracranial hemorrhage, aneurysm, or arteriovenous malformation. The usual initial diagnostic test for these is CT, but when CT is not available and the patient does not have focal neurologic findings, papilledema, or other signs of increased intracranial pressure, rule out these problems by performing a lumbar puncture (LP). Other indications for a CT scan are changes in frequency, severity, or clinical features of headaches or a new, daily, persistent headache.

✔ If the headache is accompanied by fever and stiff neck or change in mental status, rule out bacterial meningitis as soon as possible, again by performing LP.

✔ If there is a history or suspicion of head injury, especially in elderly patients or those on anticoagulants or with a bleeding diathesis, obtain a CT scan to rule out an intracranial hemorrhage. Chronic alcoholic patients must be presumed to be coagulopathic in these circumstances.

✔ **If the headache is nonspecific or was preceded by ophthalmic or neurologic symptoms that are now resolving, which is suggestive of a migraine headache, try prochlorperazine, sumatriptan, or ergotamine therapy** (see Chapter 5). If vasospastic symptoms persist into the headache phase, the cause may still be a migraine, but it becomes more important to rule out other cerebrovascular causes.

✔ If the headache follows prolonged reading, driving, or television watching and decreased visual acuity is improved when the patient looks through a pinhole, the headache may be the result of a defect in optical refraction, which is correctable with new eyeglass lenses.

✔ If the temples are tender, check for visual defects, myalgias, and an elevated erythrocyte sedimentation rate, which accompany temporal arteritis.

✔ If there is a history of recent dental work or grinding of the teeth, tenderness anterior to the tragus, or crepitus on motion of the jaw, suspect arthritis of the temporomandibular joint.

✔ If there is fever, tenderness to percussion over the frontal or maxillary sinuses, purulent drainage visible in the nose, or facial pain exacerbated by lowering the head, consider sinusitis.

✔ If pain radiates to the ear, inspect and palpate the teeth, which are a common site of referred pain.

✔ Finally, **after checking for all other causes of headache, palpate the temporalis, occipitalis, and other muscles of the calvarium and neck, looking for areas of tenderness and spasm that usually accompany muscle tension headaches. Watch for especially tender trigger points** (Figure 8-1) **that may resolve with gentle pressure, massage, or trigger point injection** (see Chapter 121).

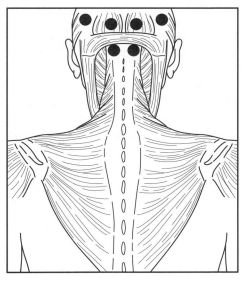

Figure 8-1 Tension headache trigger points.

✔ **Prescribe antiinflammatory analgesics (i.e., ibuprofen, naproxen), recommend rest, and have the patient try applying cool compresses** and massaging any trigger points.

✔ Explain the cause and treatment of muscle spasm of the head and neck.

✔ Tell the patient that there is no evidence of other serious disease (if this is true); especially inform him that a brain tumor is unlikely. (Often this fear is never voiced.)

✔ Arrange for follow-up. Instruct the patient to return to the emergency department or contact his own physician if symptoms change or worsen.

What Not To Do:

✘ Do not discharge the patient without providing follow-up instructions. Many serious illnesses begin with a minor cephalgia, and patients may postpone necessary early follow-up care if they believe that they were definitively diagnosed on their first visit.

✘ Do not obtain CT scans for patients who have recurrent headaches with no recent change in pattern, no history of seizures, and no focal neurologic findings.

✘ Do not overlook possible subarachnoid hemorrhage or meningitis. The majority of CT scans and LP results should be normal. If your results are usually abnormal, you may not be looking often enough. LP is more sensitive than CT for detecting subarachnoid hemorrhage within 12 hours after the onset of headache.

✘ Do not prescribe sumatriptan, ergotamine, or narcotics without knowledge of the patient's previously prescribed medications, nor without arranging appropriate follow-up.

 DISCUSSION

Headaches are common and usually benign, but any headache brought to medical attention deserves a thorough evaluation. Screening tests are of little value; a laborious history and physical examination are required.

Tension headache is not a wastebasket diagnosis of exclusion but a specific diagnosis confirmed by palpating tenderness in craniocervical muscles. (*Tension* refers to muscle spasm more than life stress.) Tension headache is often dignified with the diagnosis of "migraine" without any evidence of a vascular etiology and is often treated with minor tranquilizers, which may or may not help.

Focal tenderness over the greater occipital nerves (C2, 3) can be associated with an occipital neuralgia or occipital headache and can be secondary to cervical radiculopathy resulting from cervical spondylosis. This tends to occur in older patients and should not be confused with tension headache.

Thunderclap headache has been described with both ruptured and unruptured intracranial aneurysms. Even if a CT scan and LP are normal, magnetic resonance angiography is needed to rule out an unruptured aneurysm.

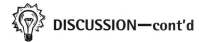 **DISCUSSION—cont'd**

Other causes of headache include carbon monoxide exposure from wood-burning heaters, fevers and viral myalgias, caffeine withdrawal, hypertension, glaucoma, tic douloureux (trigeminal neuralgia), and intolerance of foods containing nitrite, tyramine, or xanthine.

SUGGESTED READINGS

ACEP Clinical Policies Committee: Clinical policy for the initial approach to adolescents and adults presenting to the emergency department with a chief complaint of headache, *Ann Emerg Med* 27:821–844, 1996.

9

Vasovagal Syncope (Faint, Swoon)

Presentation

The patient experiences a brief loss of consciousness, preceded by a sense of warmth and nausea and awareness of passing out. First, there is a period of sympathetic tone, with increased pulse and blood pressure, in anticipation of some stressful incident, such as bad news, an upsetting sight, or a painful procedure. Immediately after or during the stressful occurrence, there is a precipitous drop in sympathetic tone, pulse, and blood pressure, causing the victim to lose postural tone, fall down, and lose consciousness.

Transient bradycardia and a few clonic limb jerks may accompany vasovagal syncope, but there are usually no sustained palpitations, dysrhythmias, seizures, incontinence, tongue biting, or injuries beyond a contusion or laceration resulting from the fall. Ordinarily the victim spontaneously revives after spending a few minutes supine, suffers no sequelae, and can recall the events leading up to the faint.

The whole process may transpire in an emergency department or clinic setting, or a patient may have fainted elsewhere, in which case the diagnostic challenge is to reconstruct what happened and rule out other causes of syncope.

What To Do:

✔ Arrange for anyone anticipating an unpleasant experience to sit or lie down and be constantly attended.

✔ If an individual faints, catch her so she will not be injured in the fall, lie her supine on the floor for 5 to 10 minutes, protect her airway, record several sets of vital signs, and be prepared to proceed with resuscitation if the episode turns out to be more than a simple vasovagal syncope.

✔ **If a patient is brought in after fainting elsewhere, ask about the setting, precipitating factors, descriptions given by several eyewitnesses, and sequence of recovery. Be alert for evidence of hyperventilation, hysteria, and seizures** (see Chapters 3, 4, and 7). **Record several sets of vital signs, including orthostatic changes, and examine carefully for signs of trauma and neurologic residua.**

Continue a more thorough evaluation of the patient suspected to have any blood loss, stroke, or pulmonary embolus.

✔ If there was no clear precipitating event or there are findings suggestive of dysrhythmia (such as age over 70 years, chest pain, palpitations, very sudden loss of consciousness, or administration of medications associated with dysrhythmia), begin a more comprehensive medical evaluation (including electrocardiography, specialty consultation, hospital admission, and monitoring).

✔ After full recovery, explain to the patient that fainting is a common physiologic reaction and that, in future recurrences, she can recognize the early lightheadedness and prevent a full swoon by lying down or putting her head between her knees.

What Not To Do:

✘ Do not allow family members to stand while being given bad news, allow parents to stand while watching their children being sutured, or allow patients to stand while being given shots or undergoing venipunctures.

✘ Do not traumatize the faint victim with ammonia capsules, slapping, or dousing with cold water.

✘ Do not discharge syncope patients who have a history of coronary artery disease, congestive heart failure, or ventricular dysrhythmia; patients who complain of chest pain; patients who have physical signs of significant valve disease, congestive heart failure, stroke, or focal neurologic disorder; or patients who have electrocardiographic findings of ischemia, bradycardia, tachycardia, increased QT interval, or bundle branch block.

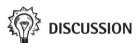 ## DISCUSSION

Most commonly, the cause of syncope in young adults is vasovagal or neurogenic. Observation of the sequence of stress, relief, and faint makes the diagnosis, but, better yet, the whole reaction can usually be prevented. Although most patients suffer no sequelae, vasovagal syncope with prolonged asystole can produce seizures and rare incidents of death. The differential diagnosis of loss of consciousness is extensive, and therefore loss of consciousness should not immediately be assumed to be caused by vasovagal syncope.

SUGGESTED READINGS

Graham DT, Kabler JD, Lunsford L: Vasovagal fainting: a diphasic response, *Psychosom Med* 6:493-507, 1961.

Lin JTY, Ziegler DK, Lai CW, et al: Convulsive syncope in blood donors, *Ann Neurol* 11:525-528, 1982.

Linzer M, Yang EH, Estes M, et al: Diagnosing syncope. I. Value of history, physical examination, and electrocardiography, *Ann Intern Med* 126:989-996, 1997.

Linzer M, Yang EH, Estes M, et al: Diagnosing syncope. II. Unexplained syncope, *Ann Intern Med* 127:76-86, 1997.

10

Vertigo (Dizziness, Lightheadedness)

Presentation

The patient may have a nonspecific complaint that must be further refined into an altered somatic sensation (giddiness, wooziness), orthostatic blood pressure changes (lightheadedness, sensation of fainting), or the sensation of the environment (or patient) spinning (true vertigo). In inner ear disease, vertigo is virtually always accompanied by nystagmus, which is the ocular compensation for the unreal sensation of spinning, but the nystagmus may cease when the eyes are open and fixed on some point. (By the same token, vertigo is usually worse with the eyes closed.) Nausea and vomiting are common accompanying symptoms, and (depending on the underlying cause) hearing changes, tinnitus, and cerebellar or adjacent cranial nerve impairment are less common. Diarrhea can be seen with episodes of severe peripheral vertigo.

What To Do:

✔ **Have the patient express how he feels in his own words (without using the word *dizzy*).** Ask about any sensation of spinning, factors that make the condition better or worse, and associated symptoms. Ask about drugs or toxins that could be responsible.

✔ **Determine whether the patient is describing vertigo (a feeling of movement of one's body or surroundings), a sensation of an impending faint, or a vague, unsteady feeling.**

✔ If the problem is near-syncope or orthostatic lightheadedness, consider potentially serious causes, such as heart disease, cardiac dysrhythmias, and blood loss.

✔ With a sensation of dysequilibrium or an elderly patient's feeling that he is going to fall, look for peripheral neuropathy, cervical spondylosis, stiff legs, and administration of vasodilator medication. These patients should be referred to their primary care physicians for management of underlying medical problems and adjustment of medications.

✔ If there is lightheadedness that is unrelated to changes in position and posture and there is no evidence of disease found on physical examination and laboratory evaluation,

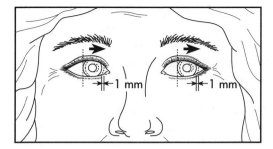

Figure 10-1 Eye should only move a few degrees to the left or right when examining for nystagmus.

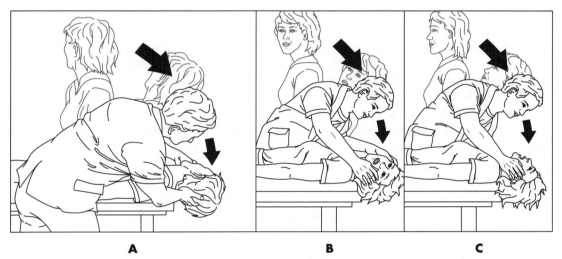

A   **B**   **C**

Figure 10-2 A, The patient's head is 30 degrees below horizontal. With her head turned to the right, quickly lower the patient to the supine position. **B,** Repeat with her head turned to the left. **C,** Repeat again with the patient facing straight ahead.

instruct the patient to hyperventilate by breathing deeply in and out 15 times. If this reproduces the symptoms, assess the patient's emotional state as a possible cause of his symptoms.

✔ **If the patient is having true vertigo, examine him for nystagmus, which can be horizontal, vertical, or rotatory** (pupils describe arcs). **Have the patient follow your finger with his eyes as it moves a few degrees to the left and then the right (not to extremes of gaze)** (Figure 10-1), and note whether there are more than the normal two to three beats of nystagmus before the eyes are still. Nystagmus may be detected when the eyes are closed by watching the bulge of the cornea moving under the lid.

✔ **If nystagmus is not clearly evident and the patient can tolerate it, attempt a provocative maneuver for positional nystagmus (the Nylen–Barany maneuver)** (Figure 10-2 *A* to *C*) by having the patient sit up, then lie back, and quickly hang his head over the stretcher side, turning his head 45 degrees to the right or left. Wait 30 seconds for the appearance of nystagmus or the sensation of vertigo. Repeat the maneuver on the other side. **When this maneuver produces positional nystagmus after a brief latent period lasting less than 30 seconds, it indicates a benign inner ear dysfunction. A normal test is not helpful in the diagnosis.**

✔ Examine ears for cerumen, foreign bodies, otitis media, and hearing loss.

✔ **Examine the cranial nerves. Test cerebellar function** (using rapid alternating movement, finger-nose, and gait tests). **Check the corneal blink reflexes** and, if absent on one side in a patient who does not wear contact lenses, consider acoustic neuroma.

✔ **Decide, on the basis of the aforementioned tests, whether the etiology is central** (brainstem, multiple sclerosis) **or peripheral** (vestibular organs, eighth nerve, cerebellopontine angle tumor). **Central lesions may require further work up,** otolaryngologic or neurologic consultation, or hospital admission, whereas **peripheral lesions, although more symptomatic, are more likely to be self-limiting.**

✔ **In the emergency department, treat moderate to severe symptoms of vertigo with IV diazepam (Valium) 5 to 10 mg or diphenhydramine (Benadryl) 25 to 50 mg. Add promethazine (Phenergan) 12.5 to 25 mg IV for nausea. If there are no contraindications (e.g., glaucoma), a patch of transdermal scopolamine (Transderm Scōp) can be worn for 3 days.** Some authors recommend hydroxyzine (Vistaril, Atarax), and others suggest corticosteroids (Solu-Medrol, prednisone). Nifedipine (Procardia) had been used to alleviate motion sickness but is no better than scopolamine patches and should not be used for patients who have postural hypotension or take beta blockers. If the patient does not respond, he may require hospitalization for further parenteral treatment.

✔ **Treat vertigo symptoms in outpatients with diazepam 5 to 10 mg qid, meclizine (Antivert) 12.5 to 25 mg qid, diphenhydramine 25 to 50 mg qid, promethazine 25 mg qid, or hydroxyzine 25 to 50 mg qid and bedrest as needed until symptoms improve.**

✔ Arrange for follow-up if there is no clear improvement within 2 days or if there is any suggestion of a central etiology.

What Not To Do:

✘ Do not attempt provocative maneuvers if the patient is symptomatic with nystagmus.

✘ Do not give antivertigo drugs to elderly patients with dysequilibrium. These medications have sedative properties that can worsen the condition.

✘ Do not make the diagnosis of Meniere's disease (endolymphatic hydrops) without the triad of paroxysmal vertigo, sensorineural deafness, and tinnitus, along with a feeling of pressure or fullness in the affected ear.

✘ Do not proceed with expensive laboratory testing or unwarranted imaging studies. Most causes of dizziness can be determined through obtaining a complete patient history and clinical examination.

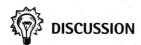 **DISCUSSION**

In general, the more violent and spinning the sensation of vertigo, the more likely the lesion is peripheral. Central lesions tend to cause less intense vertigo and more vague symptoms. Peripheral causes of vertigo or nystagmus include irritation of the ear (utricle, saccule, semicircular canals) or the vestibular division of the eighth cranial (acoustic) nerve caused by toxins, otitis, viral infection, or cerumen or a foreign body lodged against the tympanic membrane. The term *labyrinthitis* should be reserved for vertigo with hearing changes and *vestibular neuronitis* for the common, short-lived vertigo without hearing changes usually associated with viral upper respiratory tract infections. Paroxysmal positional vertigo may be related to dislocated otoconia in the utricle and saccule. If it occurs after trauma, suspect a basal skull fracture with leakage of endolymph or perilymph, and consider otolaryngologic referral for further evaluation and possible canalith repositioning maneuvers. Central causes include multiple sclerosis, temporal lobe epilepsy, basilar migraine, and hemorrhage in the posterior fossa. A slow-growing acoustic neuroma in the cerebellopontine angle usually does not present with acute vertigo but rather a progressive unilateral hearing loss with or without tinnitus. The earliest sign is usually a gradual loss of auditory discrimination.

Vertebrobasilar arterial insufficiency can cause vertigo, usually with associated nausea, vomiting, and cranial nerve or cerebellar signs. It is commonly diagnosed in dizzy patients who are older than 50 years of age, but more often than not the diagnosis is incorrect. Benign positional vertigo is the most common cause of vertigo in the elderly. The brainstem is a tightly packed structure in which the vestibular nuclei are crowded in with the oculomotor nuclei, the medial longitudinal fasciculus, and the cerebellar, sensory, and motor pathways. It would be unusual for ischemia to produce only vertigo without accompanying diplopia, ataxia, or sensory or motor disturbance. Although vertigo may be the major symptom of an ischemic attack, careful questioning of the patient commonly uncovers symptoms implicating involvement of other brainstem structures. Objective neurologic signs should be present in frank infarction of the brainstem.

Either central or peripheral nystagmus can be caused by toxins, most commonly alcohol, tobacco, aminoglycosides, minocycline, disopyramide, phencyclidine, phenytoin, benzodiazepines, quinine, quinidine, aspirin, salicylates, nonsteroidal antiinflammatories, and carbon monoxide. Nystagmus occurring in central nervous system disease may be vertical and disconjugate, whereas inner ear nystagmus never is. Central nystagmus is gaze directed (beats in the direction of gaze), whereas inner ear nystagmus is direction fixed (beats in one direction regardless of the direction of gaze). Central nystagmus is evident during visual fixation while inner ear nystagmus is suppressed.

SUGGESTED READINGS

Epley JM: Positional vertigo related to semicircular canalithiasis, *Otolaryngol Head Neck Surg* 112:154–161, 1995.

Froehling DA, Silverstein MD, Mohr DN, et al: Does this patient have a serious form of vertigo? *J Am Med Assoc* 271:385–388, 1994.

Herr RD, Zun L, Matthews JJ: A directed approach to the dizzy patient, *Ann Emerg Med* 18:664–672, 1989.

11

Weakness

Presentation

An older patient, complaining of "weakness" or an inability to carry on her usual activities or care for herself, comes to the office or emergency department (ED), often brought in by family members.

What To Do:

✔ **Obtain as much of the history as possible.** Speak to available family members or friends, as well as the patient, and ask for details. Is the patient weak before certain activities (suggests depression)? Is the weakness located in the limb girdles (suggests polymyalgia rheumatica or myopathy)? Is the weakness mostly in the distal muscles (suggests neuropathy)? Is the weakness caused by repetitive actions (suggests myasthenia gravis)? Is the weakness unilateral with slurring of speech or confusion (suggests cerebrovascular accident)?

✔ **Obtain a thorough medical history and physical examination, including a review of symptoms (e.g., headaches, weight loss, cold intolerance, change in appetite or bowel habits), strength of all muscle groups (graded on a scale of 1 to 5), deep tendon reflexes, and neurologic status. Order a head CT scan if there is an unexplained change in mental status or there are abnormal neurologic findings.**

✔ **Obtain a spectrum of laboratory tests that will yield results within the next 2 hours, including pulse oximetry, chest x-ray films, ECG, urinalysis, blood cell counts, sedimentation rate, and glucose, blood urea nitrogen, and electrolyte levels, which may disclose hypoxia, anemia, infection, diabetes, uremia, polymyalgia rheumatica, hyponatremia, or hypokalemia, common causes of "weakness." (Tests determining serum phosphate and calcium levels are also valuable, if results are immediately available.)**

✔ If no cause for weakness can be found, probe the patient, family, and friends once again for any hidden agenda, and if none is found, be sympathetic and reassure them that all the serious illnesses have been ruled out. At this time, send the patient home and make arrangements for definite follow-up.

What Not To Do:

✘ Do not order any laboratory tests that will not quickly yield results. Stick to tests that will return results while the patient is in the ED, and defer any long-term investigations to the follow-up physician. Obtaining laboratory results that will never be interpreted or acted on is worse than obtaining none at all.

✘ Do not insist on making the diagnosis in the ED in every case. The goals in the ED or during the first visit are to rule out acutely life-threatening conditions and then make arrangements for further evaluation. The primary care physician providing follow-up may consider disorders such as hyperthyroidism; hypothyroidism; chronic fatigue syndrome, or chronic Epstein-Barr virus infection; chronic parvovirus B19 infection; and Lyme disease.

 DISCUSSION

Approach the patient with "weakness" with an open mind, and be prepared to take some time with the evaluation. Demonstrable localized weakness usually points to a specific neuromuscular etiology, and generalized weakness is the presenting complaint for a multitude of ills. In young patients, weakness may be a sign of psychological depression, whereas in older patients, in addition to depression, it may be the first sign of a subdural hematoma, pneumonia, urinary tract infection, diabetes, dehydration, malnutrition, heart failure, or cancer. When a patient's weakness is probably based on a psychiatric problem, consider the somatoform disorders, such as hypochondriasis, anxiety and sleep disorders, malingering, depression, and factitious illness like Munchausen syndrome. It is important to exclude Guillain-Barré syndrome, which is one of the critical, life-threatening causes of weakness. The pattern is not always an ascending paralysis or weakness but usually does depress deep tendon reflexes. Botulism is another condition that must be excluded through the history or observation. Patients suffering from these sorts of neuromuscular weakness are in danger when they cannot breathe. Pulmonary function studies, such as pulse oximetry, capnography, blood gases, peak flow, or vital capacity, can be helpful in identifying patients who might be close to severe respiratory compromise.

part 2

Ophthalmologic Emergencies

12 Conjunctivitis

Presentation

The patient complains of a red, irritated eye; a sensation of fullness, burning, itching, or scratching around the eye; and perhaps a gritty or foreign body sensation, tearing or purulent discharge, and crusting or mattering of the eye. Examination discloses generalized injection of the conjunctiva, thinning out toward the cornea. (Localized inflammation suggests some other diagnosis, such as presence of a foreign body, episcleritis, or a viral or bacterial ulcer.) Vision and pupillary reactions should be normal, and the cornea and anterior chamber should be clear. Any discomfort should be temporarily relieved by instillation of topical anesthetic solution. Deep pain, photophobia, decreased vision, and injection more pronounced around the limbus (ciliary flush) suggest more serious involvement of the cornea and iris.

Different symptoms suggest different etiologies. Tearing, preauricular lymphadenopathy, and symptoms of upper respiratory tract infection suggest a viral conjunctivitis (Figure 12-1). Pain, lid crusting, and a copious purulent exudate present upon awakening suggest a bacterial conjunctivitis (Figure 12-2). If few symptoms are present upon awakening but discomfort worsens during the day, dry eye is probable. Minimal conjunctival injection, with a seasonal recurrence of chemosis and itching, and cobblestone hypertrophy of the tarsal conjunctiva suggest allergic (vernal) conjunctivitis (Figure 12-3). Physical and chemical conjunctivitis, caused by particles, solutions, vapors, and natural or occupational irritants that inflame the conjunctiva, should be evident from the history.

What To Do:

✔ **Instill proparacaine (Alcaine, Ophthaine) anesthetic drops** to allow for a more comfortable examination and to help determine whether the patient's discomfort is limited to the conjunctiva and cornea or, if there is no pain relief, the pain comes from deeper eye structures.

✔ **Examine the eye, including assessment of visual acuity and pupillary reaction, inspection for foreign bodies,** estimation of intraocular pressure by palpating the

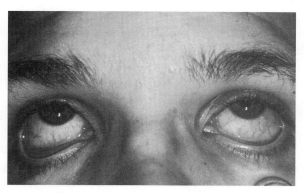

Figure 12-1 Viral conjunctivitis. *(Courtesy Dr. Kevin J. Knoop. From Knoop KJ, Stack LB, Storrow AB:* Atlas of emergency medicine, *New York, 1997, McGraw-Hill.)*

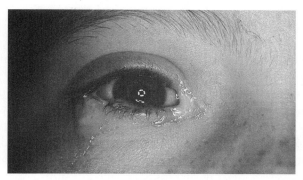

Figure 12-2 Bacterial conjunctivitis. *(Courtesty Dr. Frank Birinyi. From Knoop KJ, Stack LB, Storrow AB:* Atlas of emergency medicine, *New York, 1997, McGraw-Hill.)*

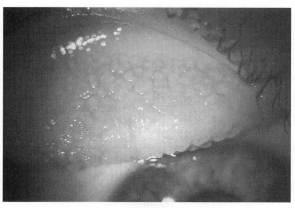

Figure 12-3 Allergic conjunctivitis. *(From Gausas RE, Raposa PA:* Hospital Medicine, *28(12):63-72, 1992.)*

globe above the tarsal plate, and examination with funduscopy, a slit lamp (when available), and **fluorescein staining and ultraviolet or cobalt blue light to assess the corneal epithelium.**

✔ Ask about and look for signs of any rash, arthritis, or mucous membrane involvement, which could point to Stevens-Johnson syndrome, Kawasaki syndrome, Reiter's syndrome, or some other syndrome that can present with conjunctivitis.

✔ **For bacterial conjunctivitis, instruct the patient to begin therapy by applying warm compresses q4h** followed by instillation under the lower lid of topical antibiotic **ointments** (which transiently blur vision), such as erythromycin (Ilotycin), sulfacetamide (Bleph-10), tobramycin (Tobrex), or gentamicin (Garamycin, Genoptic) or **instillation of ophthalmic antibiotic solutions, such as gentamicin, sulfacetamide, tobramycin, ciprofloxacin (Ciloxan), or trimethoprim plus polymyxin B (Polytrim),** q2-6h with oral analgesics as needed. No clinical sign or symptom can adequately distinguish all viral from bacterial infections, so, if it is unclear whether the problem is viral or bacterial, it is safest to treat it as bacterial. Continue therapy for 24 hours after all signs and symptoms have cleared.

✔ **For viral and chemical conjunctivitis, apply cold compresses and weak topical vasoconstrictors, such as naphazoline 0.1% (Naphcon), every 3 to 4 hours,** unless the patient has a shallow anterior chamber prone to acute angle-closure glaucoma with mydriatics.

✔ **For allergic conjunctivitis, apply cold compresses and topical decongestant-antihistamine combinations, such as drops of naphazoline with pheniramine (Naphcon A) or naphazoline with antazoline (Vasocon A), every 3 to 4 hours.** Topical corticosteroid drops provide dramatic relief, but prolonged use increases the risk of opportunistic viral, fungal, and bacterial corneal ulceration; cataract formation; and glaucoma. If a severe contact dermatitis is suspected, a short course of oral prednisone is indicated.

✔ **If the problem is dry eye (keratoconjunctivitis sicca), treat with methylcellulose (Dacriose) artificial tear drops.**

✔ Instruct the patient to follow-up with an ophthalmologist if the infection does not completely resolve within 2 days. Obtain earlier consultation if there is any involvement of the cornea or iris, impaired vision, light sensitivity, inequality in pupil size, or other signs of corneal infection, iritis, or acutely increased intraocular pressure. In addition, refer patients who have had eye surgery, have a history of herpes simplex keratitis, or wear contact lenses to an ophthalmologist.

What Not To Do:

✘ Do not forget to wash hands and equipment after examining the patient; herpes simplex or epidemic keratoconjunctivitis can be spread to clinicians and other patients. Also, do not forget to instruct the patient regarding the importance of hand washing and use of separate towels and pillows for 10 days after the onset of symptoms.

✘ Do not use ophthalmic neomycin because of the high incidence of hypersensitivity reactions. Do not use a sulfacetamide solution stronger than 10%, which can be irritating.
✘ Do not patch an infected eye; this interferes with the cleansing function of tear flow.
✘ Do not give steroids without arranging for ophthalmologic consultation, and never give steroids if a herpes simplex infection is suspected.

 DISCUSSION

Warm compresses are soothing for all types of conjunctivitis, but antibiotic drops and ointments should be used only when bacterial infection is likely. Neomycin-containing ointments and drops should probably be avoided because allergic sensitization to this antibiotic is common. Any corneal ulceration requires ophthalmologic consultation. Most viral and bacterial conjunctivitis will resolve spontaneously, with the possible exception of *Staphylococcus, Meningococcus,* and *Gonococcus* organism infections, which can produce destructive sequelae without treatment.

Most bacterial conjunctivitis is caused by *Streptococcus pneumoniae, Haemophilus aegyptius,* or *Staphylococcus aureus.* Routine conjunctival cultures are seldom of value, but Gram's method should be used to stain and culture a copious purulent exudate. A red eye in a neonate should prompt cultures for gonorrhea and chlamydia. *Neisseria gonorrhoeae* infection confirmed by gram-negative intracellular diplococci on Gram's stain requires immediate ophthalmologic consultation. Corneal ulceration, scarring, and blindness can occur in a matter of hours.

Chlamydial conjunctivitis will usually present with lid droop, mucopurulent discharge, photophobia, and preauricular lymphadenopathy. Small, white, elevated conglomerations of lymphoid tissue can be seen on the upper and lower tarsal conjunctiva, and 90% of patients have concurrent genital infection. In adults, doxycycline 100 mg bid or erythromycin 250 mg qid PO plus topical tetracycline (Achromycin Ophthalmic) for 3 weeks should control the infection (also treat sexual partners). The smear used to diagnose cervical chlamydia is not effective for an exudate from the eye because the test requires epithelial cells.

Epidemic keratoconjunctivitis is a bilateral, painful, highly contagious conjunctivitis usually caused by an adenovirus. The eyes are extremely erythematous, sometimes with subconjunctival hemorrhages. There is copious watery discharge and preauricular lymphadenopathy. Treat the symptoms with analgesics, cold compresses, and, if necessary, corticosteroids. Because the infection can last as long as 3 weeks and may result in permanent corneal scarring, provide ophthalmologic consultation and referral.

Herpes simplex conjunctivitis is usually unilateral. Symptoms include a red eye, photophobia, eye pain, and mucoid discharge. There may be periorbital vesicles, and a branching (dendritic) pattern of fluorescein staining makes the diagnosis (Figure 12-4). Treat with trifluridine

Continued

DISCUSSION—cont'd

1% (Viroptic) one drop qh, 9 ×/day for up to 21 days, analgesics, and cold compresses. Cycloplegics, such as homatropine, may help control pain resulting from iridocyclitis. Topical corticosteroids are contraindicated because they can extend duration of the infection, and ophthalmologic consultation is required.

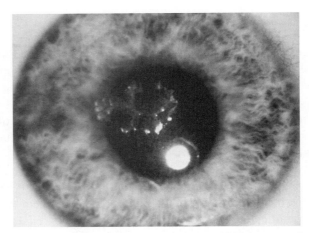

Figure 12-4 Herpetic keratitis. *(From Arffa B:* Grayson's disease of the cornea, *ed 4, 1997, St Louis, Mosby.)*

Herpes zoster ophthalmicus is shingles of the ophthalmic branch of the trigeminal nerve, which innervates the cornea and the tip of the nose. It begins with unilateral neuralgia, followed by a vesicular rash in the distribution of the nerve. Ophthalmic consultation is again required (because of frequent ocular complications), but topical corticosteroids may be used. Prescribe systemic acyclovir (Zovirax) 800 mg q4h (5 times a day) for 10 days or famciclovir (Famvir) 500 mg tid for 7 days.

13

Contact Lens Overwear and Contamination

Presentation

A patient who wears hard, impermeable contact lenses may come to the emergency department in the early morning complaining of severe eye pain after he has fallen asleep with his lenses in or stayed up late, leaving his lenses in for longer than 12 hours. Extended-wear soft contact lenses can cause a similar syndrome when worn for days or contaminated with irritants. The patient may not be able to open his eyes for examination because of pain and blepharospasm. He may have obvious corneal injury, with signs of iritis and conjunctivitis, or may have no findings visible without fluorescein staining.

What To Do:

✔ **Instill topical anesthetic drops.**

✔ **Perform a complete eye examination,** including assessment of pupillary reflexes, examination with funduscopy, and inspection of conjunctival sacs. Use a slit lamp if available.

✔ **If there are any hazy areas or ulcerations on the cornea, call for ophthalmologic consultation right away.** *Acanthamoeba* species infections resulting from overwear of soft lenses can damage the eye rapidly and may require excision and hospitalization.

✔ **Instill fluorescein dye** (use a single-dose dropper or wet a dye-impregnated paper strip and touch it to the tear pool in the lower conjunctival sac), have the patient blink, and examine the eye under cobalt blue or ultraviolet light, looking for the green fluorescence of dye bound to devitalized corneal epithelium. **This staining should demonstrate central corneal uptake of fluorescein without sharply demarcated borders.**

✔ Sketch the area of corneal injury on the patient record, rinse out the dye, and **instill tobramycin (Tobrex), gentamicin (Garamycin), or polymyxin plus bacitracin (Polysporin) ointment in the lower conjunctival sac.** Use of ophthalmic solution q2h when awake may be preferable to use of ointment q4h.

41

✔ **Prescribe analgesics (e.g., naproxen, ibuprofen, oxycodone), and administer the first dose.**

✔ Instruct the patient to avoid wearing his lenses until cleared by the ophthalmologist and to seek ophthalmologic follow-up within 1 day.

What Not To Do:

✘ Do not discharge a patient with topical anesthetic ophthalmic drops for continued administration; they potentiate serious injury.

✘ Do not let a patient reuse contaminated or infected lenses.

✘ Do not patch eyes damaged by contact lens abrasions or early ulcerative keratitis.

✘ Do not prescribe antibiotic ointments that do not provide prophylaxis against *Pseudomonas* organisms (e.g., erythromycin and sulfas).

✘ Do not use drops or ointments containing steroids.

 DISCUSSION

Hard contact lenses and extended-wear soft lenses left in place too long deprive the avascular corneal epithelium of oxygen and nutrients normally provided by the tear film. This produces diffuse ischemia, which usually heals perfectly in a day but can be exquisitely painful as soon as the lenses are removed. Soft lenses can absorb chemical irritants, allergens, bacteria, and amoebas if they soak in contaminated cleaning solution.

There are approximately 25 million contact lens wearers in the United States. Adverse reactions range from minor transient irritation to corneal ulceration and infection that may result in permanent loss of vision caused by corneal scarring. *Pseudomonas* organism infection is most commonly associated with contact lens–related keratitis. Thus the management of these cases should differ from the routine care of mechanical corneal abrasions not caused by contact lens wear. Occlusive patching and corticosteroid medications favor bacterial growth and are therefore not recommended in the setting of contact lens use.

SUGGESTED READINGS
Schein OD: Contact lens abrasions and the nonophthalmologist, *Am J Emerg Med* 11:606–608, 1993.

chapter

14

Corneal Abrasion

Presentation

The patient may complain of eye pain or a sensation of the presence of a foreign body after being poked in the eye with a finger or twig. The patient may have abraded the cornea while inserting or removing a contact lens. Removal of a corneal foreign body produces some corneal abrasion, but corneal abrasion can occur without any identifiable trauma. There is often excessive tearing and photophobia. Often the patient cannot open her eye for the examination. Abrasions are occasionally visible during sidelighting of the cornea. Conjunctival inflammation can range from nothing to severe conjunctivitis with accompanying iritis.

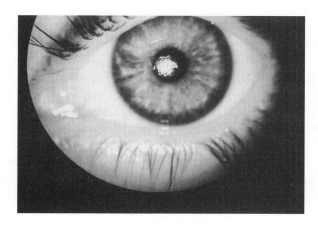

Figure 14-1 Corneal epithelial abrasion. *(From Garcia GE:* Emergency Medicine *24(4):245-256, 1992.)*

What To Do:

✔ **Instill topical anesthetic drops** (to permit examination).
✔ **Perform a complete eye examination** (including assessment of visual acuity, funduscopy, anterior chamber bright light examination, and inspection of conjunctival sacs for a foreign body).

43

✔ **Perform the fluorescein examination** by wetting a paper strip impregnated with dry orange fluorescein dye and touching this strip into the tear pool inside the lower conjunctival sac. After the patient blinks, darken the room and examine her eye under cobalt blue or ultraviolet light. (The red-free light on the ophthalmoscope does not work.) **Areas of denuded or devitalized corneal epithelium will fluoresce green.**

✔ If a foreign body is present, remove it and irrigate the eye.

✔ If iritis is present (as evidenced by consensual photophobia or, in severe cases, an irregular pupil or meiosis and a limbic blush in addition to conjunctival injection), consult the ophthalmologic follow-up physician about starting treatment with topical mydriatics and steroids (see Chapter 18).

✔ **Treat the patient with antibiotic drops such as tobramycin (Tobrex), gentamicin (Garamycin, Genoptic), or trimethoprim plus polymyxin B (Polytrim) q2-6h while awake.** Some physicians prefer ophthalmic ointment preparations, which may last longer (especially if used under an eye patch) but tend to be messy.

✔ Even when there are no signs of iritis, **one instillation of a short-acting cycloplegic, such as cyclopentolate 1% (Cyclogyl), will relieve any pain resulting from ciliary spasm.**

✔ **Analgesic nonsteroidal antiinflammatory eye drops of diclofenac (Voltaren) or ketorolac (Acular) instilled qid provide additional pain relief.**

✔ A soft, disposable contact lens (e.g., NewVue, Acuvue) in combination with antibiotic and nonsteroidal antiinflammatory drops can provide further comfort, as well as the ability to see out of the affected eye. As with any contact lens worn overnight, there is probably an increased risk of infectious keratitis.

✔ For large, deep, and painful abrasions, patch the eye with enough pressure to keep the lid closed by folding one eye patch double to rest against the lid; covering it with a second, unfolded eye patch; and taping both tightly with several strips of 1-inch tape running from the cheek to the middle of the forehead. If this patch does not improve comfort or becomes annoying, the patient can remove it.

✔ **Prescribe analgesics (e.g., oxycodone, ibuprofen, naproxen), and administer the first dose.**

✔ **Warn the patient that the pain will return when the local anesthetic wears off.**

✔ **Make an appointment for ophthalmologic follow-up to reevaluate the abrasion the next day.**

What Not To Do:

✘ Do not be stingy with pain medication. The aforementioned treatments may not provide adequate analgesia, and supplementation with systemic nonsteroidal antiinflammatory drugs (NSAIDs) or narcotic analgesics may be necessary for a day.

✘ Do not give the patient any topical anesthetic for continued instillation.

✘ Do not use a patch or soft contact lens if bacterial conjunctivitis, ulcer, or abrasions caused by contact lens overwear are present.

✘ Do not tape an eye patch up and down or across the nose.

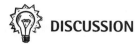

DISCUSSION

Corneal abrasions constitute a loss of the superficial epithelium of the cornea (Figure 14-1). They are generally painful because of the extensive innervation in the affected area. Healing is usually complete in 1 to 2 days unless there is extensive epithelial loss or underlying ocular disease (e.g., diabetes). Scarring will occur only if the injury is deep enough to penetrate the collagenous layer.

Fluorescein binds to corneal stroma and devitalized epithelium but not to intact corneal epithelium. Collections of fluorescein elsewhere, in conjunctival irregularities and in the tear film, are not pathologic findings.

The traditional use of eye patching has been shown to be unnecessary for both corneal reepithelialization and pain relief. It remains an option when the patient prefers it.

Continuous instillation of topical anesthetic drops can impair healing, inhibit protective reflexes, permit further eye injury, and even cause sloughing of the corneal epithelium.

With small superficial abrasions, ophthalmologic follow-up is not required if the patient is completely asymptomatic within 12 to 24 hours. With larger abrasions or with any persistent discomfort, ophthalmologic follow-up is necessary because of the risk of corneal infection or ulceration.

Hard contact lenses can abrade the cornea and cause diffuse ischemic damage when worn for more than 12 hours at a time by depriving the avascular corneal epithelium of oxygen and nutrients in the tear layer (see Chapter 13).

In follow-up examination of corneal abrasions, inspect the base of the corneal defect, ensuring that it is clear. If the base of the abrasion becomes hazy, it may indicate the early development of a corneal ulcer and demands immediate ophthalmologic consultation.

SUGGESTED READINGS

Arbour JD, Brunette I, Boisjoly HM, et al: Should we patch corneal erosions? *Arch Ophthalmol* 115:313–317, 1997.

Campanile TM, St Clair DA, Benaim M: The evaluation of eye patching in the treatment of traumatic corneal epithelial defects, *J Emerg Med* 15:769–774, 1997.

Kaiser PK, Pineda R: A study of topical nonsteroidal anti-inflammatory drops and no pressure patching in the treatment of corneal abrasions, *Ophthalmology* 104:1353–1359, 1997.

Kirkpatrick J: No eye pad for corneal abrasions, *Eye* 7:468, 1993.

Salz JJ, Reader AL, Schwartz LJ, et al: Treatment of corneal abrasions with soft contact lenses and topical diclofenac, *J Refractive Corneal Surg* 10:640–646, 1994.

15

Foreign Body, Conjunctival

Presentation

Low-velocity projectiles, such as wind-blown dust particles, can be loose in the tear film or lodged in a conjunctival sac. The patient may not be very accurate in locating the foreign body by sensation alone. On examination, normally occurring white papules inside the lids can be mistaken for foreign bodies, and transparent foreign bodies can be invisible in the tear film (until outlined by fluorescein dye).

What To Do:

✔ **Instill topical anesthetic drops.**
✔ **Perform visual acuity examination** and funduscopy, examine the anterior chamber and tear film with a bright light (best done with a slit lamp), and **examine the conjunctival sacs.**
✔ **To examine the lower sac, pull the lower lid down with your finger while the patient looks up** (Figure 15-1).
✔ **To examine the upper sac, hold the proximal portion of the upper lid down with a cotton-tipped swab while pulling the lid out and up by its lashes,** everting most of the lid, as the patient looks down. **Push the cotton swab downward to help turn the upper conjunctival sac "inside out."** The stiff tarsal plate usually keeps the upper lid everted after the swab is removed, as long as the patient continues looking downward. Looking up will reduce the lid to its usual position (Figure 15-2, *A* to *D*).
✔ **A loose foreign body usually will adhere to a swab lightly touched to the surface of the conjunctiva or can be washed out by copious irrigation with saline** (Figure 15-2, *E*).
✔ **Perform a fluorescein examination to disclose any corneal abrasions** caused by the foreign body. These vertical scratches occur when the lid closes over a coarse object and should be treated as described in Chapter 14.
✔ Follow with a brief saline irrigation to remove possible remaining fragments.

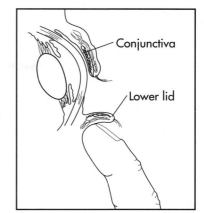

Figure 15-1 The patient looks up while the lid is pulled down.

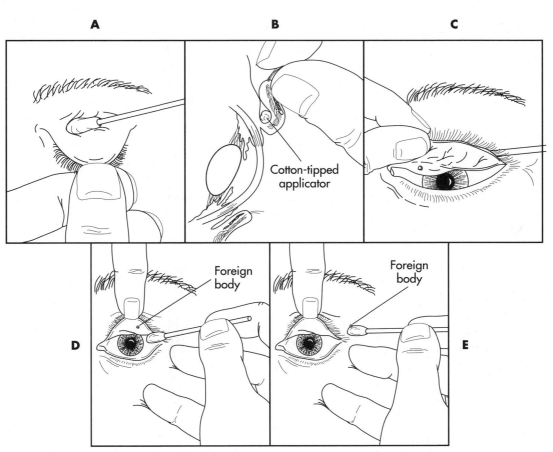

Figure 15-2 A, A cotton-tipped applicator is placed above the upper lid. **B,** Lid eversion with the patient looking downward. **C,** Push down on the applicator to reveal the foreign body hidden under the tarsal plate. **D** and **E,** The moistened applicator touches the foreign body, lifting it away.

47

What Not To Do:

✘ Do not overlook a foreign body lodged in the deep recesses of the upper conjunctival sac.

✘ Do not overlook an eyelash that has turned in and is rubbing on the surface of the eye. Sometimes a lash may be sticking out of the inferior lacrimal punctum. Extract any such lashes.

✘ Do not overlook an embedded or penetrating foreign body.

✘ Do not overlook a corneal abrasion.

DISCUSSION

Good first aid (providing copious irrigation and avoiding rubbing of the eyes) will take care of most ocular foreign bodies. The history of injury with a high-velocity fragment, such as a metal shard chipped off from a hammer or chisel, should raise suspicion of a penetrating foreign body, and x-ray films should be obtained. Techniques for conjunctival foreign body removal can also be applied to locating a displaced contact lens (see Chapter 21), but be aware that fluorescein dye absorbed by soft contact lenses fades slowly.

When eyelids become glued shut with cyanoacrylate (Crazy Glue or Super Glue) it is usually impossible to perform a complete eye examination or even gently separate the eyelids. Simply apply an antibacterial ointment and patch the eye. Spontaneous opening will occur in 1 to 4 days, and a more thorough examination can be performed at that time if any discomfort persists.

16

Foreign Body, Corneal

Presentation

The patient's eye has been struck by a falling or airborne particle, often a fleck of rust loosened while working under a car, or a foreign body has become embedded as a result of the patient rubbing his eye, thereby producing intense pain. Moderate- to high-velocity foreign bodies (fragments chipped off of a chisel when struck by a hammer or spray from a grinding wheel) can be superficially embedded or lodged deep in the vitreous. Superficial foreign bodies may be visible during simple sidelighting of the cornea or by slit-lamp examination. Deep foreign bodies may be visible only as moving shadows on funduscopy, with a trivial-appearing or invisible puncture in the sclera.

What To Do:

✔ **Instill topical anesthetic drops.**
✔ Perform visual acuity examination, funduscopy (looking for shadows), and bright light anterior chamber examination (slit lamp is best), and check pupillary reflexes (for iritis) and conjunctivae (for loose foreign bodies).
✔ **If there is any suspicion of a penetrating intraocular foreign body because there was a high-velocity mechanism of injury, obtain special orbital x-ray films or CT scans to locate it or rule it out.**
✔ **A loosely embedded foreign body might be removed by touching it with a moistened swab** as shown in Chapter 15, **but if the object is firmly embedded, it will have to be scraped off (under magnification) with an ophthalmic spud or an 18-gauge needle** (Figure 16-1). Give the patient an object to fixate on, so that he will keep his eye still; brace your hand on his forehead or cheek; and approach the eye tangentially so no sudden motion can cause a perforation of the anterior chamber. **Removal of the foreign body leaves a defect that should be treated as a corneal abrasion.** If a rust ring is present, it will appear that a foreign body remains adherent to the cornea. Use the needle to continue to scrape away this rust-impregnated corneal epithelium. A corneal burr, if available, is preferable for this task (Figure 16-2).
✔ If the extent of the corneal defect is unclear, perform a fluorescein examination.

49

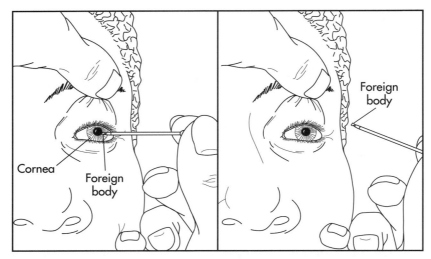

Figure 16-1 Removing a corneal foreign body with an 18-gauge needle.

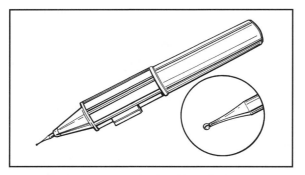

Figure 16-2 Battery-operated corneal burr for rust ring removal.

✔ **Finish treatment with further irrigation to loosen possible remaining fragments and instillation of drops of a mydriatic, antibiotic solution or ointment, and oral analgesic medication; the first dose should be given before the patient leaves the emergency department.** An eye patch is not necessary, but if there are no signs of infection, a patch may be used when it affords the patient additional comfort; the patch may be removed at the patient's discretion or at follow-up the next day.

✔ **Make an appointment for ophthalmologic follow-up the next day to evaluate healing and any residual foreign bodies.**

What Not To Do:

✘ Do not overlook a foreign body lodged deep inside the globe; the delayed inflammatory response can lead to blindness.

✘ Do not leave an iron foreign body in place without arranging for early ophthalmologic follow-up.

✘ Do not be stingy with pain medication. Large corneal abrasions resulting from foreign body removal can be quite painful even if the eye has been patched.

✘ If homatropine was instilled, do not forget to tell the patient that he will have blurred near vision and an enlarged pupil for 12 to 24 hours.

 DISCUSSION

Decide beforehand how much time will be spent (and how much trauma will be inflicted on the cornea) before removal of a corneal foreign body is given up and an ophthalmologic consultant is called. Some emergency physicians recommend using a small needle for scraping to minimize the possibility of a corneal perforation, but with a tangential approach the larger needle is less likely to cause harm.

17

Hordeolum (Sty)

Presentation

The patient complains of redness, swelling, and pain in the eyelid, perhaps at the base of an eyelash (sty or external hordeolum) or deep within the lid (meibomianitis or internal hordeolum, which is best appreciated with the lid everted) and perhaps with conjunctivitis and purulent drainage (Figure 17-1).

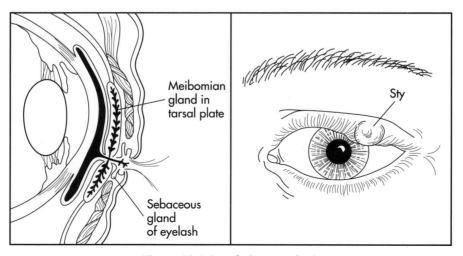

Figure 17-1 Sty of sebaceous gland.

What To Do:

✔ Examine the eye, including assessment of visual acuity and inversion of the lids (see Chapter 15 for technique).

✔ **Show the patient how to instill antibiotic drops or ointment (e.g., sulfa, tobramycin, erythromycin, gentamicin) into the lower conjunctival sac q2–6h, and instruct her to apply warm tap water compresses for 10 minutes qh or 20 minutes qid.**

✔ Instruct the patient to consult an ophthalmologist or return to the emergency department (ED) if the problem is not clearly resolving in 2 days or if it gets any worse.

✔ If the abscess does not spontaneously drain or resolve in 2 days and if it is pointing, it may be incised with the tip of a No. 11 scapel blade or small needle. Again, instruct the patient to consult an ophthalmologist or return to the ED if the problem is not clearly resolving in 2 days or if it gets any worse.

What Not To Do:

✘ Do not overlook orbital or periorbital cellulitis, which is a severe infection and requires aggressive systemic antibiotic treatment.

 DISCUSSION

The terminology describing the two types of hordeolum has become confusing. Meibomian glands run vertically within the tarsal plate, open at tiny puncta along the lid margin, and secrete oil to coat the tear film. The glands of Zeiss and Moll are the sebaceous glands opening into the follicles of the eyelashes. Either type of gland can become occluded and superinfected, producing meibomianitis (internal hordeolum) or a sty (external hordeolum). The immediate care for both acute infections is the same. A chronic granuloma of the meibomian gland is called a *chalazion*, will not drain, and requires excision.

If the patient appears to have diffuse cellulitis of the lid, check for painful or restricted extraocular movements, which would indicate extension posteriorly into an orbital cellulitis.

18 Iritis (Uveitis)

Presentation

The patient usually complains of unilateral eye pain, blurred vision, and photophobia. He may have noticed a pink-colored eye for a few days, suffered trauma during the previous day, or experienced no overt eye problems. There may be tearing, but there is usually no discharge. Eye pain is not markedly relieved after instillation of a topical anesthetic. Upon inspection of the junction of the cornea and conjunctiva (the corneal limbus), a circumcorneal injection, which on closer inspection is a tangle of fine ciliary vessels, is visible through the white sclera. This limbal blush or ciliary flush is usually the earliest sign of iritis. A slit lamp with 10 × magnification may help identification, but the injection is usually evident merely on close inspection. As the iritis becomes more pronounced, the iris and ciliary muscles go into spasm, producing an irregular, poorly reactive, constricted pupil and a lens that will not focus. The slit-lamp examination should demonstrate white blood cells or light reflection from a protein exudate in the clear aqueous humor of the anterior chamber (cells and flare) (Figure 18-1).

What To Do:

✔ **Perform a complete eye examination, using topical anesthesia if necessary, including visual acuity assessment, pupillary reflex examination, funduscopy, slit-lamp examination of the anterior chamber (including pinhole illumination to bring out cells and flare), and fluorescein staining to detect any corneal lesion.** Shining a bright light in the normal eye should cause pain in the symptomatic eye (consensual photophobia).

✔ **Attempt to ascertain the cause of the iritis.** (Is it generalized from a corneal insult or conjunctivitis, a late sequela of blunt trauma, infectious, or autoimmune?)

✔ **Explain to the patient the potential severity of the problem; this is no routine conjunctivitis, but a process that can develop into blindness.**

✔ **Arrange for ophthalmologic follow-up and agreement to immediate treatment as follows:**

  • **Dilate the pupil and paralyze ciliary accommodation with 1% cyclopentolate (Cyclogyl) drops,** which will relieve the pain of the muscle spasm and keep the

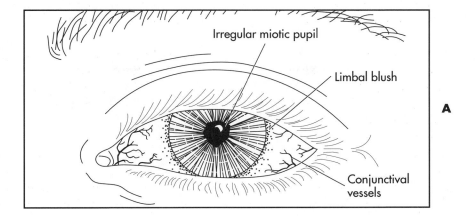

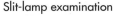

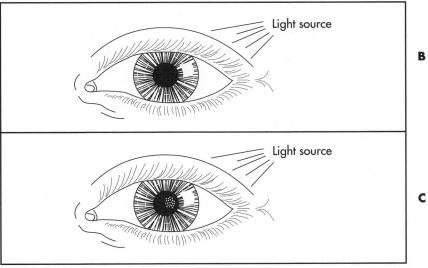

Figure 18-1 A, Early signs of iritis. **B,** Normal reflection of pinhole light from the cornea and iris. **C,** Cells and flare from iritis appear in highlight.

iris away from the lens, where miosis and inflammation might cause adhesions (posterior synechiae). **For a more prolonged effect, instill a drop of homatropine 5% before discharging the patient.**

- **Suppress the inflammation with topical steroids, such as 1% prednisolone (Inflamase) drops qid.**
- **Prescribe oral pain medicine if necessary.**

✔ Ensure that the patient is seen the next day for follow-up.

What Not To Do:

✖ Do not let the patient shrug off his "pink eye" and neglect to obtain follow-up, even if he is feeling better, because of the real possibility of permanent visual impairment.

✖ Do not overlook a possible penetrating foreign body as the cause of the inflammation.

✖ Avoid dilating an eye with a shallow anterior chamber and precipitating acute angle-closure glaucoma (Figure 18-2).

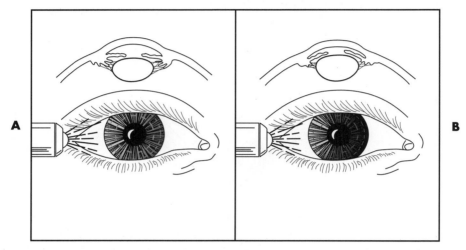

Figure 18-2 A, Normal iris. **B,** Domed iris casts a shadow. The shallow anterior chamber is prone to acute angle-closure glaucoma if the pupil is dilated.

DISCUSSION

Iritis (or anterior uveitis) always represents a real threat to vision and requires emergency treatment and expert follow-up. The inflammatory process in the anterior eye can opacify the anterior chamber, deform the iris or lens, scar them together, or extend into adjacent structures. Posterior synechiae can potentiate cataracts and glaucoma. Treatment with topical steroids can backfire if the process is caused by an infection (especially herpes keratitis); thus the slit-lamp examination is especially useful.

Iritis may have no apparent cause or may be associated with ankylosing spondylitis, Reiter's syndrome, psoriatic arthritis, sarcoidosis, malignancies, and infections, such as tuberculosis, Lyme disease, and syphilis.

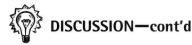 **DISCUSSION—cont'd**

Sometimes an intense conjunctivitis or keratitis may produce some sympathetic limbal blush, which will resolve as the primary process resolves and requires no additional treatment. A more definite, but still mild, iritis may resolve with administration of cycloplegics and may not require steroids. All of these conditions, however, mandate ophthalmologic consultation and follow-up.

SUGGESTED READINGS

Au YK, Henkind P: Pain elicited by consensual pupillary reflex: a diagnostic test for acute iritis, *Lancet* ii:1254–1255, 1981.

Periorbital and Conjunctival Edema

Presentation

The patient is frightened by facial distortion and itching that seem to appear spontaneously or up to 24 hours after she was bitten by a bug or came in contact with some irritant. The patient may have been rubbing her eyes; an allergen or chemical irritant, on the hand, may cause periorbital edema long before a reaction, if any, is evident on the skin of the hand. There may be minimal to marked generalized conjunctival swelling (chemosis) but little injection. Tenderness and pain should be minimal or absent, and there should be no erythema of the skin, photophobia, or fever. Visual acuity should be normal, there should be no fluorescein uptake over the cornea, and the anterior chamber should be clear (Figure 19-1).

What To Do:

✔ After completing a full eye examination, reassure the patient that this condition is not as serious as it looks.

✔ **Prescribe hydroxyzine (Atarax) 25 to 50 mg q6h for mild-to-moderate swelling and a 6-day course of steroids (Aristopak 4 mg) for more severe cases. Naphazoline (Vasocon, Naphcon) ophthalmic drops are soothing and reduce swelling when the conjunctiva is involved.**

✔ **Instruct the patient to apply cool compresses** to reduce swelling and discomfort.

✔ Inquire about possible causes, including allergies and chemical irritants.

✔ Warn the patient about the potential signs of infection.

What Not To Do:

✔ Do not apply heat; heat causes swelling and pruritus to increase.

✔ Do not confuse this condition with orbital or periorbital cellulitis, which are serious infections manifested by pain, heat, and fever. Orbital cellulitis is more posterior, involves the ocular muscles, which causes painful extraocular movements, and calls for IV antibiotic therapy.

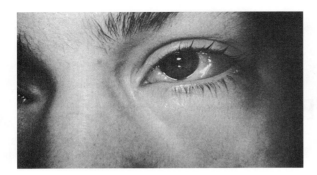

Figure 19-1 Spontaneous swelling and itching are common symptoms of periorbital and conjunctival edema.

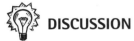 **DISCUSSION**

The dramatic swelling that often brings a patient to the emergency department or the family doctor occurs because there is loose connective tissue surrounding the orbit. Fluid quickly accumulates when a local allergic response causes increased capillary permeability, resulting in dramatic eyelid swelling. The envenomation, allergen, or irritant responsible may actually be located some distance away from the affected eye, on the scalp, face, or hand, but the loose periorbital tissue is the first to swell. If the swelling is due to contact dermatitis and the allergen is bound to the skin, oral steroids should be continued for 10 to 14 days, until the skin renews itself (see Chapter 153).

20

Periorbital Ecchymosis (Black Eye)

Presentation

The patient has suffered blunt trauma to the eye, most often resulting from a blow inflicted during a fistfight, a fall, or a car accident, and he is alarmed because of the swelling and discoloration. Family or friends may be more concerned than the patient about the appearance of the eye. There may be an associated subconjunctival hemorrhage, but the remainder of the eye examination should be normal, and there should be no palpable bony deformities, diplopia, or subcutaneous emphysema (Figure 20-1).

What To Do:

✔ **Clarify as well as possible the specific mechanism of injury.** A fist is much less likely than a baseball bat to cause serious injury.

✔ **Perform a complete eye examination, including a bright light examination to rule out an early hyphema** (blood in the anterior chamber), a funduscopic examination to rule out a retinal detachment or dislocated lens, and a fluorescein stain to rule out a corneal abrasion. **Visual acuity testing should always be performed and, with an uncomplicated injury, is expected to be normal.** All patients having contusions associated with visual loss should be referred to an ophthalmologist. **Special attention should be given to ruling out a blow-out fracture of the orbital floor or wall. Test extraocular eye movements, looking especially for restriction of eye movement or diplopia on upward gaze, and check sensation over the infraorbital nerve distribution.** Enophthalmos usually is not observed, although it is part of the classic textbook triad associated with a blow-out fracture. Subcutaneous emphysema is a recognized complication of orbital wall fracture.

✔ **Symmetrically palpate the supraorbital and infraorbital rims, as well as the zygoma, feeling for a deformity** such as that which would be encountered with a displaced tripod fracture. A unilateral deformity will be obvious if your thumbs are fixed

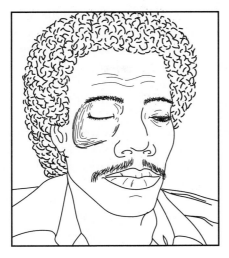

Figure 20-1 Blunt trauma to the eye.

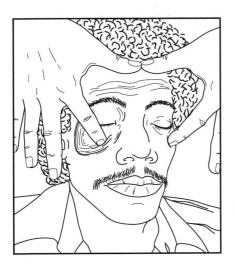

Figure 20-2 Proper hand placement for symmetrically palpating the supraorbital and infraorbital rims.

in a midline position while you use your index fingers to palpate the patient's facial bones simultaneously both left and right (Figure 20-2).

✔ **When there is a substantial mechanism of injury or if there is any clinical suspicion of an underlying fracture, obtain x-ray films of the orbit.** CT scans are more sensitive and allow visualization of subtle fractures of the orbit and small amounts of orbital air. **CT scanning is indicated for patients with abnormal physical examinations but normal routine films.**

✔ **If a significant injury is discovered, consult an ophthalmologist.** For diplopia and blow-out fracture, immediate surgical intervention is not required and follow-up may be delayed for 7 to 10 days, when the edema has subsided. On the other hand, a patient with a hyphema should see an ophthalmologist within 24 hours. The patient should be instructed to rest with his head elevated, a protective metal shield should be placed over the eye, and he should be instructed not to take aspirin or NSAIDs. Hospital admission is not required.

✔ Consider the possibility of abuse; when suspected, obtain the appropriate consultations and make the appropriate referrals.

✔ **When a significant injury has been ruled out, reassure the patient that the swelling will subside within 12 to 24 hours, if he uses a cold pack, and the discoloration will take 1 to 2 weeks to clear.** Acetaminophen should be sufficient for analgesia.

✔ Instruct the patient to follow-up with an ophthalmologist if there is any problem with vision or pain developing after the first few days. Rarely, traumatic iritis, retinal tears, or vitreous hemorrhage may develop later, secondary to blunt injury.

What Not To Do:

✗ Do not order unnecessary radiographs. For minor injuries, if the eye examination is normal and there are no palpable deformities, x-ray films are unnecessary.

✗ Do not brush off bilateral deep periorbital ecchymoses ("raccoon eyes"), especially if caused by head trauma remote to the eye. This may be the only sign of a basilar skull fracture.

 DISCUSSION

Black eyes are usually nothing more than uncomplicated facial contusions. Patients become upset about them because they are so "near the eye," because they produce such noticeable facial disfigurement, and because the patient may seek secondary gain against the person who hit him. Nonetheless, serious injury or abuse must always be considered and appropriately ruled out before the patient is discharged.

21

Removal of Dislocated Contact Lens

Presentation

The patient may know the lens has dislocated into one of the recesses of the conjunctiva and complain only of the loss of refractory correction, or he may have lost track of the lens completely, in which case the eye is a logical place to look first. Pain and blepharospasm suggest a corneal abrasion, perhaps resulting from attempts to remove an absent lens he thought was still in place.

What To Do:

✔ **If pain and blepharospasm are a problem, topically anesthetize the eye.**

✔ **Pull back the eyelids as if looking for conjunctival foreign bodies,** invert the upper lid, and, if necessary, instill fluorescein dye (a last resort with soft lenses, which absorb the dye tenaciously).

✔ **If the lens is loose, slide it over the cornea, and let the patient remove it in the usual manner.** Irrigation may loosen a dry, stuck lens.

✔ **For a more adherent hard lens, use a commercially available suction cup lens remover. Soft lenses may be pinched between the fingers, or a commercially available rubber pincer can be used** (Figure 21-1).

✔ Put the lens in a proper container with sterile saline.

✔ **Complete the eye examination, including visual acuity assessment and bright light and fluorescein examination.** Treat any corneal abrasion as explained in Chapter 14.

✔ Instruct the patient not to wear the lens until all symptoms have abated for 24 hours and to see his ophthalmologist if there are any problems.

63

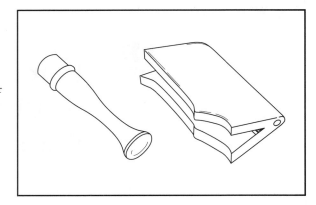

Figure 21-1 A, Rubber suction cup used for extracting hard lenses. **B,** Rubber pincer used for extracting soft lenses.

What Not To Do:

✘ Do not give up on locating a missing lens too easily. Lost lenses have been excavated from under scar tissue in the conjunctival recesses years after they were first dislocated.

✘ Do not omit examination with fluorescein stain for fear of ruining a soft contact lens. The dye may take a long time to elute out, but it is most important to find the dislocated lens.

 DISCUSSION

The deepest recess in the conjunctiva is under the upper lid, but lenses can lodge anywhere; in rare cases lenses have perforated the conjunctival sac and migrated posterior to the globe. Be sure to evert the upper conjunctival sac by pushing down with a cotton-tipped applicator (see Chapter 15).

Often no lens can be found because the lens was missing from the start due to actual loss or forgetfulness.

22

Subconjunctival Hemorrhage

Presentation

This condition may occur spontaneously or may follow a minor trauma, coughing episode, vomiting, or drinking binge. There is no pain or visual loss, but the patient may be frightened by the appearance of her eye and have some sensation of superficial fullness or discomfort. Often a friend or family member insists that the patient see a physician. This hemorrhage usually appears as a bright red area covering part of the sclera but contained by the conjunctiva. It may cover the whole visible globe, sparing only the cornea (Figure 22-1).

What To Do:

✔ **Look for associated trauma or other signs of a potential bleeding disorder, including overmedication with anticoagulants.**

✔ **Perform a complete eye examination** that includes (1) visual acuity assessment, (2) conjunctival sac inspection, (3) bright light examination of the anterior chamber, (4) extraocular movement testing, (5) fluorescein staining, and (6) funduscopic examination.

✔ **Reassure the patient that there is no serious eye damage; explain that the blood may continue to spread but the redness should resolve in 2 to 3 weeks.**

What Not To Do:

✘ Do not neglect to warn the patient that the redness may spread during the next 2 days.

✘ Do not ignore any significant finding discovered during the complete eye examination. Penetrating injuries and ruptured globes also present with subconjunctival hemorrhage, obscuring the damage beneath.

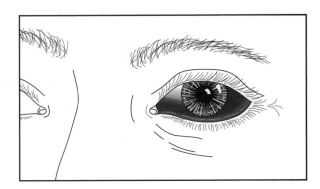

Figure 22-1 A bright red area covering part of the sclera.

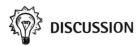 **DISCUSSION**

Although this condition looks serious, it is usually caused by a leak in a superficial blood vessel resulting from trivial trauma. Recurrent hemorrhage or evidence of other bleeding sites, however, should prompt evaluation of a vasculitis or clotting disorder.

23 Ultraviolet Keratoconjunctivitis (Welder's or Tanning Bed Burn)

Presentation

The patient arrives in the emergency department or clinic complaining of burning eye pain, which is usually bilateral, beginning 6 to 8 hours after a brief exposure to a high-intensity ultraviolet light source, such as a sunlamp or welder's arc, without eye protection. The eye examination shows conjunctival injection; fluorescein staining may be normal or may show diffuse superficial uptake (discerned as a punctate keratopathy under slit-lamp examination). The patient may also have first-degree burns on his skin.

What To Do:

✔ **Apply topical anesthetic ophthalmic drops (once, to permit examination).**

✔ **Perform a complete eye examination,** including visual acuity assessment, funduscopy, anterior chamber bright light examination, fluorescein staining, and conjunctival sac inspection.

✔ **Instill an antibiotic ointment and patch the eyes; the eyes should remain patched for approximately 12 hours. Prescribe cold compresses, rest, and analgesics (e.g., oxycodone, codeine, ibuprofen, naproxen) to control pain.**

✔ Warn the patient that pain will return when the local anesthetic wears off but that the oral medication prescribed should help to relieve it.

What Not To Do:

✘ Do not give the patient a topical anesthetic for continued instillation, which can slow healing, blunt protective reflexes, and allow damage to the corneal epithelium.

✘ Do not be stingy with pain medications. This is a painful, albeit short-lived, injury.

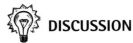 **DISCUSSION**

The history of brief exposure to a welder's arc torch may be difficult to elicit because of the long asymptomatic interval. Longer exposures to lower-intensity ultraviolet light sources may resemble a sunburn. Some physicians find it quite acceptable to substitute a one-time instillation of an ophthalmic anesthetic ointment (Tetracaine), which allows longer-lasting topical anesthesia, for the antibiotic ointment. Some patients do not tolerate bilateral patching. Use of cold compresses or ophthalmic nonsteroidal antiinflammatory drops, such as diclofenac or ketorolac, may be substituted for patches. Healing should be complete in 12 to 24 hours. If the patient continues to experience discomfort, an ophthalmologist should be consulted.

Ear, Nose, and Throat Emergencies

24

Cerumen Impaction (Earwax Blockage)

Presentation

The patient may complain of "wax in the ear," a "stuffed up" or foreign body sensation, pain, itching, decreased hearing, tinnitus, or dizziness. On physical examination the dark brown, thick, dry cerumen, which is perhaps packed down against the eardrum (where it does not occur normally), obscures further visualization of the ear canal.

What To Do:

✔ First, explain the procedure to the patient. Inquire about any possibility of an eardrum perforation, then cover her with a waterproof drape; have her hold a basin or thick towel below her ear and tilt the affected ear slightly over it.

✔ **Fill a 5- to 10-ml syringe with warm, approximately 98.6° F (37° C), water and fit it with a short soft tubing catheter. Aim along the anterior superior wall of the external ear canal (visualize directly and do not occlude the whole canal) and squirt quickly with as much strength as possible.**

✔ Repeat irrigation until all of the cerumen is gone. Dry the canal. A final rinse with hydrogen peroxide is effective.

✔ **If multiple attempts at irrigation prove to be unsuccessful, gentle use of a cerumen spoon (ear curette) may be necessary to extract the excess wax.** Warn the patient about potential discomfort or minor bleeding before using the ear curette; this will obviate the need for lengthy explanations and apologies later.

✔ Reexamine the ear and test the patient's hearing.

✔ Warn the patient that she has thick earwax, she may require this procedure again someday, and she should never use swabs in her ear.

What Not To Do:

✘ Do not irrigate an ear in which there is suspected or known tympanic membrane perforation or myringotomy tubes.

✘ Do not waste time attempting to soften wax with ceruminolytic detergents.

✘ Do not irrigate with a cold (or hot) solution.

✘ Do not blindly insert a rigid instrument into the canal.

✘ Do not irrigate the ear using a stiff over-needle catheter. It can cause a painful abrasion and bleeding or even perforate the tympanic membrane.

✘ Do not leave water pooled in the canal, which can cause an external otitis. A final instillation of 2% acetic acid (Acetasol, Domboro Otic, half-strength vinegar) will also prevent iatrogenic swimmer's ear.

 ## DISCUSSION

This technique almost always works within 5 to 10 squirts. If the irrigation fluid used is at body temperature, it will soften the cerumen just enough that it floats out as a plug. If the fluid is too hot or cold, it can produce vertigo, nystagmus, nausea, and vomiting.

A conventional blood-drawing syringe fitted with a butterfly catheter or IV extension tubing (J-loop), with its tubing cut 1 cm from the hub, seems to work better than the big chrome-plated syringes manufactured for irrigating ears. An alternative technique is to use a WaterPik. Metal cerumen spoons can be dangerous and painful, especially for children, for whom this irrigation technique has proven more effective in cleaning the ear canal and allowing assessment of the tympanic membrane. If a cerumen spoon is required, use the soft, disposable plastic variety.

Cerumen is produced by the sebaceous glands of the hair follicles in the ear canal, and it naturally flows outward along these hairs. One of the problems associated with ear swabs is that they can push wax inward, away from these hairs, and against the eardrum, where the wax can then stick and harden. Patients may ask about "ear candles" to remove wax, but these are not very effective compared with the aforementioned technique.

SUGGESTED READINGS

Robinson AC, Hawke M: The efficacy of cerumenolytics: everything old is new again, *J Otolaryngol* 18:263–267, 1989.

25

Epistaxis (Nosebleed)

Presentation

The patient generally arrives in the emergency department (ED) with active bleeding from his nose, or he may be spitting up blood that is draining into his throat. There may or may not be a report of minor trauma, such as sneezing, nose blowing, or nasal manipulation. On occasion the hemorrhage has stopped, but the patient is concerned because the bleeding has been recurring over the past few hours or days. Bleeding is most commonly present on the anterior aspect of the nasal septum within Kiesselbach's area. The anterior end of the inferior turbinate is another site where bleeding can be seen. Often, especially with posterior hemorrhaging, a specific bleeding site cannot be determined.

What To Do:

✔ If significant blood loss is suspected, gain vascular access and administer crystalloid IV solution.

✔ Have the patient maintain compression on the nostrils by pinching with a gauze sponge while all equipment and supplies are being assembled at the bedside. Inform the patient that the bleeding will be controlled in a stepwise fashion.

✔ Have the patient sit upright (unless he is hypotensive). If necessary, sedate the patient with a mild tranquilizer, such as hydroxyzine (Vistaril), lorazepam (Ativan), or midazolam (Versed). Cover the patient and yourself to protect clothing. Follow universal precautions by using gloves and wearing protective eyewear.

✔ **Prepare 5 ml of 4% cocaine solution or a 1:1 mixture of tetracaine 2% (Pontocaine) for local anesthesia and epinephrine 1:1000 or pseudoephedrine 1% (Neo-Synephrine) for vasoconstriction.**

✔ **Form two elongated cotton pledgets and soak them in the solution.**

✔ **Use a bright headlight or head mirror to free up hands and help ensure good visualization.**

✔ **Instruct the patient to blow the clots from his nose, and then quickly inspect for a bleeding site using a nasal speculum and Frazier suction tip. Clear out any additional clots or foreign bodies** (Figure 25-1).

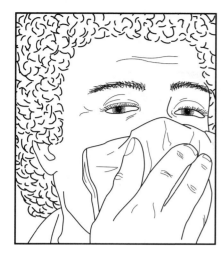

Figure 25-1 The patient must blow the clots from his nose prior to the insertion of medicated cotton pledgets.

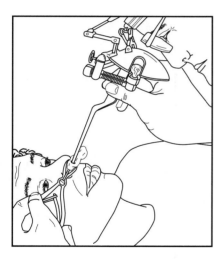

Figure 25-2 Insertion of medicated cotton pledgets.

✔ **Insert the medicated cotton pledgets as far back as possible into both nostrils** (Figure 25-2).

✔ **Allow the patient to relax with the pledgets in place for approximately 5 to 10 minutes.** During this lull, inquire about the patient's history of nosebleeds or other bleeding problems, the pattern of this nosebleed, which side the bleeding seems to be coming from, use of any aspirin or blood-thinning medication, and any significant medical or surgical problems.

✔ In the majority of cases, active bleeding will stop with this treatment. **The cotton pledgets can be removed, and the nasal cavity can be inspected** using a nasal speculum and head lamp. If bleeding continues, insert another pair of medicated cotton pledgets.

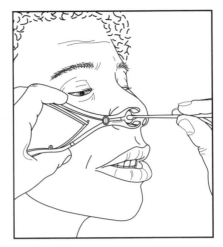

Figure 25-3 Cauterize mucosa with a silver nitrate stick.

✔ **If the bleeding point can be located, cauterize a 0.5-cm area of mucosa around the bleeding site with a silver nitrate stick, and then cauterize the site itself.** If there is an individual vessel bleeding briskly, hold the tip of the cautery stick against that vessel with pressure until the bleeding stops (Figure 25-3). Observe the patient for 15 minutes. If this stops the bleeding, cover the cauterized area with antibiotic ointment and instruct the patient about prevention (avoid picking the nose, bending over, sneezing, and straining) and treatment of recurrences (compress below the bridge of the nose with thumb and finger for 5 minutes).

✔ **If the bleeding point cannot be located or if bleeding continues after cauterization, insert an anterior pack. The best is a 1- × 10-cm stick of compressed cellulose (Merocel, Rhino Rocket)** that expands to conform. A shorter pack may be used for purely anterior bleeding. To prevent putrefaction of the pack, partly cover it with antibiotic ointment before insertion. Leave some cellulose exposed to allow for water absorption. Instill several drops of saline if the compressed cellulose does not expand spontaneously.

✔ **An alternative anterior pack can be made from up to 6 feet of ½–inch ribbon gauze impregnated with petroleum jelly** (Vaseline). Cover the gauze with antibiotic ointment, and insert it with bayonet forceps. Start with three to four layers placed in accordion fashion on the floor of the nasal cavity, placing the gauze as far posteriorly as possible and pressing it down firmly with each subsequent layer. Continue inserting the gauze until the affected nasal cavity is tightly filled (expect to use about 3 to 5 feet per nostril). If unilateral anterior nasal packing does not provide enough pressure, packing the opposite side of the nose anteriorly can sometimes increase the pressure by preventing the septum from bowing over into the side of the nose that is not packed (Figure 25-4).

✔ **Observe the patient for 15 to 30 minutes. If no further bleeding occurs in the nares or the posterior oropharynx, discharge him on a regimen of antibiotics**

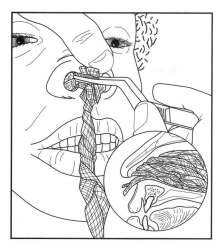

Figure 25-4 Packing the nasal cavity with ribbon gauze.

(amoxicillin 250 mg tid) for 5 days to help prevent a secondary sinusitis. The packing should be removed in 2 to 4 days.

✔ Tape a small folded-gauze pad beneath the nose to catch any minor drainage. The patient can replace this from time to time if necessary.

✔ Warn the patient about sneezing with his mouth closed, bending over, straining, and picking his nose. The patient should keep his head elevated for 24 to 48 hours. Provide detailed printed instructions regarding home care.

✔ If the hemorrhage is suspected to have been severe, determine the patient's orthostatic blood pressure, pulse, and hematocrit level before sending him home.

✔ If the hemorrhage does not stop after adequate packing anteriorly, one or two posterior packs or nasal balloons should be inserted, and the patient should be admitted to the hospital under the care of an otolaryngologist.

What Not To Do:

✘ Do not waste time trying to locate a bleeding site if brisk bleeding is obscuring your vision in spite of vigorous suctioning. Have the patient blow out any clots, and insert the medicated cotton pledgets.

✘ Do not order routine clotting studies unless there is other evidence of an underlying bleeding disorder.

✘ Do not cauterize or use instruments in the nose before providing adequate topical anesthesia. (However, some initial blind suctioning may be required to clear the nose of clots before anesthetics are instilled.)

✘ Do not discharge a patient as soon as the bleeding stops, but keep him in the ED for 15 to 30 minutes more. Look behind the uvula. If it is dripping blood, the bleeding has not been controlled adequately. Posterior epistaxis typically stops and starts cyclically and may not be recognized until all of the aforementioned treatments have failed.

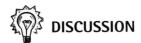 **DISCUSSION**

Nosebleeds are more common in winter, no doubt reflecting the low, ambient humidity indoors and outdoors and the increased incidence of upper respiratory tract infections. Troublesome nosebleeds are more common in middle-aged and elderly patients.

Causes are numerous; dry nasal mucosa, nose picking, and vascular fragility are the most common causes, but others include foreign bodies, blood dyscrasias, nasal or sinus neoplasm or infection, septal deformity, atrophic rhinitis, hereditary hemorrhagic telangiectasis, and angiofibroma. High blood pressure makes epistaxis difficult to control but is rarely the sole precipitating cause.

Drying and crusting of the bleeding site, along with nose picking, may result in recurrent nasal hemorrhage. Instruct the patient that it may be helpful to gently apply petroleum jelly onto his nasal septum once or twice a day to prevent future drying and bleeding.

Other useful techniques include electrocautery down a metal suction catheter, ophthalmic electrocautery tips (see Chapter 150), submucosal injection of lidocaine with epinephrine, and application of hemostatic collagen (Gelfoam). There are also several balloon devices that provide anterior and posterior tamponade, some with a channel to maintain a patent nares. Additional topical anesthesia and lubrication can be obtained before packing by injecting lidocaine jelly into the nose using a Uroject syringe (as used before placement of a Foley catheter).

Because of the nasopulmonary reflex, arterial oxygen pressure will drop about 15 mm Hg after the nose is packed, which can be troublesome in a patient with heart or lung disease and often requires hospitalization and supplemental oxygen.

When removing a compressed cellulose pack on a follow-up visit, soften it with 10 to 15 ml of water and wait 5 minutes, thereby reducing trauma, pain, and rebleeding.

SUGGESTED READINGS

Pringle MB, Beasley P, Brightwell AP: The use of Merocel nasal packs in the treatment of epistaxis, *J Laryngol Otol* 110:543-546, 1996.

Viducich RA, Blanda MP, Gerson LW: Posterior epistaxis: clinical features and acute complications, *Ann Emerg Med* 25:592-596, 1995.

26

Foreign Body, Ear

Presentation

Sometimes a young child admits to putting something, such as a bead or a bean, in her ear, or an adult may witnesses the act. Sometimes the history is not revealed, and the child simply presents with a purulent discharge, pain, bleeding, or hearing loss. Most dramatically, a panic-stricken adult patient arrives at the emergency department because she feels and hears a bug "crawling around" in her ear.

What To Do:

✔ **If there is a live insect in the patient's ear, simply fill the canal with mineral oil** (e.g., microscope immersion oil). Instruct the patient to lay on her side, and then drop the oil down the canal while pulling on the pinna to remove air bubbles. This will suffocate the intruder so that it can be removed using one of the techniques described later (Figure 26-1). The least invasive methods should be attempted first.

✔ **If a tympanic membrane perforation is not suspected, water irrigation is often an effective way to safely remove a foreign body that is not tightly wedged in the ear canal.** This can be accomplished with an irrigation syringe, WaterPik, or standard syringe and scalp vein needle catheter that has been cut short (Figure 26-2). **Tap water or saline solution at body temperature can be used to flush out the foreign body.** Direct the stream along the wall of the ear canal and around the object, thereby flushing it out (Figure 26-3).

✔ **If the object is light and moves easily, attempt to suction it *out* with a standard metal suction tip or specialized flexible tip,** whichever can make a vacuum seal on the foreign body (Figure 26-4).

✔ **If a hard or spherical foreign body remains in the ear canal and if the patient is able to hold still, attempt to roll the foreign body out with a right-angle hook, ear curette, or wire loop. Stabilize the patient's head and fix your hand against it, holding the instrument loosely between your fingers to reduce the risk of injury should the patient move suddenly.** While looking through an ear speculum, slide the tip of the right-angle hook, ear curette, or wire loop behind the

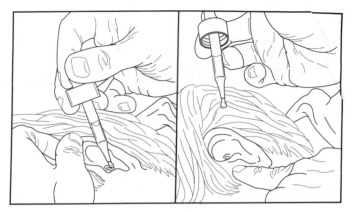

Figure 26-1

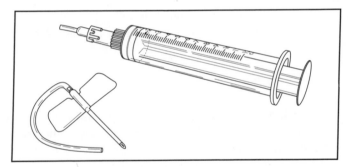

Figure 26-2

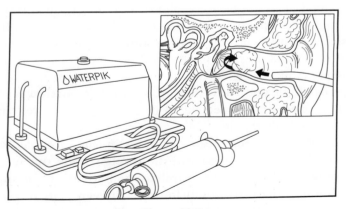

Figure 26-3

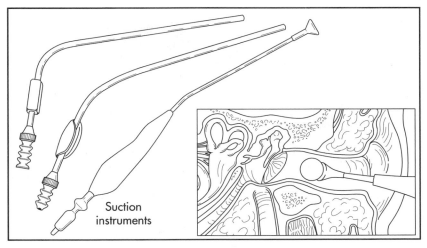

Figure 26-4

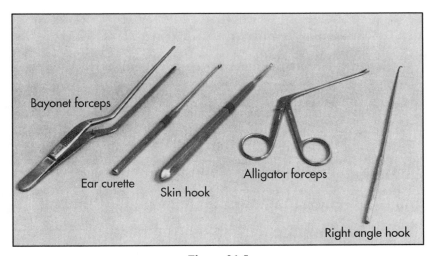

Figure 26-5

object, rotate the hook to catch it, and then roll or slide the foreign body out of the ear (Figures 26-5 and 26-6).

✔ **Alligator forceps are best for grasping soft objects, such as cotton or paper.** One drop of cyanoacrylate (Super Glue) can be applied to the wooden shaft of a long cotton swab, which will then adhere to a smooth, clean, dry foreign body. Touch the swab to the foreign body, hold for 10 seconds, then pull. Try not to glue the stick to the wall of the ear canal, but if this happens, be thankful for cerumen.

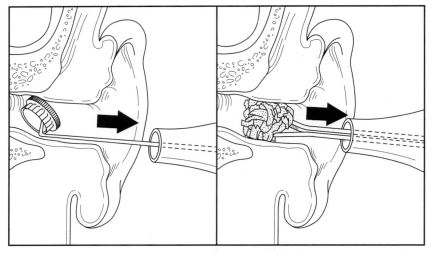

Figure 26-6

What Not To Do:

✘ Do not use a rigid instrument to remove an object from an uncooperative patient's ear. An unexpected movement might cause serious injury to the middle ear.

✘ Do not attempt to remove a large bug or insect without killing it first. They tend to be wily, evasive, and well equipped for fighting in tunnels. In the heat of battle, the patient can become terrorized by the noise and pain, and the instrument being used is likely to damage the ear canal.

✘ Do not attempt to irrigate a tightly wedged bean or seed from an ear canal. The water may cause the bean to swell.

✘ Do not attempt to remove a large or hard object with bayonet or similar forceps. The bony canal will slowly close the forceps as they are advanced, and the object will be pushed farther into the canal. Alligator forceps are designed for use in the canal, but even they will push a large, hard foreign body farther into the ear.

 DISCUSSION

The cutaneous lining of the bony canal of the ear is very sensitive and is not affected much by topical anesthetics. If the patient is an uncooperative child, one cautious attempt can be made to remove the object while the patient is under conscious sedation with firm head restraint. The most prudent strategy, however, is to schedule elective removal under general anesthesia by a specialist.

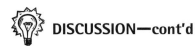

DISCUSSION—cont'd

Irrigation techniques and the use of the ear curette can also be effective in removing excess cerumen from the ear canal (see Chapter 24). Whenever an instrument is used in an ear canal, warn the patient or parents beforehand that there may be a small amount of bleeding.

There should be no delay in removing an external auditory canal foreign body when there is an obvious infection or when the foreign body is a disk battery. On contact with moist tissue, this type of alkaline battery is capable of producing a liquefactive necrosis extending into deep tissues. After removal of the battery, irrigate the canal to remove alkali residue.

Styrofoam beads instantly dissolve when sprayed with a small amount of ethyl chloride. Application of lidocaine has been shown to make cockroaches exit the ear canal, but this may be unpleasant for the patient. On telephone consultation, patients can be instructed to use cooking or baby oil to kill an insect, which can then be removed in a subsequent office visit.

Complications of foreign body removal include trauma to the skin of the canal; less commonly, canal hematoma, otitis externa, tympanic membrane perforations, or ossicular dislocations; and rarely, facial nerve palsy.

SUGGESTED READINGS

Bressler K, Shelton C: Ear foreign-body removal: a review of 98 consecutive cases, *Laryngoscope* 103:367-370, 1993.

Brunskill AJ, Satterwaite K: Foreign bodies, *Ann Emerg Med* 24:757, 1994.

Leffler S, Cherney P, Tandberg D: Chemical immobilization and killing of intra-aural roaches: an in-vitro comparative study, *Ann Emerg Med* 22:1795-1798, 1993.

O'Toole K, Paris PM, Stewart RD, et al: Removing cockroaches from the auditory canal: controlled trial, *N Engl J Med* 312:1197, 1985.

Skinner DW, Chui P: The hazard of button-sized batteries as foreign bodies in the nose and ear, *J Laryngol Otol* 100:1315-1319, 1986.

27 Foreign Body, Nose

Presentation

A child may admit to his parents that he has inserted something into his nose. Sometimes, however, the history is obscure, and the child presents with a purulent unilateral nasal discharge, a voice change (with a "nasal" character), or a secondary pharyngeal infection causing bad breath. The most commonly encountered nasal foreign bodies are beans or other foodstuffs, beads, pebbles, paper wads, and eraser tips. These objects usually lodge on the floor of the anterior or middle third of the nasal cavity. Occasionally, the child has sniffed caustic material into his nose, or it was coughed up into the posterior nasopharynx (e.g., a ruptured tetracycline capsule). In this case the patient experiences much discomfort and tearing, and inspection reveals mucous membranes covered with particulate debris.

What To Do:

✔ Explain the procedure in detail to the patient and parents beforehand. Explain that it will be a little uncomfortable and that aspiration of the foreign body into the trachea is a remote possibility. Reassure them that the procedure will not injure the nose, but it may cause a little bleeding.

✔ **After initial inspection with a nasal speculum and bright light, suction out any purulent discharge and insert a cotton pledget soaked in 4% cocaine or a solution of one part phenylephrine (Neo-Synephrine) or oxymetazoline (Afrin) and one part tetracaine (Pontocaine),** which will shrink the nasal mucosa and provide local anesthesia. Be careful to avoid pushing the foreign body posteriorly. **Remove the pledget after approximately 5 to 10 minutes.** If you cannot safely insert a saturated pledget, drip or spray the same solution around the foreign body and onto the nasal mucosa.

✔ **If the patient is able to cooperate, instruct him to blow his nose in an attempt to remove the foreign body.** With an infant, sometimes the parent can blow a sharp puff of air into the baby's mouth while holding the opposite nostril closed and blow the object out of the nose.

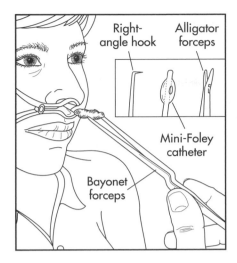

Figure 27-1 Remove foreign bodies with bayonet forceps, right-angle hook, mini-Foley catheter, or alligator forceps.

✔ Before attempting any removal using surgical instruments, a potentially uncooperative child must be firmly restrained and sedated.

✔ **Alligator forceps should be used to remove cloth, cotton, or paper foreign bodies. Pebbles, beans, and other hard foreign bodies are most easily grasped using bayonet forceps or Kelly clamps. If the object cannot be grasped, it may be rolled out of the nose by using an ear curette, single skin hook, or right-angle ear hook to get behind it.** A soft-tipped hook can be made by bending the tip of a metal shaft of a calcium alginate swab (Calgiswab) to a 90-degree angle. **A less intrusive approach is to bypass the object with a Fogarty, biliary, or small Foley catheter (passing it superior to the foreign body), inflate the balloon with approximately 1 ml of air, and pull the object out through the nose.** A drop of cyanoacrylate (Super Glue) can be applied to the wooden end of a regular cotton-tipped applicator, which is then touched to the foreign body, held there for 1 minute, and used to pull the attached foreign body out of the nose (Figure 27-1).

✔ Any bleeding can be stopped by reinserting a cotton pledget soaked in the topical solution used initially.

✔ To irrigate loose foreign bodies and particulate debris from the nasal cavity and posterior nasopharynx, simply insert the bulbous nozzle of an irrigation syringe into one nostril while the patient is sitting up and facing forward. Then ask the patient to repeat the sound *eng* several times, which will close off the back of his throat, and flush the irrigating solution out through the opposite nostril into an emesis basin (Figure 27-2).

✔ **After the foreign body is removed, inspect the nasal cavity again, checking for additional objects that may have been placed in the nose. Look also for unsuspected foreign bodies in the ears.**

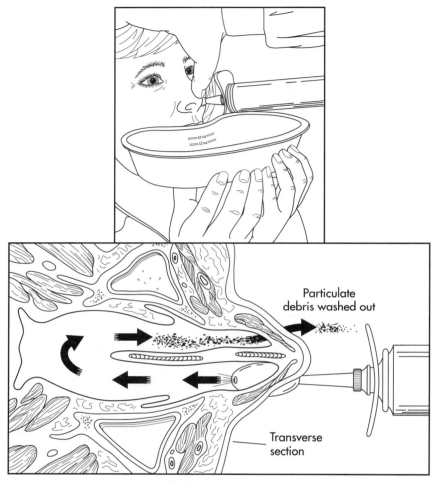

Figure 27-2 Nasal irrigation.

What Not To Do:

✗ Do not ignore a unilateral nasal discharge in a child. It must be assumed to be caused by the presence of a foreign body until proved otherwise.

✗ Do not push a foreign body down the back of a patient's throat, where it may be aspirated into the trachea.

✗ Do not attempt to remove a foreign body from the nose without first using a topical anesthetic and vasoconstrictor.

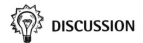 **DISCUSSION**

The mucous membrane lining the nasal cavity allows the tactical advantages of vasoconstriction and topical anesthesia. The patient who has unsuccessfully attempted to blow a foreign body out of his nose may be successful after instillation of an anesthetic vasoconstrictive solution. If a patient has swallowed a foreign body that was pushed back into the nasopharynx, it is usually harmless and the patient and parents can be reassured (see Chapter 69). If the object has been aspirated into the tracheobronchial tree, it may produce coughing and wheezing, and bronchoscopy under anesthesia is required for retrieval. Button batteries can cause serious local damage and should be removed quickly.

SUGGESTED READINGS

Backlin SA: Positive-pressure technique for nasal foreign body retrieval in children. *Ann Emerg Med* 25:554–555, 1995.

Noorily AD, Noorily SH, Otto RA: Cocaine, lidocaine, tetracaine: which is best for topical nasal anesthesia? *Anesth Analg* 81:724–727, 1995.

chapter
28
Foreign Body, Throat

Presentation

The patient is usually convinced that there is a foreign body stuck in her throat because she recently swallowed something, such as a fish or chicken bone, and she can still feel a "sensation" in her throat, especially (perhaps painfully) when swallowing. She may be able to localize the foreign body sensation to precisely above the thyroid cartilage (which implies a foreign body in the hypopharynx that may be visible), or she may only vaguely localize the foreign body sensation to the suprasternal notch (which could imply a foreign body anywhere in the esophagus). A foreign body lodged in the tracheobronchial tree usually stimulates coughing and wheezing. Obstruction of the esophagus produces drooling and causes the patient to spit up whatever fluid is swallowed.

What To Do:

✔ Establish exactly what was swallowed, when, and the progression of symptoms since then. Patients can accurately tell if a foreign body is on the left or right side.

✔ **With the patient sitting in a chair, inspect the oropharynx with a tongue depressor, looking for foreign bodies or mucosal abrasions.**

✔ If symptoms are mild, test the patient's ability to swallow, first using a small cup of water and then a small piece of bread. See what symptoms are reproduced or if the bread eliminates the foreign body sensation.

✔ Percuss and auscultate the patient's chest. A foreign body sensation in the throat can be produced by a pneumothorax, pneumomediastinum, or esophageal disease, all of which may show up on a chest x-ray examination.

✔ **Inspect the hypopharynx using a good light or headlamp mirror, paying special attention to the base of the tongue, tonsils, and vallecula,** where foreign bodies are likely to lodge. **Maximize visibility and minimize the patient's urge to gag by holding her tongue out (use a washcloth or 4- × 4-inch gauze strip for traction** and take care not to lacerate the frenulum of the tongue on the lower incisors), and then instruct the patient to raise her soft palate by panting "like a dog." This may be

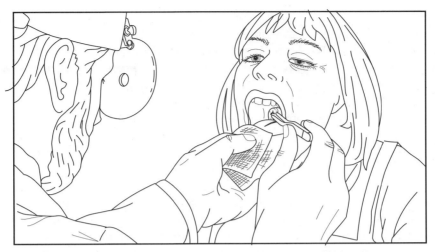

Figure 28-1 Carefully grasp and remove any foreign body that can be seen in the throat.

accomplished without topical anesthesia, but if the patient is skeptical or tends to gag, **the soft palate and posterior pharynx can be anesthetized by spraying them (Cetacaine, Hurricaine, or 10% lidocaine)** or by having the patient gargle with lidocaine (viscous Xylocaine) diluted 1:1 with tap water. Some patients may continue to gag even with the entire pharynx anesthetized. If the gag reflex is minimal, a foreign body may sometimes be palpated with a gloved finger.

✔ If a foreign body that can be plucked out or an abrasion of the mucosa is found, then the problem has been revealed. A small fish bone is frequently difficult to see. It may be overlooked entirely except for the tip, or it may look like a strand of mucus. **If the object can been seen directly, carefully grasp and remove it with bayonet forceps or a hemostat** (Figure 28-1). Objects lodged in the base of the tongue or the hypopharynx require a mirror or indirect laryngoscope for visualization. Fiberoptic nasopharyngoscopy is preferred when available. **Further treatment is probably not required, but the patient should be instructed to seek follow-up care if pain worsens, fever develops, breathing or swallowing is difficult, or the foreign body sensation has not totally resolved in 2 days.**

✔ If you and the patient are not yet satisfied, obtain a soft tissue lateral x-ray film of the neck. This examination probably will not show radiolucent or small foreign bodies, such as fish bones or aluminum pop tops, but may point out other pathologic findings, such as a retropharyngeal abscess, Zenker's diverticulum, or severe cervical spondylosis, which might account for symptoms. (Obtaining x-ray films also allows some time for the patient's gag reflex to settle down so that, if previously impossible, the hypopharynx can now be inspected.) **Lateral soft tissue x-ray films can be very misleading because ligaments and cartilage in the neck calcify at various rates and patterns. The foreign body visible on a plain x-ray film may simply be normal calcification of thyroid cartilage.**

✔ A barium swallow, if available, can be used to demonstrate with fluoroscopy any problems involving swallowing motility or perhaps to coat and thus allow visualization of a radiolucent foreign body. **Remember that endoscopy is technically difficult after barium has coated the mucosa and possibly obscured a foreign body.** It may be preferable to use a water-soluble contrast (e.g., Gastrografin); but even under the best of circumstances, contrast studies are of limited value.

✔ Reserve rigid laryngoscopy, esophagoscopy, and bronchoscopy performed under general anesthesia for the few cases in which suspicion of a perforating foreign body remains high (e.g., when the patient has moderate to severe pain, is febrile or toxic, cannot swallow, is spitting up blood, or has respiratory involvement).

✔ **If x-ray films are normal, careful inspection does not reveal a foreign body, and the patient is afebrile with only mild discomfort, the patient may be sent home. Reassure her that a scratch on the mucosa can produce a sensation that the foreign body is still there. Also inform her that if the symptoms worsen the next day or fail to resolve within 2 days she may need further endoscopic studies.** If there are any continued symptoms, the patient should be referred to an otolaryngologist for consultation within 2 to 3 days.

What Not To Do:

✗ Do not assume that a foreign body is absent just because the pain disappears after a local anesthetic is applied.

✗ Do not reassure the patient that the presence of a foreign body has been ruled out if it has not. Explain what is likely and why invasive evaluation is more dangerous than careful follow-up.

✗ Do not overlook preexisting pathologic conditions incidentally discovered during swallowing.

✗ Do not attempt to blindly remove a foreign body from the throat using a finger or instrument because the object may be pushed farther down into the airway and obstruct it or cause damage to surrounding structures.

 DISCUSSION

During swallowing, as the base of the tongue pushes a bolus of food posteriorly, any sharp object hidden in that bolus may become embedded in the tonsil, the tonsillar pillar, the pharyngeal wall, or the tongue base itself. In one study, the majority of patients with symptoms of an embedded fish bone had no demonstrated pathologic findings, and their symptoms resolved in 48 hours. Only 20% actually had an embedded fish bone, and the majority of these were easily identified and removed on the initial visit.

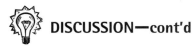 **DISCUSSION—cont'd**

All patients who complain of a foreign body in the throat should be taken seriously. Even relatively smooth or rounded objects that remain impacted in the esophagus have the potential to cause serious problems. A fish bone can perforate the esophagus in only a few days, and chicken bones carry even greater risk for serious injury. An impacted button battery represents a true emergency and requires rapid intervention and removal because leaking alkali produces liquefactive necrosis. A tablet composed of irritating medicine, if swallowed without adequate liquid, may stick to the mucosa of the pharynx or esophagus and cause an irritating ulcer. Bay leaves, which are invisible on x-ray films and laryngoscopy, can lodge in the esophagus at the cricopharyngeus and produce severe symptoms until removed via rigid endoscope.

The sensation of a lump in the throat, unrelated to swallowing food or drink, may be globus hystericus, which is related to cricopharyngeal spasm and anxiety. The initial work up is the same as that for any foreign body sensation in the throat.

29

Mononucleosis (Glandular Fever)

Presentation

The patient is usually of school age (nursery through high school) and complains of several days of fever, malaise, lassitude, myalgias, and anorexia, culminating in a severe sore throat. The physical examination is remarkable for generalized lymphadenopathy, including the anterior and posterior cervical chains, and huge tonsils, perhaps meeting in the midline and covered with a dirty-looking exudate. There may also be palatal petechiae and swelling, periorbital edema, splenomegaly, hepatomegaly, and a diffuse maculopapular rash.

What To Do:

✔ Perform a complete physical examination, looking for signs of other ailments and the rare complications of airway obstruction, encephalitis, hemolytic anemia, thrombocytopenic purpura, myocarditis, pericarditis, hepatitis, and rupture of the spleen.

✔ **Send blood samples to be tested. Obtain a differential white cell count (looking for atypical lymphocytes) and a heterophil or monospot test.** Either of these tests, along with the generalized lymphadenopathy, will confirm the diagnosis of mononucleosis, but atypical lymphocytes are less specific, being present in several viral infections.

✔ **Culture the throat. Patients with mononucleosis harbor group A streptococcus and require penicillin with about the same frequency as anyone else with a sore throat.**

✔ **Warn the patient that the period of convalescence for mononucleosis is longer than that of most other viral illnesses (typically 2 to 4 weeks, occasionally more) and that he should seek attention if he experiences lightheadedness, abdominal or shoulder pain, or any other sign of the rare complications mentioned earlier.**

✔ **Despite controversy, prednisone is widely used for symptomatic relief of infectious mononucleosis, usually 40 mg of prednisone qd for 5 days. Such therapy is particularly helpful in young adults with severe pharyngeal pain,**

odynophagia, or marked tonsillar enlargement with impending oropharyngeal obstruction. Dexamethasone in doses up to 10 mg has also been used to treat impending airway obstruction caused by markedly enlarged "kissing tonsils."

✔ Arrange for medical follow-up.

What Not To Do:

✘ Do not routinely begin therapy with penicillin for the pharyngitis, and certainly do not use ampicillin. In a patient with mononucleosis, ampicillin can produce an uncomfortable rash, which incidentally does not imply that the patient is allergic to ampicillin.

✘ Do not unnecessarily frighten the patient about possible splenic rupture. If the spleen is clinically enlarged, he should avoid contact sports, but spontaneous ruptures are rare.

 DISCUSSION

All of the instructions provided here probably apply to treatment of cytomegalovirus as well, although the severe tonsillitis and positive heterophil test are both less likely in the latter condition. Some patients who report having mononucleosis twice probably actually had cytomegalovirus once and mononucleosis once.

30 Nasal Fracture

Presentation

After a direct blow to the nose, the patient usually arrives at the emergency department concerned that her nose is broken. There is usually minimal continued hemorrhage along with tender ecchymotic swelling over the nasal bones or the anterior maxillary spine; inspection and palpation may or may not disclose a nasal deformity.

What To Do:

✔ Examine the patient for any associated injuries (e.g., blow-out fractures, zygoma fractures, and eye injuries).

✔ **Explain to the patient that, for minor injuries, x-ray examinations are not routinely used and usually are not helpful because all therapeutic decisions are made on the basis of the physical examination.** If there is a fracture, but it is stable and in good position clinically, the nose need not be reset. Conversely, a broken and displaced cartilage may obstruct breathing and require operation but may never show up on the film. Send the patient for x-ray films of the nasal bones only if there is a good reason.

✔ If bleeding continues, instill cotton pledgets soaked in 4% cocaine or 2% tetracaine (Pontocaine) mixed 1:1 with 1% phenylephrine (Neo-Synephrine) or 1:1000 epinephrine into both nasal cavities.

✔ After removing the cotton pledgets, **inspect the nasal mucosa for large lacerations or a septal hematoma.**

✔ **Patients with nondisplaced fractures and no nasal deformity should be sent home with analgesics, cold packs, and instructions to avoid contact sports and related activities for 6 weeks.**

✔ **Patients with displaced fractures, nasal deformity, or both should be referred for otolaryngologic or plastic surgery consultation to discuss immediate or delayed reduction. Patients can be instructed that reduction is more accurate after the swelling subsides and that there is no greater difficulty if it is done within 6 days of the injury.**

✔ Septal hematomas should be drained to prevent septal necrosis and the development of a saddle-nose deformity. Otolaryngologic consultation is advisable.

✔ An isolated fracture of the anterior nasal spine (in the columella of the nose) does not necessitate restriction of activities. Such fractures hurt only when the patient smiles.

✔ A laceration over a nasal fracture should probably be closed with antibiotic prophylaxis such as cefadroxil (Duricef) 500 mg bid for 3 to 5 days.

What Not To Do:

✘ Do not automatically obtain x-ray films of every injured nose. Patients may expect this because it used to be standard practice, but routine films have turned out to be useless.

✘ When a deformity is apparent, do not assume that a normal x-ray examination means there is no fracture. X-ray films can often be inaccurate in determining the presence and nature of a nasal fracture. Rely on the clinical assessment. When there is swelling, arrange for reexamination in 3 to 4 days when the swelling has subsided, and then look for subtle deformities.

✘ Do not pack an injured nose that does not continue to bleed. Packing is generally unnecessary and will only add to the patient's discomfort.

 DISCUSSION

The two most common indications for reducing a nasal fracture are an unacceptable appearance and the patient's inability to breathe through the nose. Regardless of x-ray findings, if neither breathing nor cosmesis is a concern, it is not necessary to reduce the fracture.

Nasal fractures are uncommon in young children because their noses are composed of mostly pliable cartilage.

Suspect septal hematoma when a patient's nasal airway is completely occluded. Within 48 to 72 hours a hematoma can compromise the blood supply to the cartilage and cause irreversible damage.

SUGGESTED READINGS

Altreuter RW: Facial form and function: film versus physical examination, *Ann Emerg Med* 15:240-244, 1986.

Li, S, Papsin B, Brown DH: Value of nasal radiographs in nasal trauma management, *J Otolaryngol* 25:162-164, 1996.

31

Otitis Externa
(Swimmer's Ear)

Presentation

The patient complains of ear pain, which is always uncomfortable and sometimes unbearable, often accompanied by drainage and a blocked sensation and sometimes by fever. When the condition is mild or chronic there may be itching rather than pain. Pulling on the auricle or pushing on the tragus of the ear classically causes increased pain (Figure 31-1). The tissue lining the canal may be swollen, and in severe cases the swelling can extend into the soft tissue surrounding the ear. Tender erythematous swelling or an underlying furuncle may be present, and it may be pointing or draining. The canal may be erythematous and dry, or it may be covered with fuzzy cottonlike grayish or black fungal plaques. Most often, the canal lining is moist and covered with purulent drainage and debris, and cerumen is characteristically absent. The canal may be so swollen that it is difficult or impossible to view the tympanic membrane, which when visible often looks dull.

What To Do:

✔ Suction out the debris and drainage present in the canal. Irrigation can be very effective in cleaning out the canal. Inspect the ear for the presence of any foreign body.

✔ **Incise and drain any furuncle that is pointing or fluctuant.**

✔ **If the ear canal is too narrow to allow medication to flow freely, insert a wick. The best wick is the Pope ear wick (Merocel), which is about 1- $\times$ 10-mm of compressed cellulose;** it is thin enough to slip into an occluded canal but expands when wet. If this wick is not available, try using alligator forceps to insert a 1 cm strip of ¼-inch plain gauze. (This method is more painful.) **After a wick is inserted, water must be kept out of the ear, and the patient must be instructed to use soft wax earplugs while showering.**

✔ **Prescribe a topical antimicrobial steroid solution (Cipro HC Otic, Otic Tridesilon Solution, VōSol HC, or Acetasol HC) to be instilled down the wick every 6 to 8 hours for the next 7 to 14 days.** Clear solutions are used most often because they do not obscure follow-up examination, but if there might be a perforation

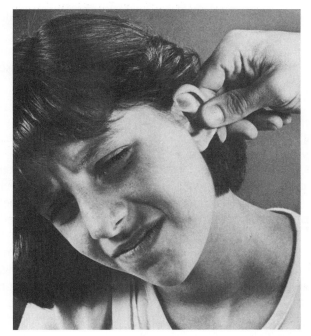

Figure 31-1 Pulling on the ear causes increased pain.

of the tympanic membrane, use a less irritating suspension. Ophthalmic gentamicin solution (Garamycin) is a good choice for treatment of *Pseudomonas* infections but should be avoided if a tympanic membrane perforation is suspected. The antifungal cresyl acetate solution (Cresylate) may be prescribed for a purely fungal infection.

✔ **For moderate to severe pain and soft tissue swelling or other signs of cellulitis, prescribe an appropriate analgesic (e.g., acetaminophen, ibuprofen, naproxen, hydrocodone, or oxycodone) and an antibiotic such as trimethoprim plus sulfamethoxazole (Bactrim) or ciprofloxacin (Cipro), and instruct the patient to use warm, moist compresses to help relieve any pain or swelling.**

✔ **Provide follow-up in 2 to 3 days to remove the wick and any remaining debris from the ear canal.**

✔ Instruct the patient to use a prophylactic 2% acetic acid solution (e.g., Otic Domeboro Solution or half-strength vinegar) after swimming or bathing after the initial therapy has been completed. Also, instruct her to avoid the use of Q-tips within her ear canals.

What Not To Do:

✗ Do not use oral antibiotics to treat simple otitis externa without evidence of cellulitis or concurrent otitis media.

✗ Do not use topical antibiotics for prophylaxis. Long-term use of any topical antibiotics can lead to a fungal superinfection.

✘ Do not instill medication without first cleansing the ear canal, unless restricted because of pain.

✘ Do not expect medicine to enter a canal that is swollen shut without a wick.

✘ Do not use ear drops containing neomycin, which sometimes causes allergic dermatitis.

 DISCUSSION

Otitis externa has a seasonal occurrence, being more frequently encountered in the summer months when the climate and contaminated water will most likely precipitate a fungal or *Pseudomonas aeruginosa* bacterial infection. Various dermatoses, diabetes, aggressive ear cleaning with cotton-tipped swabs, previous external ear infections, and furunculosis also predispose patients to developing otitis externa.

The healthy ear canal is coated with cerumen and sloughed epithelium. Cerumen is water repellent and acidic and contains a number of antimicrobial substances. Repeated washing or cleaning can remove this defensive coating. Moisture retained in the ear canal is readily absorbed by the stratum corneum. The skin becomes macerated and edematous, and the accumulation of debris may block gland ducts, preventing further production of the protective cerumen. Finally, endogenous or exogenous organisms invade the damaged canal epithelium and cause the infection.

Malignant or necrotizing external otitis is a life-threatening condition that occurs primarily in elderly diabetic patients and immunocompromised individuals. Early consultation should be obtained if there is any suspicion of this condition in a susceptible patient with a draining ear.

The ear is innervated by the fifth, seventh, ninth, and tenth cranial nerves and the second and third cervical nerves. Because of this rich nerve supply, the skin is extremely sensitive. Otalgia may arise directly from the seventh cranial nerve (geniculate ganglion), ninth cranial nerve (tympanic branch), external ear, mastoid air cells, mouth, teeth, or esophagus. Ear pain can result from sinusitis, trigeminal neuralgia, and temporomandibular joint dysfunction or may be referred from disorders of the pharynx and larynx. A mild pain referred to the ear may be felt as itching, may cause the patient to scratch the ear canal, and may present as an external otitis. When the source of ear pain is not readily apparent, the patient should be referred for a more complete otolaryngologic investigation.

SUGGESTED READINGS
Wong DLH, Rutka JA: Do aminoglycoside otic preparations cause ototoxicity in the presence of tympanic membrane perforations? *Otolaryngol Head Neck Surg* 116:404-410, 1994.

32

Otitis Media

Presentation

Adults and older children will complain of ear pain. There may or may not be accompanying symptoms of upper respiratory tract infection. In younger children and infants, parents may report that their child is irritable and sleepless, with or without fever, and possibly pulling at her ears. The tympanic membrane shows marked redness, distinct fullness, or bulging. It may be dull or opacified with reduced mobility on pneumatic otoscopy, and there may or may not be accompanying otorrhea.

What To Do:

✔ Investigate for any other underlying illness. When clinical evidence of otitis media is obscure or absent, consider other sources of ear pain, such as dental or oral disease, temporomandibular joint dysfunction, or disorders of the mastoid, pharynx, or larynx.

✔ Inquire as to whether the patient has had a recent or unresponsive ear infection and whether the patient has recently been on an antibiotic.

✔ **If the patient has no recent history of otitis media or antibiotic use, then prescribe an appropriate dose of amoxicillin for 10 days. Trimethoprim plus sulfamethoxazole (Bactrim) may be substituted in the penicillin-allergic patient. It may be reasonable to prescribe 5 days of antibiotics instead of 10 for children at lower risk for complications (e.g., those older than 2 years of age, those experiencing a milder episode, and those with no previous history of otitis media). When there is reliable follow-up and the parents are responsible, mild cases may be treated initially with analgesics alone; adding antimicrobials is an option if symptoms persist or worsen.** Follow-up by telephone or office visit within 3 days or less to reassess.

✔ More expensive antibiotics, such as amoxicillin plus clavulanate (Augmentin), erythromycin plus sulfamethoxazole (Pediazole), azithromycin (Zithromax), and cephalosporins, should be reserved for cases in which treatment has failed and those in which there is associated illness requiring a beta-lactamase–stable antimicrobial. **Ceftriaxone (Rocephin) can be used in a dose of 50 mg/kg IM when compliance problems are anticipated.**

✔ **Provide pain and fever control with acetaminophen or ibuprofen elixir. Additional pain relief may be obtained using antipyrine, benzocaine, oxyquinoline, and glycerine (Auralgan) otic drops.**

✔ Advise parents that pacifier use, exposure to tobacco smoke, and bottle feeding an infant in a reclining rather than an upright position all increase the risk of acute otitis media.

✔ **Recommend a 10-day follow-up examination for all patients younger than 2 years of age,** in those cases in which the parents do not feel the infection has resolved or the child's symptoms persist, and when there is a family history of recurrent otitis or the accuracy of the parental observations may be in doubt. Because otitis media is much less common in adults, these patients also require follow-up with possible otolaryngologic consultation.

What Not To Do:

✗ Do not overlook serious underlying illnesses, such as meningitis.

✗ Do not prescribe antihistamines or decongestants. These drugs do not decrease the incidence or hasten the resolution of otitis media. Antihistamines can make children drowsy, as well as thicken the middle ear fluid, and decongestants can cause irritability.

✗ Do not prescribe ear drops to treat acute otorrhea resulting from spontaneous perforation and drainage. The standard oral therapy is sufficient.

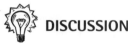 **DISCUSSION**

Most otitis is caused by a viral infection, and most patients do well regardless of the antibiotic chosen. Despite the increase in antimicrobial resistance of community-acquired *Streptococcus pneumoniae*, *Haemophilus influenzae*, and *Moraxella catarrhalis* and the plethora of alternative antibiotics available, amoxicillin remains the drug of choice.

SUGGESTED READINGS

Culpepper L, Froom J: Routine antimicrobial treatment of acute otitis media: is it necessary? *JAMA* 278:1643-1645, 1997 (editorial).

Del Mar C, Glaszion P, Hayem M: Are antimicrobials indicated as initial treatment for children with acute otitis media? A meta-analysis, *Br Med J* 314:1526-1529, 1997.

Froom J, Culpepper L, Jacobs M, et al: Antimicrobials for acute otitis media? A review for the international primary care network, *Br Med J* 315:98-102, 1997.

Niemela M, Uhari M, Jounio-Ervasti K, et al: Lack of specific symptomology in children with acute otitis media, *Pediatr Infect Dis J* 13:765-768, 1994.

Paradise JL: Managing otitis media: a time for change, *Pediatrics* 96:712-715, 1995 (editorial).

Rosenfeld RM, Vertrees JE, Carr J, et al: Clinical efficacy of antimicrobial drugs for acute otitis media: meta-analysis of 5400 children from thirty-three randomized trials, *J Pediatr* 124:355-367, 1994.

33

Perforated Tympanic Membrane (Ruptured Eardrum)

Presentation

The patient experiences ear pain after barotrauma, such as a blow or slap on the ear or a fall while water skiing or during a deep water dive, or after direct trauma inflicted with a stick or other sharp object. Hemorrhage is often noticed within the external canal, and the patient will experience some partial hearing loss and pain. Tinnitus or vertigo may also be present. Otoscopic examination reveals a defect in the tympanic membrane that may or may not be accompanied by disruption of the ossicles (Figure 33-1). The presence of blood may make assessment difficult.

What To Do:

✔ Clear any debris from the canal, using gentle suction.

✔ Test for nystagmus and gross hearing loss.

✔ **Place a protective cotton plug inside the ear canal, and instruct the patient to keep the canal dry by using soft wax earplugs and to avoid submerging his head under water.**

✔ **Prescribe an appropriate analgesic,** such as ibuprofen (Motrin), naproxen (Anaprox), or acetaminophen with hydrocodone (Lorcet) or with oxycodone (Percocet).

✔ **Prescribe systemic antibiotics only if the lacerated tympanic membrane and middle ear were contaminated with lake water, seawater, or a dirty object, such as a tree branch.**

✔ **Ensure that the patient gets early follow-up with an otolaryngologist.**

What Not To Do:

✘ Do not instill any fluid into the external canal or allow the patient to get water into his ear. Water in the middle ear is painful and irritating and may introduce bacteria. Wax earplugs or a cotton plug covered with petroleum jelly will allow the patient to shower safely.

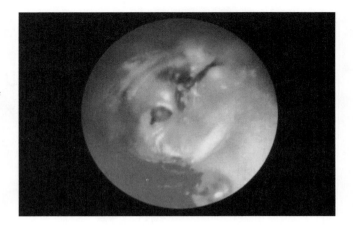

Figure 33-1 Acute tympanic membrane perforation. *(From Knoop KJ, Stack LB, Storrow AB:* Atlas of emergency medicine, *New York, 1997, McGraw-Hill.)*

 DISCUSSION

Small uncomplicated perforations usually heal without sequelae. When there is nystagmus, vertigo, profound hearing loss, or disruption of the ossicles, early otolaryngologic consultation is advisable.

34

Pharyngitis (Sore Throat)

Presentation

The patient with a bacterial pharyngitis complains of a rapid onset of throat pain worsened by swallowing. There is usually a fever; pharyngeal erythema; purulent, patchy, yellow, gray, or white exudate; tender anterior cervical adenopathy; headache; and absence of cough. Viral infections are typically accompanied by conjunctivitis, nasal congestion, hoarseness, cough, aphthous ulcers on the soft palate, and myalgias. It is helpful to differentiate pain on swallowing (odynophagia) from difficulty swallowing (dysphagia); the latter is more likely to be caused by obstruction or abnormal muscular movement.

What To Do:

✔ First examine the ears, nose, and mouth, which are, after all, connected to the pharynx and often contain clues to the diagnosis.

✔ Depress the tongue with a blade, and then instruct the patient to say "ah," thereby raising her soft palate. Inspect the posterior pharynx, and swab both tonsillar pillars for a culture. (It can be decided later whether or not the culture should be planted. Rapid strep tests may provide results in a few minutes, while cultures may take 1 to 2 days to incubate and interpret.)

✔ **If there is a current epidemic of group A streptococcal pharyngitis or if the patient is between 3 and 25 years of age, has a history of rheumatic fever and recurrent "strep throats," has recently been exposed to the bacteria, or has a red throat, fever, tender anterior cervical nodes, and no symptoms of a viral upper respiratory tract infection (or any convincing subset of the above), begin therapy with antibiotics. Throat culture is optional,** at the preference of the follow-up physician. **The recommended dosage for the treatment for streptococcal pharyngitis is oral penicillin VK 250 mg q8h for 10 days. Injectable penicillins are preferable for patients who are unlikely to finish 10 days of pills**

and for those with a personal or family history of rheumatic fever. Patients weighing less than 60 lbs (30 kg) should be given one IM injection of benzathine penicillin G 600,000 units and those weighing more than 60 lbs given 1,200,000 units IM. **For those allergic to penicillin, prescribe erythromycin 250 mg qid** (or 333 mg of erythromycin base tid) for 10 days. Amoxicillin offers no significant advantage for treating group A streptococcal infections.

✔ **If the infection is not clearly bacterial or the need for antibiotic therapy is questionable (or you or the patient "need to know" if this is really a strep infection), obtain a rapid strep test.** If the results of the rapid strep test are positive, then treat with antibiotics as described earlier. **If the results are negative or unavailable and clinical suspicion of a viral pharyngitis is high, provide symptomatic treatment** (as described later), **send for the throat culture, and hold off treatment with antibiotics pending the results.**

✔ For resistant or recurrent infections with possible beta-lactamase–producing copathogens, consider instead 10 days of treatment with cephalexin (Keflex), cefadroxil (Duricef, Ultracef), cefaclor (Ceclor), or cefuroxime (Ceftin, Zinacef).

✔ If mononucleosis is suspected, draw blood to test for atypical lymphocytes and perform a heterophile antibody or monospot test to confirm the diagnosis (see Chapter 29).

✔ **Relieve pain with acetaminophen, ibuprofen, aspirin, warm saline gargles, and gargles or lozenges containing phenol as a mucosal anesthetic (e.g., Chloraseptic, Cepastat).** A 1:1 mixture of diphenhydramine and kaolin–pectin suspension can also provide temporary relief of throat pain. Lidocaine (Viscous Xylocaine) gargles anesthetize the throat, but patients may still have difficulty swallowing because of the lack of sensation. **For severe pain in patients without contraindications, one dose of dexamethasone 10 mg IM has been used in conjunction with antibiotics.**

What Not To Do:

✘ Do not overlook acute epiglottic or supraglottic inflammation. In children this presents as a sudden, severe pharyngitis, with a guttural rather than hoarse voice (because it hurts to speak), drooling (because it hurts to swallow), and respiratory distress (because swelling narrows the airway). Adults usually have a more gradual onset over several days and are not as prone to a sudden airway occlusion, unless they present later in the progression of the swelling and are already experiencing some respiratory distress.

✘ Do not give ampicillin to a patient with mononucleosis. Although the resulting rash helps make the diagnosis, it does not imply ampicillin allergy and can be uncomfortable.

✘ Do not overlook abscesses, which usually require hospitalization and IV penicillin, and perhaps drainage. Peritonsillar abscesses or cellulitis cause the tonsillar pillar to bulge toward the midline. Retropharyngeal abscesses (and epiglottitis) may be visible only on soft tissue lateral neck films.

✘ Do not overlook gonococcal pharyngitis in patient at risk. This can produce a mild clinical syndrome and requires special cultures on Thayer-Martin medium.

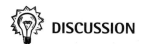

DISCUSSION

Be aware of the rare but deadly causes of sore throat. A patient with paresthesia at the site of an old, healed bite and painful spasms when she even thinks of swallowing may have rabies. A patient with facial palsy, myocarditis, and a tough, white, membrane adherent to the posterior pharynx may have diphtheria. Squamous cell carcinoma should be considered in high risk patients whose symptoms do not resolve as expected. If they are not considered, these conditions may go undiagnosed.

Members of the general public know to see a doctor for a sore throat, but the actual benefit of this visit is unclear. Rheumatic fever is a sequela of about 1% of group A streptococcal infections, and only about 10% of sore throats seen by physicians represent group A streptococcal infections. Poststreptococcal glomerulonephritis is usually a self-limiting illness and is not prevented with antibiotic treatment. Penicillin therapy does prevent acute rheumatic fever and may sometimes reduce symptoms or shorten the course of a sore throat. Antibiotics probably inhibit the infection from progressing into tonsillitis, peritonsillar and retropharyngeal abscesses, adenitis, and pneumonia.

Group A streptococcal infection cannot be diagnosed reliably based on clinical signs and symptoms. Typically a quarter of throat cultures grow group A streptococcus, and half of those represent carriers who do not raise antistreptococcal antibodies and risk rheumatic fever. Rapid strep screens are less sensitive than cultures. The best approach to the identification and treatment of streptococcal pharyngitis depends on the prevalence of group A streptococcal infection in the patient population, the cost and availability of culture and rapid test methods, the reliability of communication and follow-up, and the relative values of cost, antibiotic overuse, and adverse outcomes.

SUGGESTED READINGS

Bisno AL, Gerber MA, Gwaltney JM, et al: Diagnosis and management of group A streptococcal pharyngitis: a practice guideline, *Clin Infect Dis* 25:574-583, 1997.

Coonan KM, Kaplan EL: In vitro susceptibility of recent North American group A streptococcal isolates to eleven oral antibiotics, *Pediatr Infect Dis J* 13:630-635, 1994.

Huovinen P, Lahhtonen R, Ziegler T et al: Pharyngitis in adults: the presence and coexistence of viruses and bacterial organisms, *Ann Intern Med* 110:612-616, 1989.

O'Brien JF, Meade JL, Falk JL: Dexamethasone as adjuvant therapy for severe acute pharyngitis, *Ann Emerg Med* 22:212-214, 1993.

Pichichero ME: Group A streptococcal tonsillopharyngitis: cost-effective diagnosis and treatment, *Ann Emerg Med* 25:390-403, 1995 (editorial 404-406).

35

Serous (Secretory) Otitis Media

Presentation

After an upper respiratory tract infection, an episode of acute otitis media, or an airplane flight or during a bout with allergies, an adult may complain of a feeling of fullness in his ears, an inability to equalize middle ear pressure, decreased hearing, and hearing clicking, popping, or crackling sounds, especially when he moves his head. There is little pain or tenderness. When viewed through the otoscope, the tympanic membrane appears retracted, with a dull to normal light reflex, minimal if any injection, and poor motion on insufflation. An air-fluid level or bubbles through the eardrum may be visible (Figure 35-1). Hearing may be decreased, and the Rinne test may show decreased air conduction (i.e., a tuning fork is heard no better through air than through bone).

What To Do:

✔ **Instruct the patient to lie supine, with his head tilted back and toward the affected side, and then instill vasoconstrictor nose drops such as phenylephrine 1% (Neo-Synephrine) or oxymetazoline 0.05% (Afrin). Allow 2 minutes for the nasal mucosa to shrink, and instill nose drops again. Wait an additional 2 minutes for the medicine to seep down to the posterior pharyngeal wall and around the opening of the eustachian tube. Have the patient repeat this procedure with drops (not spray) every 4 hours during the day for no more than 3 days.**

✔ **Instruct the patient to insufflate his middle ear via his eustachian tube after each treatment with nose drops by closing his mouth, pinching his nose shut, and blowing until his ears "pop."**

✔ **When treating adults, unless contraindicated by hypertension or other medical conditions, add a systemic vasoconstrictor (pseudoephedrine 60 mg qid).**

✔ When treating children or adults, if a middle ear effusion is associated with an upper respiratory tract infection that has not improved after more than 2 weeks, consider administering antibiotics as for treatment of acute otitis media.

✔ Instruct the patient to seek otolaryngologic follow-up if the condition does not improve within 1 week.

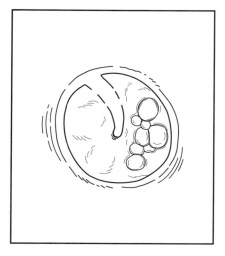

Figure 35-1 Bubbles inside the tympanic membrane.

What Not To Do:

✗ Do not allow the patient to become habituated to vasoconstrictor nose drops. After a few days of use, the drops become ineffective, and then the nasal mucosa develops a rebound swelling known as *rhinitis medicamentosa* when the medicine is withdrawn.

✗ Do not prescribe antihistamines (which dry out secretions) unless clearly indicated by an allergy.

 ## DISCUSSION

Acute serous otitis media is probably caused by obstruction of the eustachian tube, creating negative pressure in the middle ear that then draws a fluid transudate out of the middle ear epithelium. Most such episodes resolve spontaneously within 1 to 2 months. The treatment described here is directed solely at reestablishing the patency of the eustachian tube, but further treatment includes insufflation of the eustachian tube or myringotomy. Fluid in the middle ear is more common in children because of frequent viral upper respiratory tract infections and an underdeveloped eustachian tube. Children are also more prone to bacterial superinfection of the fluid in the middle ear, and when accompanied by fever and pain, this condition merits treatment with analgesics and antibiotics (e.g., ibuprofen and amoxicillin) (see Chapter 32). Repeated bouts of serous otitis, especially if unilateral, in an adult should raise suspicion regarding obstruction of the eustachian tube by tumor or lymphatic hypertrophy.

SUGGESTED READINGS

Csortan E, Jones J, Haan M, et al: Efficacy of pseudoephedrine for the prevention of barotrauma during air travel, *Ann Emerg Med* 23:1324-1327, 1994.

36

Sinusitis

Presentation

After a viral infection, the patient may complain of a dull facial pain, which is usually unilateral, gradually increases over a couple of days, is exacerbated by sudden motion of the head or the patient bending over and holding her head dependent, may radiate to the upper molar teeth (via the maxillary antrum), and may increase with eye movement (via the ethmoid sinuses). Often there is a sensation of facial congestion and stuffiness. The child with sinusitis often has a cough and fetid breath. The patient's voice may have a resonance similar to that of an individual with a "stopped up" nose, and she may complain of a foul taste in her mouth. Stuffy ears and impaired hearing are common because of associated serous otitis media and eustachian tube dysfunction. A colored nasal discharge is a particularly sensitive finding. Fever is present in only half of all patients with acute infection and is usually low grade. A high fever usually indicates a serious complication, such as meningitis, or another diagnosis altogether. Transillumination of sinuses in the emergency department (ED) is usually unrewarding, but tenderness may be elicited on gentle percussion or firm palpation over the maxillary or frontal sinuses or between the eyes (ethmoid sinuses). Swelling and erythema may exist (Figure 36-1), and pus may be visible draining below the nasal turbinates, with a purulent, yellow-green, and sometimes foul-smelling or bloody discharge from the nose, or running down the posterior pharynx.

What To Do:

✔ Rule out other possible causes of facial pain or headache via the patient's history (determine whether she woke up with a typical migraine) and physical examination (palpate the scalp muscles, temporal arteries, temporomandibular joints, eyes, and teeth).

✔ **Shrink swollen nasal mucosa (and thereby open the ostia, draining the sinuses) with 1% phenylephrine (Neo-Synephrine) or 0.05% oxymetazoline (Afrin) nose drops. Instill 2 drops in each nostril, allow the patient to lie supine for 2 minutes, and then repeat the process** (Figure 36-2). (Repeating the process allows the first application to open the anterior nose so the second dose gets farther back.) **Have the patient repeat this process every 4 hours but for no more than 3 days** (to avoid rhinitis medicamentosa).

✔ Examine the nose for purulent drainage before and after shrinking the nasal mucosa with a topical vasoconstrictor.

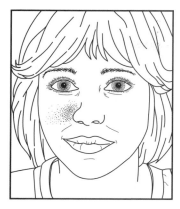

Figure 36-1 Swelling and erythema may exist with sinusitis.

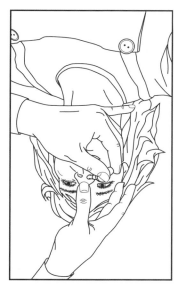

Figure 36-2 Procedure for applying nose drops.

✔ **Prescribe systemic sympathomimetic decongestants such as pseudoephedrine (Sudafed) 60 mg q6h or phenylpropanolamine (Entex LA) 75 mg q12h.**

✔ **If there is fever, pus, heat, or any other sign of a bacterial superinfection or if symptoms have been prolonged, administer a 10-day course of antibiotics such as amoxicillin plus clavulanate (Augmentin), trimethoprim plus sulfamethoxazole (Bactrim), cefuroxime (Ceftin), or clarithromycin (Biaxin).**

✔ **Provide pain relief** (e.g., ibuprofen, naproxen, acetaminophen, oxycodone, hydrocodone) when necessary.

✔ **For symptomatic relief, recommend that the patient try hot water vapor inhalation** using a simple teakettle, a hot shower, a steam vaporizer, or a home facial sauna device, if available.

✔ Arrange for follow-up within 1 to 7 days, depending on the severity of the initial findings.

What Not To Do:

✗ Do not ignore signs of an orbital cellulitis with swelling, erythema, decreased extraocular movements, and possible proptosis. These patients require consultation and hospital admission for IV antibiotic therapy.

✗ Do not ignore the toxic patient who has marked swelling, high fever, severe pain, profuse drainage, or other signs and symptoms of a serious infection. See the potential complications described later. These patients require immediate consultation and intervention.

✗ Do not order routine x-ray films. Reserve them for difficult diagnoses and treatment failures.

✗ Do not prescribe antihistamines, which can make mucous secretions dry and thick and interfere with necessary drainage. Antihistamines cure sinusitis only on television or when it is due to allergic rhinitis.

✗ Do not allow the patient to use decongestant nose drops for more than 3 days, which will prevent her nasal mucosa from becoming habituated to sympathomimetic medication. If she uses the drops for more than 3 days, the patient will suffer a rebound nasal congestion (rhinitis medicamentosa) when use of the drops is discontinued; resolution of this condition requires time, topical steroids, and reeducation.

✗ Do not prescribe long-term topical or systemic sympathomimetic decongestants to a patient who suffers from hypertension, tachycardia, or difficulty initiating urination, all of which may be exacerbated.

 DISCUSSION

Sinusitis is the most common health care complaint in the United States. The paranasal sinuses drain through tiny ostia under the nasal turbinates. Occlusion of these ostia allows secretions and pressure differences to build up, resulting in the pressure and pain of acute sinusitis and the air-fluid levels sometimes visible on upright x-ray films. Early mild cases do not require treatment with antibiotics. However, congested sinuses can become a site for bacterial superinfection.

Most sinusitis begins with ostial obstruction caused by mucosal swelling associated with a viral upper respiratory tract infection. Other causes include dental infection; allergic rhinitis; barotrauma caused by flying, swimming, or diving; nasal polyps and tumors; and foreign bodies, including nasogastric and endotracheal tubes placed in hospitalized patients. Abscessed teeth can be the source of a maxillary sinusitis. If there is tenderness on percussion of the bicuspids or molars, arrange for dental referral.

Complications such as orbital cellulitis, osteomyelitis, epidural abscess, meningitis, cavernous sinus thrombosis, and subdural empyema can be devastating, and therefore patients must be instructed to seek early follow-up when signs and symptoms worsen or do not improve in 48 to 72 hours or if there is any change in mentation. Frontal sinusitis has the greatest potential for serious complications, particularly in adolescent boys, the group at greatest risk for intracranial complications.

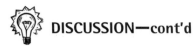

DISCUSSION—cont'd

Sinusitis can sometimes be demonstrated on x-ray films, but usually films are not necessary or helpful on an emergency basis. If symptoms and physical findings of sinusitis are classic, plain sinus radiographs need not be obtained before treatment is begun. If an acute attack does not resolve with medical treatment or if the diagnosis of sinusitis is in doubt, plain films are helpful as the primary imaging study. A single upright Water's view will usually allow adequate visualization of maxillary, frontal, and ethmoid sinuses. Chronic sinusitis appears as thickened mucosa, and acute sinusitis appears as an air-fluid level or complete opacification.

CT scans of the sinuses are more accurate than plain x-ray films, particularly when evaluating the ethmoid or sphenoid sinuses, but CT scans are needed by the ED only in unusual circumstances. Most patients can receive initial treatment on the basis of the history and physical examination findings alone. Anyone who has facial pain, headache, purulent nasal discharge, and nasal congestion persisting for more than 10 days, with or without fever, should probably be treated empirically for sinusitis.

Many patients have been conditioned by the advertising of over-the-counter antihistamines for "sinus" problems (usually meaning "allergic rhinitis") and may relate a history of "sinuses," which on closer questioning turns out to have been rhinitis.

SUGGESTED READINGS

Gwaltney J: Acute community-acquired sinusitis, *Clin Infect Dis* 23:1209-1223, 1996.

Low DE, Desrosiers M, McSherry J, et al: A practical guide for the diagnosis and treatment of acute sinusitis, *Can Med Assoc J* 156(suppl 6):S1-S14. 1997.

Van Buchem FL, Knottnerus JA, Schrijnemaekers VJ: Primary-care-based randomized placebo-controlled trial of antibiotic treatment in acute maxillary sinusitis, *Lancet* 349:683-687, 1997.

Williams JW, Simel DL: Does this patient have sinusitis? Diagnosing acute sinusitis by history and physical examination, *J Am Med Assoc* 270:1242-1246, 1993.

37   Split Earlobe

Presentation

A patient comes to the emergency department or clinic with an earlobe split by a sudden pull on an earring (Figure 37-1).

What To Do:

✔ **Excise the skin edges on both sides of the wound, leaving the apical epithelium intact. Suture these freshened wound edges together using a fine monofilament material.**

✔ **If the patient wants to maintain a pierced earlobe, tie a loop of sterile suture material through the hole to maintain a tract while the rest of the lobe heals.**

✔ Provide tetanus prophylaxis if needed.

What Not To Do:

✘ Do not suture the wound primarily. The edges may epithelialize, resulting in the split re-developing after the sutures are removed.

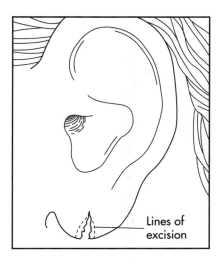

Figure 37-1 Excision lines for a split earlobe.

 DISCUSSION

There are many techniques for the repair of split earlobes. Some methods, including this one, attempt to preserve the earring hole, whereas others use a Z-plasty on the free margins of the lobes to prevent notching at the points of reunion. Depending on the specific circumstances, it may be advisable to consult with a plastic surgeon before attempting to repair this type of earlobe injury.

Oral and Dental Emergencies

38

Aphthous Ulcer
(Canker Sore)

Presentation

The patient complains of a painful lesion in her mouth and may be worried about having herpes. A pale yellow, flat, even-bordered ulcer surrounded by a red halo may be seen on the buccal or labial mucosa, lingual sulci, soft palate, pharynx, tongue, or gingiva. Lesions are usually solitary but can be multiple and recurrent. The pain is usually greater than the size of the lesions would suggest, and major aphthae (larger than 1 cm) indicate a severe form of the disease that may last for weeks or months (Figure 38-1).

What To Do:

✔ Attempt to differentiate these sores from lesions of **herpes simplex** (see Chapter 52), **and reassure the patient of the benign nature of most canker sores.**

✔ **Inform the patient that these lesions usually last 1 to 2 weeks, and that she should avoid hot, acidic, or irritating food and drink.**

✔ **Prescribe amlexanox (Aphthasol Oral Paste) to be applied qid. This medication may sting, but it is the first drug to be approved by the FDA for aphthous ulcers in healthy people.**

✔ **An alternative treatment that can be used for transient pain relief is a tablet of sucralfate crushed in a small amount of warm water and swirled in the mouth or gargled.** Another alternative is tetracycline elixir (or a capsule dissolved in water) not swallowed but applied to cauterize lesions or used as a mouth wash. This also stings but sometimes can relieve pain after one or more applications. Diphenhydramine (Benadryl) elixir mixed 1:1 with kaolin-pectin (Kaopectate), lidocaine (Xylocaine 2% Viscous Solution), and **benzocaine (Orabase HCA) applied topically can also provide symptomatic relief.**

✔ **For more severe cases, prescribe triamcinolone acetonide (Kenalog) 0.1% suspension** (add injectable triamcinolone to sterile water without preservatives) **in a 5-ml oral rinse; instruct the patient to rinse qid, after meals and before bed,** spit the rinse out, and take nothing by mouth for an hour afterward. An alternative treatment

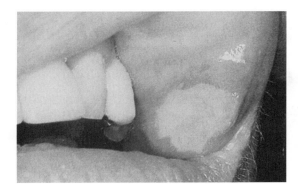

Figure 38-1 Major recurrent aphthous ulcer. *(From Ship JA: Recurrent aphthous stomatitis: an update,* Oral Surg Oral Med Oral Pathol *81(2):141-147, 1996.)*

regimen is dexamethasone elixir 1.5 mg in a 15-ml rinse, which should be taken qid and swallowed, tapering to 3 days of 0.5 ml in a 5-ml rinse, swallowing each dose, then 3 days, swallowing every other dose. The regimen should be discontinued as soon as the mouth becomes comfortable.

✔ **In very severe cases, try a burst dose of prednisone 40 to 60 mg qd for 5 days** (no tapering).

✔ Warn patients that a detergent and foaming agent, sodium laurel sulfate, found in most toothpastes can aggravate canker sores.

 ## DISCUSSION

Aphthous stomatitis has been studied for many years by numerous investigators. Although many exacerbating factors have been identified, the cause as yet remains unknown. Lesions can be precipitated by minor trauma, food allergy, stress, nutritional deficiencies (e.g., iron, folic acid, vitamin B_{12}), and systemic illness. Recurrent aphthous ulcers may accompany malignancy or autoimmune disease. At present, the treatment is only palliative and may not alter the course of the syndrome. Aphthous ulcers may be an immune reaction to damaged mucosa or altered oral bacteria.

Herpangina and hand-foot-and-mouth disease can produce ulcers resembling aphthous ulcers, but these ulcers are instead part of coxsackie viral exanthems, usually occurring with fever and in clusters among children. Behçet's syndrome is an idiopathic condition characterized by oral ulcers that are clinically indistinguishable from aphthae but are accompanied by genital ulcers, conjunctivitis, retinitis, iritis, leukocytosis, eosinophilia, and increased erythrocyte sedimentation rate (ESR).

SUGGESTED READINGS

Ship JA: Recurrent aphthous stomatitis: an update, *Oral Surg Oral Med Oral Pathol* 81:141-147, 1996.
Vincent SD, Lilly GE: Clinical, historic and therapeutic features of aphthous stomatitis, *Oral Surg Oral Med Oral Pathol* 74:79-86, 1992.

39

Avulsed Tooth

Presentation

After a direct blow to the mouth, the patient may have a permanent tooth that has been knocked out of its socket. The tooth is intact down to its root, from which hangs the delicate periodontal ligament that used to attach to alveolar bone and provide the tooth with its blood supply.

What To Do:

- ✔ **If the tooth is only partially avulsed and is just protruding farther out of its socket than normal, simply push it back in until it sits in its proper position.**
- ✔ **In the field, fully avulsed teeth may be stored under the tongue or in the buccal vestibule** between the gums and the teeth. **If the patient is unconscious, the tooth can be stored in saline solution, milk, or water** until a better preservation solution is available. **A child's permanent tooth might be preserved, if necessary, in the parent's mouth.**
- ✔ **If the tooth has been out of its socket for less than 15 minutes, take it by the crown, drop it in a tooth-preservation solution (Hank's solution, Sav-A-Tooth kit), and flush the socket with the same solution. Then reimplant the tooth firmly, instruct the patient to bite down hard on a piece of gauze to help stabilize the tooth, and when possible secure the tooth to adjacent teeth with wire, arch bars, or a temporary periodontal pack (Coe-Pak).** Coe-Pak is a periodontal dressing that comes in the form of a base and a catalyst. Mix together the two parts, and mold the resulting paste, which will eventually set semi-hard, over the gingival line and between the teeth. **Put the patient on a liquid diet, prescribe penicillin VK 500 mg qid for 2 weeks, and schedule a dental appointment.**
- ✔ **If the tooth has been out of its socket for 15 minutes to 2 hours, soak it for 30 minutes to replenish nutrients. Local anesthesia will probably be needed before the tooth can be reimplanted as described earlier.**
- ✔ If the tooth has been out of its socket for longer than 2 hours, the periodontal ligament is dead and should be removed, along with the pulp. Soak the tooth for 30 minutes in 5% sodium hypochlorite (Clorox) and 5 minutes each in saturated citric acid, 1% stannous fluoride, and 5% doxycycline before reimplanting. The dead tooth should ankylose into the alveolar bone of the socket like a dental implant.

✔ **Even when the tooth has been out less than 2 hours, if the patient is between 6 and 10 years of age, also soak the tooth for 5 minutes in 5% doxycycline to kill bacteria that could enter the immature apex and form an abscess.**

✔ **If all this cannot be done right away, simply keep the tooth soaking in the preservation solution until a dentist can get to it. The solution should preserve the tooth safely for up to 4 days.**

✔ **If a tooth is lost, obtain a chest x-ray film to rule out bronchial aspiration.**

✔ Add **tetanus prophylaxis** to the treatment protocol if required (see Chapter 151).

What Not To Do:

✘ Do not touch a viable root with fingers, forceps, gauze, or anything else, and do not try to scrub or clean it. The periodontal ligament will be injured and unable to revascularize the reimplanted tooth.

✘ Do not overlook fractures of teeth and alveolar ridges.

✘ Do not substitute the calcium hydroxide composition (Dycal) used for covering fractured teeth for the temporary periodontal pack (Coe-Pak) used to stabilize luxated teeth. They are different products.

✘ Do not replace primary deciduous or baby teeth. Reimplanted primary teeth heal by ankylosis; they literally fuse to the bone, which can lead to cosmetic deformity because the area of ankylosis will not grow at the same rate as the rest of the dentofacial complex. Ankylosis can also interfere with eruption of the permanent tooth.

✘ Do not confuse an avulsed adult tooth with a child's deciduous tooth that would fall out soon anyway. Normal developmental shedding of primary decidual teeth is preceded by absorption of the root, so that if such a tooth is brought in by mistake, there is no root to reimplant and little or no empty socket; instead, a new permanent tooth may be visible or palpable underneath.

 DISCUSSION

Before commercially available 320-mOs, 7.2-pH reconstitution solutions (e.g., Hank's solution), the best treatment that could be offered the avulsed tooth was rapid reimplantation. Without a preservation solution, the chances of successful reimplantation decline 1 percentage point every minute the tooth is absent from the oral cavity. In mature teeth (those more than 10 years old) the pulp will not survive avulsion even if the periodontal ligament does, and at the 1-week follow-up visit with the dentist the necrotic pulp will be removed to prevent a chronic inflammatory reaction from interfering with the healing of the periodontal ligament.

SUGGESTED READINGS

Krasner P: Modern treatment of avulsed teeth by emergency physicians, *Am J Emerg Med* 12:241-246, 1994.

40

Bleeding After Dental Surgery

Presentation

The patient who had an extraction or other dental surgery performed earlier in the day now has excessive bleeding at the site and is unable to contact her dentist.

What To Do:

✔ Ask the patient what procedure was done. Inquire about ingestion of antiplatelet drugs such as aspirin, underlying coagulopathies, and previous experiences with unusual bleeding.

✔ **Using suction and saline irrigation, clear any packing and clot from the bleeding site.**

✔ **Roll a 2- × 2-inch gauze pad, insert it over the bleeding site, and have the patient apply constant pressure on it (biting down usually suffices) for 20 minutes.**

✔ **If the site is still bleeding after 20 minutes** of gauze pressure, infiltrate the extraction area and **inject a local anesthetic and vasoconstrictor, such as 2% lidocaine with 1:100,000 or 1:200,000 epinephrine, into the socket until the tissue blanches. Again, have the patient bite on a gauze pad for 20 minutes.** The anesthetic allows the patient to bite down harder, and the epinephrine helps restrict the bleeding.

✔ **If this injection does not stop the bleeding, pack the bleeding site with Gelfoam or gauze soaked in topical thrombin. Then place the gauze pad on top, and apply pressure again.**

✔ An arterial bleeder resistant to all the aforementioned treatments may require ligation with a figure-eight stitch.

✔ Assess any possible large blood loss by obtaining orthostatic vital signs.

✔ When the bleeding stops, remove the overlying gauze and instruct the patient to leave the site alone for a day and see her dentist for follow-up.

What Not To Do:

✗ Do not routinely obtain laboratory clotting studies or hematocrit levels, unless there is reason to suspect that they will be abnormal.

 DISCUSSION

Occasionally this problem can be handled with telephone consultation alone. Some say a tea bag works even better than a gauze pad.

chapter

Burning Tongue

Presentation

The patient is very uncomfortable because of a burning sensation of the tongue or mouth. There may be xerostomia (reduced salivary flow), dental disease, geographic tongue, candidiasis (see Chapter 51), or no visible explanation for the pain.

What To Do:

✔ **Treat specific causative factors such as *Candida* infections or dental problems.**
✔ **Provide symptomatic relief with a 1:1 mixture of diphenhydramine (Benadryl) elixir and kaolin-pectin (Kaopectate), or prescribe viscous lidocaine (Xylocaine).**
✔ If the etiology is uncertain, refer the patient for a comprehensive medical evaluation.

 DISCUSSION

Burning tongue or burning mouth symptoms are usually caused by xerostomia, candidiasis or another chronic infection, referred pain from the tongue muscles, dental disease, reflux of gastric acid, reaction to medications, noxious oral habits, blood dyscrasias, nutritional deficiencies, allergies, inflammatory disorders, psychogenic factors, or unknown causes. Geographic tongue results from loss of filiform papillae from patches on the dorsal surface of the tongue. The location of the patches may appear to shift over a period of weeks. Usually this condition is not painful and does not require specific treatment.

42

Dental Pain, Periapical Abscess

Presentation

The patient complains of dull, constant facial or dental pain, often associated with facial swelling and cellulitis and accompanied by signs of systemic toxicity. Dental caries may or may not be apparent. Percussion of the offending tooth causes increased pain (Figure 42-1). Hot and cold sensitivity may no longer be present because of necrosis of the pulp. There may be increased mobility of the tooth, and an examining finger in the soft tissues of the mouth, face, or neck may even palpate a fluctuant abscess.

What To Do:

✔ **Adequate pain medication should be administered and prescribed for continued pain relief.** A combination of acetaminophen with hydrocodone or oxycodone usually suffices. Add NSAIDs for synergistic analgesia.

✔ **Depending on the level of toxicity, the patient initially should be treated with either parenteral or oral penicillin, and a 10-day course of penicillin VK 500 mg qid should be prescribed. Erythromycin or clindamycin may be substituted if the patient is allergic to penicillin.**

✔ **If a fluctuant abscess cavity is present, perform incision and drainage** at the most dependent location, and, when possible, insert a drain for 24 hours.

✔ **Instruct the patient to apply warm compresses to the affected area and seek follow-up care from a dentist within 24 hours.**

What Not To Do:

✘ Do not insert an obstructing pack (i.e., cotton soaked with oil of cloves) into a tooth cavity when an abscess or cellulitis is present.

✘ Do not prescribe aspirin if it is possible that a tooth will need to be extracted.

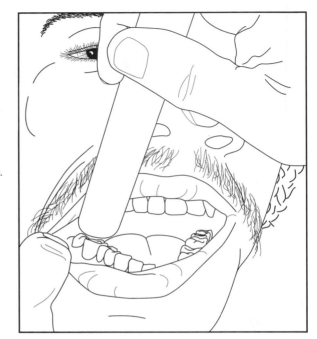

Figure 42-1 Percussion of tooth with tongue blade.

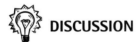 **DISCUSSION**

Dental pain may be referred to the ear, temple, eye, neck, or other teeth. Conversely, what appears to be dental pain may in fact be caused by overlying maxillary sinusitis or otitis. Diabetes and valvular heart disease increase the risk from bacteremia, and local extension of infection can lead to retropharyngeal abscess, Ludwig's cellulitis, cavernous sinus thrombosis, osteomyelitis, mediastinitis, and pulmonary abscess.

An acute periodontal (as opposed to periapical) abscess causes localized, painful, fluctuant swelling of the gingiva, either between the teeth or laterally, and is associated with vital teeth that are not sensitive to percussion. Treatment consists of local infiltrative anesthesia and drainage by subgingival curettage. In severe cases or cases in which there is fever, prescribe doxycycline 100 mg bid for 10 days. Also, instruct the patient to rinse his mouth with warm salt water and consult a dentist for further treatment.

43

Dental Pain, Pericoronitis

Presentation

The patient is between the ages of 17 and 25 and seeks help because of painful swelling and infection around an erupting or impacted third molar (wisdom tooth). Occasionally there can be trismus or pain on biting. The site appears red and swollen, with a flap that may reveal a partial tooth eruption and purulent drainage when pulled open. There is no pain on percussion of the tooth (Figure 43-1).

What To Do:

✔ **Irrigate with a weak (2%) hydrogen peroxide solution.** Purulent material can be released by placing the catheter tip of the irrigating syringe under the tissue flap overlying the impacted molar.

✔ **Prescribe oral analgesics for comfort and penicillin to be taken over the next 10 days (penicillin VK 500 mg qid).**

✔ Instruct the patient regarding the importance of cleansing away any food particles that collect beneath the gingival flap. This can be accomplished simply by using a soft toothbrush or by using water jet irrigation.

✔ **A follow-up visit with a dentist should be arranged** so that the resolution of the acute infection can be observed and the need to remove the gingival flap or molar can be evaluated.

What Not To Do:

✗ Do not undertake any major blunt dissection while draining pus. This could spread a superficial infection into the deep spaces of the head and neck or follow a deep abscess posteriorly into the carotid sheath.

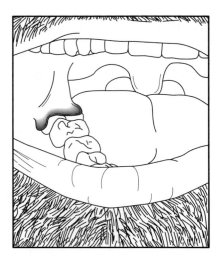

Figure 43-1 Painful swelling and infection around an erupting or impacted third molar.

 DISCUSSION

Pericoronitis is a special type of acute periodontal abscess that occurs when gingival tissue (operculum) overlies an erupting tooth (usually a third molar, also known as a wisdom tooth). Recurring acute symptoms are usually initiated by trauma inflicted by the opposing tooth or by impaction of food or debris under the flap of tissue that partially covers the erupting tooth.

When dental referral is not readily available, one procedure that can relieve the pain is surgical removal of the operculum. Inject local anesthetic directly into the overlying tissue, and then cut it away using the outline of the tooth as a guide for the incision. Sutures are not required.

Dental Pain, Postextraction (Dry Socket)

Presentation

The patient develops severe, dull, throbbing pain 2 to 4 days after a tooth extraction. The pain is often excruciating, may radiate to the ear, and is not relieved by oral analgesics. There may be associated foul odor and taste. The extraction site is filled with necrotic tissue that is delaying wound healing.

What To Do:

✔ **Consider an anesthetic nerve block (see Appendix D) before initiating any treatment.**

✔ **Irrigate the socket with warm normal saline solution.**

✔ **Pack the socket with ¼-inch iodoform gauze soaked in oil of cloves (eugenol).**

✔ **Prescribe oxycodone (Percocet, Tylox) and NSAIDs for additional pain relief.**

✔ **Refer the patient back to her dentist for follow-up.** The gauze packing should be removed and replaced every 24 hours until symptoms subside.

What Not To Do:

✗ Do not prescribe antibiotics unless there is a systemic infection. Resolution of the problem depends on granulation in the socket rather than elimination of infection.

✗ Do not try to create a new clot by stirring up bleeding. Scraping the socket can implant bacteria in the alveolar bone, setting the stage for osteomyelitis.

DISCUSSION

Dry socket results from a pathologic process combining loss of the healing blood clot with a localized inflammation (alveolar osteitis). It most commonly occurs with extraction of the mandibular molars. This condition may be encouraged by smoking, spitting, or drinking through a straw, which create negative pressure in the oral cavity. Intractable pain usually responds to a nerve block with long-acting local anesthetics.

45

Dental Pain, Pulpitis

Presentation

The patient develops an acute toothache with sharp, throbbing pain that is often worse with recumbent position. The patient may or may not be aware that he has a cavity in the affected tooth. Initially the pain is decreased by heat application and increased by cold application, but as the condition progresses, heat application worsens the pain, whereas application of ice dramatically relieves it. (The patient might come to the emergency department with his own cup of ice and may not allow examination unless ice can be kept on the tooth.) Oral examination may reveal dental cavities (caries) or an extensive tooth restoration, without facial or gingival swelling.

What To Do:

✔ **Administer a strong analgesic, such as oxycodone in combination with acetaminophen or (Percocet), and prescribe additional medication, including NSAIDs, for home use. Severe pain may necessitate a nerve block** (see Appendix D).

✔ **If a cavity is present, insert a small cotton pledget soaked in oil of cloves (eugenol).** The cotton should fill the cavity loosely without rising above the opening (where it would strike the opposing tooth). **An alternative to eugenol is a pearl of benzonatate (Tessalon Perles) opened so the contents can soak the cotton pledget.** Or benzonatate pearls can be prescribed and the patient can bite them for repeated topical anesthesia.

✔ Refer the patient to a dentist for definitive therapy (removal of caries, removal of pulp, or removal of the tooth) within 12 hours.

What Not To Do:

127

✘ Do not prescribe antibiotics if there are no signs of cellulitis or abscess formation.

✘ Do not pack a tooth cavity tightly with eugenol-soaked cotton. If an abscess develops, this cavity may serve as a route for drainage.

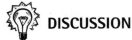 **DISCUSSION**

As the patient's condition progresses from pulpitis to pulpal necrosis, he experiences excruciating pain caused by fluid and gaseous pressure within a closed space. Heat increases the pressure and pain, whereas cold reduces it.

Intractable pain usually responds to nerve block techniques with injection of long-acting local anesthetics. If a patient refuses a nerve block or a nerve block fails to relieve the pain, consider the possibility that the patient is seeking drugs. At the same time, remember that some people have extreme phobias about dental injections. When in doubt, err on the side of compassion.

46

Dental Trauma (Fracture, Subluxation, and Displacement)

Presentation

After a direct blow to the mouth, a portion of the patient's tooth may be broken off or a tooth may be loosened to a variable degree. **Ellis class I** dental fractures involve only enamel and are a problem only if they have left a sharp edge, which can be filed down. **Ellis class II** fractures expose yellow dentin, which is sensitive, can become infected, and should be covered. **Ellis class III** fractures expose pulp, which bleeds and hurts. A tooth that is either impacted inward or partially avulsed outward is recognizable because its occlusal surface is out of alignment compared with adjacent teeth. There is also usually some hemorrhaging at the gingival margin. If several teeth move together, suspect a fracture of the alveolar ridge (Figure 46-1).

What To Do:

✔ Assess the patient for any associated injuries, such as facial or mandibular fractures. Clean and irrigate the mouth to expose all injuries. Touch injured teeth with a tongue depressor, or grasp them between gloved fingers to see if they are loose, sensitive, painful, or bleeding.

✔ Consider possible locations of any tooth fragments. Broken tooth fragments may be embedded in the soft tissue, swallowed, or aspirated. **A chest x-ray examination can disclose tooth fragments that have been aspirated into the bronchial tree.**

✔ **For sensitive Ellis class II fractures exposing dentin, cover the exposed surface with a calcium hydroxide composition (Dycal), tooth varnish (copal ether varnish), a strip of Stomahesive, or clear nail polish to decrease sensitivity. Provide pain medications,** instruct the patient to avoid hot and cold food or drink, and arrange for follow-up with a dentist.

✔ **Patients with Ellis class III fractures exposing pulp should be seen by a dentist immediately. Calcium hydroxide or moist cotton covered with foil can be used as a temporary covering.** Provide analgesics as needed.

✔ **Minimally subluxed (loosened) teeth may require no emergency treatment. Very loose teeth should be pressed back into their sockets and wired or covered with a temporary periodontal splint (Coe-Pak) for stability,** and the patient

129

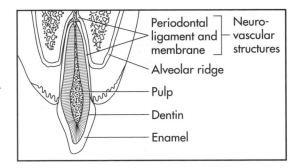

Figure 46-1 Anatomy of the tooth.

should be scheduled for dental follow-up and a possible root canal. **These patients should be placed on a soft-food or liquid diet to prevent further tooth motion. Antibiotic prophylaxis with penicillin should be provided.**

✔ **Intruded primary teeth and permanent teeth of young patients can be left alone and allowed to reerupt.** Intruded teeth of adolescents and older patients are usually repositioned by an oral surgeon. An extruded primary or permanent tooth can be readily returned to its original position by applying firm pressure using your fingers. **Both intrusive and extrusive injuries require early dental follow-up and antibiotic prophylaxis such as penicillin VK 250 mg qid.**

What Not To Do:

✗ Do not overlook associated injuries of the alveolar ridge, mandible, facial bones, or neck.

 DISCUSSION

Exposure of dentin leads to variable sequelae, depending on the age of the patient. Because it is composed of microtubules, dentin can serve as a conduit for pathogenic microorganisms.

In children the exposed dentin in an Ellis class II fracture lies nearer the neurovascular pulp and is more likely to lead to a pulp infection. Therefore, in patients younger than 12 years of age, this injury requires a dressing such as a calcium hydroxide composition (Dycal). Mix a drop of resin and catalyst over the fracture, and cover it with dry aluminum foil. When in doubt, consult a dentist.

In older patients with Ellis class II fractures, however, treatment including administration of analgesics, avoidance of hot and cold foods, and follow-up with a dentist within 24 hours is quite adequate. If a temporary periodontal splint (Coe-Pack) or wire is not available to stabilize loose teeth, spread soft wax over palatal and labial tooth surfaces and neighboring teeth as a temporary splint.

47 Gingivitis

Presentation

The patient complains of generalized severe pain of the gums, often with a foul taste or odor. The gingiva will appear edematous and red, with a grayish necrotic membrane between the teeth. The gums bleed on gentle touch, and there is loss of gingival tissue, especially the interdental papillae. The patient is usually afebrile and shows no sign of systemic disease.

What To Do:

✔ **Prescribe (in order of preference) tetracycline, penicillin VK, or erythromycin 250 mg qid for 10 days.**

✔ **Instruct the patient to rinse with warm saline every 1 to 2 hours, floss, and gently brush with sodium bicarbonate toothpaste.**

✔ **For comfort, prescribe viscous lidocaine.**

✔ For definitive care and the prevention of periodontal disease, refer the patient for dental follow-up care. With appropriate treatment, patients usually respond dramatically in 48 to 72 hours.

 DISCUSSION

Acute necrotizing ulcerative gingivitis is also known as *Vincent's angina* or *trench mouth*. This condition is usually seen in those patients who practice poor oral hygiene, those who are under stress, those who smoke, and sometimes those who have immune deficiencies. Systemic diseases that may simulate the appearance of acute necrotizing ulcerative gingivitis include infectious mononucleosis, leukemia, aplastic anemia, and agranulocytosis.

48

Jaw Dislocation

Presentation

The patient's jaw is "out" and will not close, usually after yawning or perhaps after laughing, a dental extraction, a jaw injury, or a dystonic drug reaction. The patient has difficulty speaking and may have severe pain anterior to the ear. A depression can be seen or felt in the preauricular area, and the jaw may appear prominent.

What To Do:

✔ If there was no trauma (and especially if the patient's jaw is dislocated often), attempt reduction immediately. If there is any possibility of an associated fracture, however, obtain x-ray films first.

✔ Have the patient sit on a low stool, with his back and head braced against something firm, either against the wall (facing you) or against your body (facing away from you).

✔ **With gloved hands, wrap your thumbs in gauze, place them on the lower molars, grasp both sides of the mandible, lock your elbows, and, bending from the waist, exert slow, steady pressure downward and posteriorly.** The mandible should be at or below the level of your forearm (Figure 48-1).

✔ In a bilateral dislocation, attempt to reduce one side at a time.

✔ **If the jaw does not relocate easily** or convincingly, it may be necessary to reassess the dislocation with x-ray films and **reattempt relocation using IV midazolam to overcome the muscle spasm and 1 to 2 ml of intraarticular 1% lidocaine to overcome the pain.** Inject medication directly into the palpable depression left by the displaced condyle.

✔ **After the dislocation is reduced, application of a soft cervical collar will reduce the range-of-motion at the temporomandibular joint,** which will comfort the patient. Recommend a soft-food diet, and instruct the patient to refrain from opening her mouth too widely. **Prescribe analgesics if needed.**

✔ If reduction cannot be accomplished using the aforementioned techniques, consider admitting the patient to the hospital for reduction under general anesthesia.

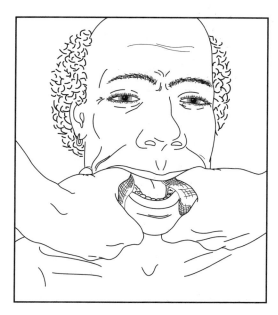

Figure 48-1 Dislocation reduction of the jaw.

What Not To Do:

✘ Do not allow your thumbs to be bitten when the jaw snaps back into position. Maintain firm, steady traction, and protect your thumbs with gauze.

✘ Do not apply pressure to oral prostheses, which could cause them to break.

✘ Do not attempt to reduce a temporomandibular joint dislocation with the patient's jaw at the level of your shoulders or higher. Having the patient in a lower position will provide the necessary leverage. Do not try to force the patient's jaw shut.

 ## DISCUSSION

The mandible usually dislocates anteriorly and subluxes when the jaw is opened wide. Other dislocations imply that a fracture is present and require referral to a surgeon. Dislocation is often a recurring problem (avoided by limiting motion) and is associated with temporomandibular joint dysfunction. If dislocation is not obvious, consider other possible conditions, such as fracture, hemarthrosis, closed lock of the joint meniscus, and myofascial pain.

133

SUGGESTED READINGS
Luyk NH, Larsen PE: The diagnosis and treatment of the dislocated mandible, *Am J Emerg Med* 7:329-335, 1989.

49

Lacerations of the Mouth

Presentation

Because of the rich vascularity of the soft tissues of the mouth, impact injuries often lead to dramatic hemorrhages that bring patients with relatively trivial lacerations to the emergency department (ED). Blunt trauma to the face can cause secondary lacerations of the lips, frenulum, buccal mucosa, gingiva, and tongue. Active bleeding has usually stopped by the time a patient with a minor laceration has reached the ED.

What To Do:

✔ Provide appropriate tetanus prophylaxis, and check for associated injuries, such as loose teeth and mandibular or facial fractures.

✔ **When only small lacerations are present and only minimal gaping of the wound occurs, reassurance and simple aftercare are all that is required.** Inform the patient that the wound will become somewhat uncomfortable and covered with pus over the next 48 hours, and **instruct him to rinse with lukewarm water or half-strength hydrogen peroxide** for 1 week **after meals and every 1 to 2 hours** while awake.

✔ **If there is continued bleeding, if the wound edges gape significantly (especially on the edge of the tongue), or if there is a flap or deformity when the underlying musculature contracts, the wound should be anesthetized using lidocaine with epinephrine, cleansed thoroughly with saline, and loosely approximated using a 5-0 or 6-0 absorbable suture.** Consider using conscious sedation when suturing children who cannot cooperate. **A traction stitch or special rubber-tipped clamp can be very helpful when attempting to suture the tongue** of a small child or intoxicated adult (Figure 49-1). The same aftercare as described earlier applies here as well.

✔ **When the exterior surface of the lip is lacerated, any separation of the underlying musculature must be repaired with buried absorbable sutures.** To avoid an unsightly scar when the lip heals, **precise skin approximation is very important. First, approximate the vermilion border, making this the key suture.** Fine non-

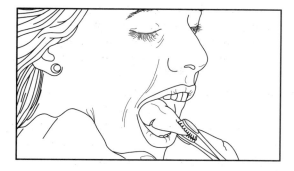

Figure 49-1 Proper use of a rubber-tipped clamp.

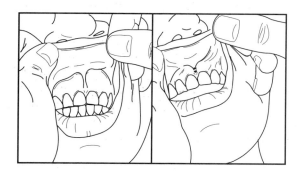

Figure 49-2 A, Normal frenulum. **B,** Lacerated frenulum.

absorbable suture material (e.g., 6-0 nylon or Prolene) is most appropriate for the skin surfaces of the lip, whereas a fine absorbable suture (e.g., 6-0 Dexon or Vicryl) is quite acceptable for use on the mucosa and vermilion.

✔ **For deep lacerations of the mucosa or lip or for any sutured laceration in the mouth, prescribe prophylactic penicillin (penicillin VK 500 mg tid for 3 to 4 days)** to prevent deep tissue infections. (Erythromycin may be substituted in penicillin-allergic individuals.) Recommend acetaminophen or ibuprofen for pain.

✔ Instruct patients to return in 48 hours for a wound reevaluation.

✔ Recommend that the patient consume only cool liquids and soft foods beginning 4 hours after the repair.

What Not To Do:

✘ Do not bother to repair a simple laceration or avulsion of the frenulum of the upper lip. It will heal quite nicely on its own (Figure 49-2).

✘ Do not use nonabsorbable suture material on the tongue, gingiva, or buccal mucosa. There is no advantage, and suture removal on a small child will be an unpleasant struggle at best.

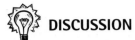 **DISCUSSION**

Imprecise repair of the vermilion border will lead to a "step-off" or puckering that is unsightly and difficult to repair later. Fortunately, the tongue and oral mucosa usually heal with few complicating infections, and there is a low risk of subsequent tissue necrosis.

50

Mucocele
(Mucous Cyst)

Presentation

A patient may be alarmed by the rapid development of a soft, rounded cyst, most often found inside the lower lip. The cyst varies from 2 to 10 mm in diameter, and the surface is made up of pearly or translucent mucosa (Figure 50-1). The patient may be aware of previous trauma to the lip.

What To Do:

✔ Reassure the patient that this is not a serious tumor.
✔ Refer the patient to an appropriate oral surgeon who can perform laser ablation or total cyst excision.

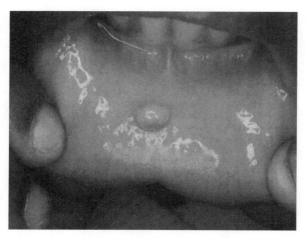

Figure 50-1 Traumatic mucous cyst. *(From Kolenik SA III, Ehrustrom PG, Kohn SR: A pictorial guide to lip lesions,* Emergency Medicine, *24[14]:265, 1992.)*

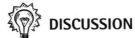 **DISCUSSION**

This cyst is caused by traumatic rupture of the mucous gland duct with extravasation of sialomucin into the submucosa. It usually occurs inside the lower lip but may also occur under the tongue or in the buccal mucosa. These traumatic mucous retention cysts rupture easily, releasing sticky, straw-colored fluid.

51

Oral Candidiasis (Thrush)

Presentation

An infant (who usually has a concurrent diaper rash) has white patches in his mouth, or an older patient (who usually has poor oral hygiene, diabetes, a hematologic malignancy, or some immunodeficiency or is on antibiotic, cytotoxic, or steroid therapy) complains of a sore mouth and sensitivity to foods that are spicy or acidic. On physical examination, painless, white patches are found in the mouth and on the tongue; the patches wipe off easily with a swab, leaving an erythematous base that may bleed. There also may be intense, dark red inflammation throughout the oral cavity.

What To Do:

✔ If there is any doubt about the etiology, confirm the diagnosis by smearing, Gram staining, and examining the exudate under a microscope for large, gram-positive pseudohypha and spores. A fungal culture may also confirm the diagnosis but is usually unnecessary.

✔ **For topical treatment, prescribe an oral suspension of nystatin (Mycostatin) 100,000 u/ml; place 1 ml in each cheek for infants and 4 to 6 ml in each cheek for children and adults.** Instruct the patient to gargle and swish the liquid in his mouth as long as possible before swallowing, **4 times a day, for at least 2 days beyond resolution of symptoms.** Nystatin is also available in pastilles of 200,000 u; one or two pastilles can be dissolved in the mouth 4 to 5 times daily. **Alternatively, prescribe clotrimazole (Mycelex) in 10-mg troches to be dissolved slowly in the mouth 5 times a day for 7 to 14 days.**

✔ **For adults, a single dose of fluconazole 200 mg followed by 100-mg doses qd PO for 7 to 14 days may be a better regimen.** Sometimes a single oral dose is effective, but the longer course decreases the risk of recurrence.

✔ Have patients with removable dental appliances or dentures soak them overnight in a nystatin suspension to prevent reinfection with these contaminated objects.

✔ Look elsewhere for *Candida* infection (e.g., esophagitis, intertrigo, vaginitis, diaper rash). All of these conditions should respond to topical treatment with nystatin or clotrimazole.

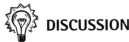 **DISCUSSION**

In the healthy newborn, thrush is a self-limited infection, but it should be treated to avoid feeding problems. Infants who fail to respond to treatment with nystatin oral suspension can be given nystatin or clotrimazole vaginal suppositories placed in a split pacifier, which will provide a more prolonged topical application.

In adults, oral candidiasis is found in a variety of acute and chronic forms. Localized erythema and erosions with minimal white exudate may be caused by candidal colonies beneath dentures and are commonly called *denture sore mouth*. When treating diabetics, remember that nystatin suspension has a high sugar content. Maintenance prophylaxis may be required in patients with AIDS.

52

Oral Herpes Simplex (Cold Sore)

Presentation

Patients have swelling, burning, or soreness at the vermilion border of the lips followed by the appearance of clusters of small vesicles on an erythematous base (see Figure 52-1). The vesicles then rupture to produce red, irregular ulcerations, with swollen borders and crusting, and eventually heal without leaving a scar. These lesions can also occur on the hard palate or gingiva. Episodes last 7 to 14 days and recur after exposure to sunlight or emotional or physical stress. The initial episode is usually the worst, and recurrences are milder and shorter.

What To Do:

✔ When there is any doubt about the diagnosis, scrape the base of a vesicle (warn the patient that this hurts), smear it on a slide, stain it with Wright's or Giemsa solution, and examine it for multinucleate giant cells (look for nuclear molding). This is called a *Tzanck prep* and establishes the diagnosis of herpes. Alternatively the swab can be sent for viral cultures, which may take days to grow.

✔ **Prescribe penciclovir 1% cream (Denavir) 2 g. Have the patient apply every 2 waking hours for 4 days.** This treatment has been shown to hasten the resolution of lesions and pain in immunocompetent adults with recurrent herpes simplex labialis regardless of whether it is applied early or late in the course of the eruption. **An alternative treatment is oral acyclovir (Zovirax) 400 mg tid for 5 days.** This therapy reduces viral shedding, appearance of new lesions, severity of pain, and time to heal. Treat recurrences early, if possible during the prodrome or at the first sign of the first skin lesion.

✔ **For topical treatment, an equal mixture of kaolin-pectin (Kaopectate) and diphenhydramine (Benadryl) elixir can coat and dry the area and reduce pain. Topical lip salves (Orabase, Blistex), lidocaine (Xylocaine 2% Viscous Solution), diphenhydramine elixir, and application of cold compresses will also relieve the pain. Prescribe NSAIDs or even narcotics and mild sedation for the most severe pain.**

✔ Instruct the patient to keep lesions clean and to avoid touching lesions, which will prevent spreading the virus to the eyes, unaffected skin, and other people. Instruct the patient on the benefits of thorough hand washing and avoiding kissing and other close

141

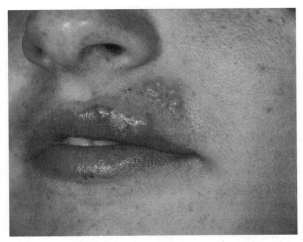

Figure 52-1 Herpes simplex labialis. *(From Habif TP:* Clinical dermatology: a color guide to diagnosis and therapy, *ed 3, St Louis, 1996, Mosby.)*

contact while lesions are apparent. Inform the patient that oral herpes need not be related to genital herpes, that the vesicles and pain should resolve over about 2 weeks (barring superinfection), that they are infectious during this period (and perhaps at other times as well), and that the herpes simplex virus, residing in sensory ganglia, can be expected to cause recurrences from time to time (especially during periods of illness or stress).

What Not To Do:

✗ Do not prescribe topical acyclovir or corticosteroids. They are ineffective. Do not use topical anesthetics on keratinized skin. They are effective only on oral mucosa and lip vermilion.

 DISCUSSION

In most cases, herpes labialis is caused by herpes simplex virus type 1 (HSV-1). Primary herpes usually appears as gingivostomatitis, pharyngitis, or a combination of the two, whereas recurrent infections usually occur as intraoral or labial ulcers.

Primary infection is acquired mainly by direct person-to-person contact, such as kissing, wrestling, sexual intercourse, and inadvertent touching of lesions. Health care workers are at particular risk of finger or hand infections (whitlows). Primary infection tends to be a disease of childhood or young adulthood; is more severe than recurring episodes; is preceded by a temperature to 105° F, sore throat, and headache; and is followed by red, swollen gums that bleed easily.

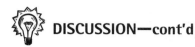

DISCUSSION—cont'd

This gingivostomatitis may need to be differentiated from herpangina, acute necrotizing ulcerative gingivitis, Stevens-Johnson syndrome, Behçet's syndrome, and hand-foot-and-mouth disease. Herpangina is caused by coxsackievirus group A and involves the posterior pharynx. Acute necrotizing ulcerative gingivitis, also known as *Vincent's angina* or *trench mouth,* is bacterial in origin, causes characteristic blunting of the interdental gingival papillae, and responds rapidly to treatment with penicillin. Stevens-Johnson syndrome is a severe form of erythema multiforme. In this syndrome there are characteristic lip lesions, the gingiva is only rarely affected, and there may be bull's-eye skin lesions on the hands and feet. Behçet's syndrome is thought to be an autoimmune response and is associated with genital ulcers and inflammatory ocular lesions. Hand-foot-and-mouth disease is also caused by coxsackievirus group A and is associated with concurrent lesions of the palms and soles.

Secondary recurrences are due to reactivation of latent infection in the trigeminal ganglion. Possible causes of HSV-1 reactivation include stress, fever, menstruation, gastrointestinal disturbance, infection, fatigue, and exposure to cold or sunlight.

Home remedies for cold sores include application of ether, lecithin, lysine, and vitamin E. Because herpes is a self-limiting affliction, all of these therapies work, but in controlled studies, none has outperformed placebos (which also do very well).

SUGGESTED READINGS

Raborn GW, Dip MS, McGaw WT, et al: Treatment of herpes labialis with acyclovir, *Am J Med* 85(suppl 2A):39-42, 1988.

Spruance SL, Rea TL, Thoming C, et al: Penciclovir cream for the treatment of herpes simplex labialis: a randomized, multicenter, double-blind, placebo-controlled trial, *JAMA* 277:1374-1379, 1997.

53

Orthodontic
Complications

Presentation

Someone wearing braces on his teeth was struck on the mouth or his orthodontic appliances broke spontaneously, puncturing, hooking or otherwise entrapping some oral mucosa. There may be pain, blood, lacerations, a confusing tangle of wires and elastic bands, and panic on the part of the patient and family. Other problems involve food, candy, or chewing gum becoming stuck and causing gingival infection.

What To Do:

✔ Irrigate and cleanse the mouth so the nature of the problem can be clearly visualized.

✔ **Inject local anesthetic into entrapped or punctured mucosa to ease the patient's discomfort and allow necessary manipulation.**

✔ **Release mucosa from hooklike attachments by pushing the lip against the teeth and moving it (usually upward) to unhook it.**

✔ **Bend any sharp wire end so that it points toward the teeth rather than toward sensitive lips and gums. Use a hemostat to grasp the wire. If a brace wire has popped out of the bands around the molars and the grooves the wire fits in are visible, just slide it back in place.**

✔ **When a sharp wire cannot be moved, cover the point with soft wax, cotton, or chewing gum.**

✔ Release foreign objects by sacrificing them.

✔ Treat gingival infections with frequent warm saline rinses and penicillin or erythromycin 250 mg qid for 10 days.

✔ **Arrange for early orthodontic follow-up.**

What Not To Do:

✘ Do not cut a protruding wire, which would only create another sharp edge.

✘ Do not administer antibiotics for minor oral abrasions, punctures, or small lacerations.

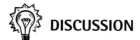

DISCUSSION

Fortunately, after orthodontic trauma, the tongue and oral mucosa usually heal with few complicating infections and little tissue necrosis.

54 Perlèche (Angular Cheilitis)

Presentation

The patient complains of inflammation and soreness of the skin and contiguous labial mucous membranes at the angles of the mouth. On examination, there is erythema, fissuring, and maceration of the oral commissures.

What To Do:

✔ Attempt to identify a precipitating cause, and advise corrective action when possible.

✔ **Prescribe an antifungal cream, such as naftifine 1% tid, followed in a few hours by a corticosteroid in a nongreasy base, such as triamcinolone 1%, and discontinue the steroids when the inflammation subsides in favor of a protective lip balm, such as ChapStick.**

DISCUSSION

Perlèche is associated with the collection of moisture at the corners of the mouth, which encourages invasion by *Candida albicans,* staphylococci, streptococci, and other organisms. In children this collection of moisture is often caused by lip licking, drooling, thumb sucking, and mouth breathing. Adults may be troubled by age-related changes in oral architecture and poorly fitting dentures. The differential diagnosis includes **impetigo** (see Chapter 171) and **herpes simplex** (see Chapter 52) infections. Vitamin B deficiency can cause perlèche, but this is rare and should not be treated presumptively.

55

Sialolithiasis (Salivary Duct Stones)

Presentation

Patients of any age may develop salivary duct stones. The majority of such stones occur in Wharton's duct from the submaxillary gland. The patient is alarmed by the rapid swelling that suddenly appears beneath his jaw while he is eating. The swelling may be painful but is not hot or red and usually subsides within 2 hours. This swelling may only be intermittent and may not occur with every meal. Infection can occur and will be accompanied by increased pain, exquisite tenderness, erythema, and fever. Under these circumstances, pus can sometimes be expressed from the opening of the duct when the gland is pressed on (Figure 55-1).

What To Do:

✔ **Bimanually palpate the course of the salivary duct, feeling for stones.**

✔ **When a small superficial stone can be felt, anesthetize the tissue beneath the duct and ampule with a small amount of lidocaine 1% with epinephrine. If available, a punctum dilator can be used to widen the orifice of the duct. Then milk the gland and duct with your fingers to express the stone or stones.**

✔ If the stone cannot be palpated, try to locate it through x-ray examination. Standard x-ray films of the mandible are likely to demonstrate only large stones. Dental x-ray films shot at right angles to the floor of the mouth are much more likely to demonstrate small stones in Wharton's duct. Place the film between the cheek and the gum to visualize Stensen's duct.

✔ When a stone cannot be demonstrated or manually expressed, the patient should be referred for contrast sialography or surgical removal of the stone. Often, sialography, ultrasound, CT scan, or MRI will show whether an obstruction is due to stenosis, a stone, or a tumor.

✔ **Begin treatment of any infection with cephalexin (Keflex) or dicloxacillin (Dynapen) 500 mg PO tid for 10 days after obtaining cultures.**

✔ **Treat pain with appropriate analgesics and have the patient use lemon drops to promote the flushing effect of salivation.**

147

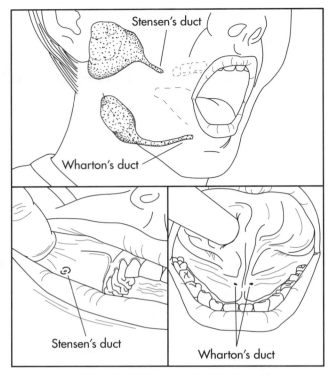

Figure 55-1 The majority of salivary duct stones occur in Wharton's duct.

What Not To Do:

✗ Do not attempt to dilate a salivary duct if the patient has a suspected case of mumps. Acute, persistent pain and swelling of the parotid gland along with inflammation of the papilla of Stensen's duct, fever, lymphocytosis, hyperamylasemia, and malaise should raise suspicion regarding the probability of mumps.

 DISCUSSION

Salivary duct stones are generally composed of calcium carbonate and calcium phosphate. Uric acid stones may form in patients with gout. Although the majority form in Wharton's duct in the floor of the mouth, approximately 10% occur in Stensen's duct in the cheek, and 5% in the sublingual ducts. Depending on the location and the size of the stone, the presenting symptoms will vary. As a rule, the onset of swelling is sudden and associated with salivation during a meal.

56

Temporomandibular Joint Pain

Presentation

Patients usually complain of poorly localized facial pain or headache that does not appear to conform to a strict anatomic distribution. The pain is generally dull and unilateral, centered in the temple, above and behind the eye, and in and around the ear. The pain may be associated with instability of the temporomandibular joint (TMJ), crepitus, or clicking with movement of the jaw. It is often described as an earache. Other less obvious symptoms include radiation of pain down the carotid sheath, tinnitus, dizziness, decreased hearing, itching, sinus symptoms, a foreign body sensation in the external ear canal, and trigeminal, occipital, and glossopharyngeal neuralgias. Patients may have been previously diagnosed as suffering from migraine headaches, sinusitis, or recurrent external otitis. Predisposing factors include malocclusion, recent extensive dental work, or a habit of grinding the teeth (bruxism), all of which put unusual stress on the TMJ. Clinical signs include tenderness of the chewing muscles, the ear canal, or the joint itself; restricted opening of the jaw or lateral deviation on opening; and a normal neurologic examination.

What To Do:

✔ Examine the head thoroughly for other causes of the pain, including assessment of visual acuity, examination of the cranial nerves, and palpation of the scalp muscles and the temporal arteries. **Pain and popping with movement of the TMJ are useful but not infallible signs.** Look for signs of bruxism, such as ground-down teeth. If the patient has a headache, perform a complete neurologic examination, including funduscopy. If the temporal artery is tender, swollen, or inflamed, send blood to be tested for an erythrocyte sedimentation rate (see Chapters 8 and 121).

✔ **If pain is severe, try injecting the TMJ, just anterior to the tragus, with 1 to 2 ml of plain lidocaine (Xylocaine) or bupivacaine (Marcaine), along with 10 mg (0.25 ml) of methylprednisolone (Depo-Medrol) or 1.5 mg (0.5 ml) of betamethasone (Celestone Soluspan)** (Figure 56-1). **If this helps, the diagnosis may have been made and long-term relief may have been provided.**

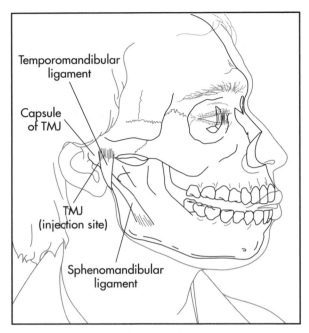

Figure 56-1 Proper TMJ injection site.

✔ Explain to the patient the pathophysiology of the syndrome, including how many different symptoms may be produced by inflammation at one joint, how TMJ pain is not necessarily related to arthritis at other joints, and how common it is (some estimates are as high as 20% of the population).

✔ **Prescribe antiinflammatory analgesics (e.g., aspirin, ibuprofen, naproxen), a soft diet, application of heat, and muscle relaxants (e.g., diazepam) if necessary for muscle spasm.**

✔ Refer the patient for follow-up with a dentist or otolaryngologist who has some interest in and experience with TMJ problems. Long-term treatments include orthodontic correction, physical therapy, and sometimes psychotherapy and treatment with antidepressants.

What Not To Do:

✗ Do not rule out TMJ arthritis simply because the joint is not tender on examination. This syndrome typically fluctuates, and the diagnosis often is made based on the history alone.

✗ Do not omit the TMJ in the work up of any headache.

✗ Do not administer narcotics unless there is going to be early follow-up.

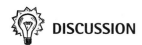 **DISCUSSION**

The relative etiologic roles of inadequate dentition, unsatisfactory occlusion, dysfunction of the masticatory muscles, and emotional disorders remain controversial. To stress the role played by muscles, it has been suggested that the term *myofascial pain-dysfunction syndrome* is more accurate than the term *TMJ arthritis.* There is also much debate as to the indications for and the efficacy of treatment modalities aimed at the presumed etiologies. At the least, irreversible treatments such as surgery should be replaced by more conservative therapy. The use of bite blocks for bruxism was based on outdated information and may serve only to alter normal dental occlusion with deleterious effects.

Perhaps everyone suffers pain in the TMJ occasionally, and only a few require treatment or modification of lifestyle to reduce symptoms. In the emergency department the diagnosis of TMJ pain is often suspected but seldom made definitively. It can be gratifying, however, to see patients with a myriad of seemingly unrelated symptoms respond dramatically after only conservative measures and advice are offered.

SUGGESTED READINGS

Guralnick W, Kaban LB, Merrill RG: Temporomandibular joint afflictions, *N Engl J Med* 299:123-128, 1978.

57

Uvular Edema

Presentation

The patient complains of a foreign body sensation or fullness in the throat, possibly associated with a muffled voice and gagging. On examination of the throat, the uvula is swollen, pale, and somewhat translucent (uvular hydrops). If greatly enlarged, the uvula might rest on the tongue and move in and out with respiration. There might be an associated rash or a history of exposure to physical stimuli or allergens, a recurrent seasonal incidence, or a prescription for an ACE inhibitor.

What To Do:

✔ Because of the known association of uvular edema with hypopharyngeal edema, watch for signs of airway compromise. **If the patient complains of respiratory difficulty or breathes with stridor, commence treatment with IV lines, intubation, and cricothyrotomy equipment at the bedside, and obtain a lateral soft tissue neck x-ray examination to rule out epiglottic swelling.** Begin medical treatment immediately.

✔ If there is no acute respiratory difficulty, ask the patient about precipitating events. Consider foods, drugs, physical agents, inhalants, insect bites, and hereditary angioedema.

✔ **When fever, sore throat, and pharyngeal injection are present, swab the throat for a rapid strep screen and administer an antibiotic effective against *Haemophilus influenzae*,** such as clarithromycin (Biaxin), amoxicillin plus clavulanate (Augmentin), or trimethoprim plus sulfamethoxazole (Bactrim).

✔ If the presentation is confusing, it is reasonable to obtain a complete blood count with a manual differential to demonstrate eosinophilia, which would support the possibility of an allergic reaction, or a high leukocyte count with increased granulocytes and bands, which would support a bacterial infection.

✔ **When an allergic reaction is suspected, the patient should initially receive parenteral H_1 and H_2 blocking antihistamines, such as hydroxyzine (Vistaril) 50 to 100 mg IM or diphenhydramine (Benadryl) 25 to 50 mg IV along with cimetidine (Tagamet) 300 mg IV or PO or ranitidine (Zantac) 50 mg IV or 150 mg PO.**

✔ **For more severe cases, give repeated doses of epinephrine 0.3 ml of 1:1000 SC every 20 minutes for up to three doses. Nebulized isomeric or racemic epinephrine or albuterol is also effective. Topical application of a vasoconstrictor, such as cocaine gel, works very well.**

✔ **Parenteral corticosteroids, such as methylprednisolone (Solu-Medrol) 125 mg IV, are also typically used,** although their efficacy remains unproved.

✔ **If the patient is on an ACE inhibitor,** such as lisinopril (Prinivil, Zestril), captopril (Capoten), enalapril (Vasotec), fosinopril (Monopril), benazepril (Lotensin), moexipril (Univasc), quinapril (Accupril), ramipril (Altace), or trandolapril (Mavik), **use of that medication should be discontinued and therapy with an alternative antihypertensive should begin. The patient should be held for several hours of observation, and hospital admission should be considered if the swelling worsens.**

✔ If the patient has a history of recurrent episodes of edema and there is a family history of the same, consider ordering tests to determine the C4 complement level or the C1 esterase inhibitor level to screen for hereditary angioedema. In this condition the edema often involves the uvula and soft palate together.

✔ Uvular decompression may be useful in patients who are resistant to medical therapy or who have rapidly progressing symptoms. This procedure consists of grasping the uvula with forceps and either making several lacerations with a sterile needle or snipping the distal centimeter as a partial uvulectomy.

✔ **All patients should be observed for an adequate period of time to ensure that there is either improvement or no further increase in the swelling before being sent home. When discharged, the patient should be given a 4- to 5-day supply of H_1 and H_2 blockers and steroids if required.**

What Not To Do:

✘ Do not perform a comprehensive and costly laboratory evaluation on every patient. Order only those specific tests that are clearly indicated and will provide results that can be followed up.

 ## DISCUSSION

The uvula (Latin for "little grape") is a small, conical, peduncular process hanging from the middle of the lower border of the soft palate. The soft palate is composed of muscle, connective tissue, and mucous membrane, and the bulk of the uvula consists of glandular tissue with diffuse muscle fibers interspersed throughout. During the acts of deglutition and phonation, the uvula and soft palate are directed upward, thereby walling off the nasal cavity from the pharynx. During swallowing, this prevents ingested substances from entering the nasal cavity.

153

Continued

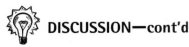

DISCUSSION—cont'd

Angioedema, also known as *angioneurotic edema* and *Quincke's disease,* is defined as a well-localized edematous condition that may variably involve the deeper skin layers, subcutaneous tissues, and mucosal surfaces of the upper respiratory and gastrointestinal tracts.

Immediate hypersensitivity type I reactions, seen with atopic states and specific allergen sensitivities, are the most common causes of angioedema. These reactions involve the interaction of an allergen with IgE antibodies bound to the surface of basophils or mastocytes. Physical agents, including cold, pressure, light, and vibration or other processes that increase core temperature, may also cause edema through the IgE pathway.

Hereditary angioedema, a genetic disorder of the complement system, is characterized by either an absence or a functional deficiency of C1 esterase inhibitor. This absence or deficiency allows unopposed activation of the first component of complement, with subsequent breakdown of its two substrates, the second (C2) and fourth (C4) components of the complement cascade. This process, in the presence of plasmin, generates a vasoactive kininlike molecule that causes angioedema. Acquired C1 esterase inhibitor deficiency and other complement consumption states have been described in patients with malignancies and immune complex disorders, including serum sickness and vasculitides.

Other causes of angioedema include certain medications and diagnostic agents (e.g., opiates, d-tubocurarine, curare, radiocontrast materials) that have a direct degranulation effect on mast cells and basophils; substances such as aspirin, NSAIDs, azo dyes, and benzoates that alter the metabolism of arachidonic acid, thus increasing vascular permeability; and ACE inhibitors, implicated presumably by promoting the production of bradykinin.

The known infectious causes of uvulitis include group A streptococci, *H. influenzae,* and *Streptococcus pneumoniae.* An associated cellulitis may contiguously involve the uvula and the tonsils, posterior pharynx, or epiglottis.

SUGGESTED READINGS

Evans TC, Roberge RJ: Quincke's disease of the uvula, *Am J Emerg Med* 5:211-216, 1987.

Goldberg R, Lawton R, Newton E, et al: Evaluation and management of acute uvular edema, *Ann Emerg Med* 22:251-255, 1993.

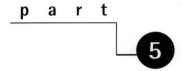

part

5

Pulmonary and Thoracic Emergencies

58 Costochondritis

Presentation

The patient, usually between the ages of 15 and 39, complains of a day or more of steady aching with intermittent stabbing chest pain. The pain may follow a period of frequent coughing or unusual physical stress; may be localized to the left or right of the sternum, without radiation; and may worsen when the patient takes a breath, changes position, or moves her arm overhead. She may be concerned about the possibility of a heart attack (though she may not voice her fear), but there is no associated nausea, vomiting, diaphoresis, or dyspnea. The middle anterior costal cartilages (connecting the ribs to the sternum) are diffusely tender to palpation, without swelling or erythema, exactly matching the patient's complaint. The rest of the physical examination is normal, along with normal vital signs and pulse oximetry.

What To Do:

✔ Obtain a thorough history and physical examination. Pay special attention to the character of the pain (e.g., onset, severity, quality, radiation, duration, relationship to movement), associated symptoms (e.g., shortness of breath, nausea, vomiting, diaphoresis, cough), and history of preexisting cardiac risk factors (e.g., family history of coronary artery disease, smoking, hypertension, diabetes mellitus, elevated cholesterol levels, cocaine use, age older than 33 years for men and 40 years for women). Read the nurse's note, checking for critical details the patient may not have repeated to you. Look for pleural or pericardial rubs and dysrhythmias, and obtain a cardiogram and chest x-ray examination if there is any suspicion of a cardiac or pulmonary disorder. **The presence of costochondritis does not exclude the possibility of myocardial infarction, pericarditis, pulmonary embolus, pneumothorax, pneumonia, or pleural effusion.**

✔ **If there is any suggestion of cardiac or pulmonary disease, if there are complaints of chest tightness or pressure, or if there are significant cardiac risk factors, obtain appropriate consultation and consider admission and further diagnostic evaluation.**

✔ **If there is no evidence of other disease, prescribe antiinflammatory analgesics, have the patient apply heat to ease discomfort,** explain the condition and the lack of other disease, direct the patient to seek follow-up, and instruct the patient to return if she experiences any fever, shortness of breath, diaphoresis, change in character of pain, or radiation to the arm, shoulder, or jaw.

What Not To Do:

✗ Do not rule out myocardial infarction, especially in the middle-aged or elderly patient, simply because there is tenderness over the costal cartilage, which could represent a co-incidental finding, skin hypesthesia, or contiguous inflammation secondary to the infarct.

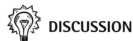

DISCUSSION

This local inflammatory process is probably related to minor trauma and would not be brought to medical attention so often if it did not resemble the pain of a heart attack. Careful reassurance of the patient is therefore most important. This disorder is self-limited, but there may be remissions and exacerbations. The pain usually resolves in weeks to months. Tietze's syndrome is a rare variant that is generally less diffuse and is associated with local swelling. Exquisite tenderness localized over the xiphoid cartilage represents a xiphoiditis or xiphoidalgia and can often be treated immediately with an injection of methylprednisolone (Depo-Medrol) 40 mg along with 5 ml of 0.5% bupivacaine (Marcaine) and a course of NSAIDs as described earlier. Injection of the xiphoid cartilage is similar to that of other trigger points; use a fine needle and fan out around the point of maximum tenderness. While injecting the xiphoid, use caution to avoid causing a pneumothorax or injecting the myocardium.

SUGGESTED READINGS

Disla E, Rhim HR, Reddy A, et al: Costochondritis: a prospective analysis in an ED setting, *Arch Intern Med* 154:2466–2469, 1994.

59 Inhalation Injury

Presentation

The patient was trapped in an enclosed space for some time with toxic gases or fumes (produced by a fire, a leak, evaporation of a solvent, a chemical reaction, fermentation of silage, etc.) and comes to the emergency department complaining of some combination of coughing, wheezing, shortness of breath, irritated or runny eyes or nose, chest or abdominal pain, or skin irritation. More severe symptoms include confusion and narcosis. Symptoms may develop immediately or after a lag of as much as 1 day. On physical examination the victim may smell of the agent or be covered with soot or burns. Inflammation of the eyes, nose, mouth, or upper airway may be visible, and pulmonary irritation may be evident as coughing, rhonchi, rales, or wheezing, although these signs may also take up to 1 day to develop.

What To Do:

✔ Separate the victim from the toxic agent by having him remove his clothes, hose himself down, or wash with soap and water.

✔ **Make sure the victim is breathing adequately, and then add oxygen at 6 to 12 liters per minute via mask with humidification. Oxygen helps treat most inhalation injuries and is essential in treating carbon monoxide poisoning.**

✔ Look for evidence that may identify the exposure: Was there a fire? What was burning? What was the estimated length of exposure? Was the patient in an open or a closed space? What is the status of any other victims? Was there an associated blast? What material is on the victim? What does he smell of? What are his current signs and symptoms? Is there soot in the posterior pharynx, singed nasal hair, hoarseness, or stridor to indicate significant injury to the airway? There may be evidence of exposure to a specific toxin that calls for a specific antidote (e.g., muscle fasciculations, small pupils, and wet lungs may imply inhalation of organophosphates, which should be treated with atropine).

✔ **Unless the patient is asymptomatic, obtain a chest x-ray examination, pulse oximetry, and arterial blood gases.** (Record the percentage of oxygen being inhaled.) An increased alveolar-arterial partial pressure of oxygen (Po_2) difference may be the earliest sign of pulmonary injury, but even if the chest x-ray film and arterial blood gases are normal, they can serve as a baseline for evaluation of possible later pulmonary problems. Consider obtaining a carboxyhemoglobin level, if only as a marker of other combustion products. Obtain a cyanide level if there is any suspicion of exposure or ingestion. (Some burning plastics give off cyanide). Serum cholinesterase levels help document organophosphate poisoning.

✔ Determine whether there are significant preexisting conditions, such as cardiac or cerebrovascular disease, chronic obstructive pulmonary disease, asthma, or other chronic illness.

✔ **If the patient has difficulty breathing or if he has any abnormality evidenced by the x-ray examination or arterial blood gases, suggesting acute pulmonary injury, administration of oxygen should be continued and he should be admitted to the hospital,** even if only overnight. **Wheezing and bronchospasm may be allergic reactions and may respond to conventional doses of aerosolized bronchodilators** but, if not promptly reversible, are probably signs of pulmonary injury. Arrange for diagnostic bronchoscopy.

✔ **If no signs or symptoms of inhalation injury develop or if all have resolved in 1 hour, it may be safe to send the patient home with instructions to return for reevaluation** the next day or sooner if any pulmonary signs or symptoms (e.g., coughing, wheezing, shortness of breath) occur.

✔ In 12 to 24 hours, repeat the physical examination, check the patient's vital signs, and consider obtaining additional chest x-ray films and arterial blood gases. Look for any changes indicative of late pulmonary injury.

What Not To Do:

✘ Do not assume that the patient has not suffered any inhalation injury simply because there are no symptoms or abnormalities evidenced by chest x-ray films or arterial blood gases in the first few hours after exposure. Some agents produce pulmonary inflammation that develops over 12 to 24 hours.

✘ Do not wait until carboxyhemoglobin levels have been determined before giving 100% oxygen to treat suspected carbon monoxide poisoning. Begin oxygen administration as soon as possible; 100% oxygen (which requires a tight-fitting mask and a reservoir for administration) reduces the half-life of carboxyhemoglobin from 6 to 1½ hours.

✘ Do not insist that the patient breathe room air for a long period before obtaining arterial blood gases. If oxygen administration is helping, its withdrawal is a disservice, and the alveolar-arterial Po_2 gradient can still be estimated while the patient is being given supplemental oxygen.

✘ Do not prescribe corticosteroids unless there is a history of asthma or allergy.

✘ Do not prescribe antibiotics unless there is a proven infection.

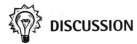 **DISCUSSION**

One type of inhalation injury is caused by relatively **inert** gases, such as carbon dioxide and fuel gases (e.g., methane, ethane, propane, acetylene), that displace air and oxygen, producing asphyxia. Treatment consists of removing the victim from the gas, allowing him to breathe fresh air or oxygen, and attending to any damage (e.g., myocardial infarction, cerebral injury) caused by the period of hypoxia.

A second category of inhalation injury is caused by **irritant** gases, including ammonia (NH_3), formaldehyde (HCHO), chloramine (NH_2Cl), chlorine (Cl_2), nitrogen dioxide (NO_2), and phosgene ($COCl_2$). When dissolved in the water lining the respiratory mucosa, irritant gases produce a chemical burn and an inflammatory response. The first gases listed, being more soluble in water, tend to produce more upper airway burns, irritating the eyes, nose, and mouth, whereas the last gases, being less water soluble, produce more pulmonary injury and respiratory distress.

A third type of inhalation injury is caused by gases that are systemic **toxins,** such as carbon monoxide (CO), hydrogen cyanide (HCN), and hydrogen sulfide (H_2S), all of which interfere with the delivery of oxygen for use in cellular energy production and aromatic and halogenated hydrocarbons, which can result in later liver, kidney, brain, lung, and other organ damage.

A fourth cause of inhalation injury is allergic; inhaled gases, particles, or aerosols produce bronchospasm and edema similar to that caused by asthma or spasmodic croup.

A fifth cause of inhalation injury is direct thermal burns. They are usually limited to the upper airway and produce varying degrees of local edema.

60

Rib Fracture and Costochondral Separation

Presentation

A patient with an isolated rib fracture or a minor costochondral separation usually has recently fallen, injuring the side of the chest; been struck by a blunt object; coughed violently; or leaned over a rigid edge. The initial chest pain may subside, but over the next few hours or days the pain increases with movement, interferes with sleep and activity, and becomes severe when the patient coughs or breathes deeply. The patient is often worried about having a broken rib and may have a sensation of bony crepitus or abnormal rib movement. Breath sounds bilaterally should be normal unless there is substantial splinting or a pneumothorax or hemothorax is present. There is point tenderness over the site of the injury, and occasionally bony crepitus can be felt.

What To Do:

✔ Examine the patient for possible associated injuries, and palpate the abdomen for any signs of a splenic or hepatic injury. If there was a significant mechanism of injury, a comprehensive evaluation may be necessary to rule out life- and limb-threatening injuries.

✔ **When there is a history of minor trauma, check for pain by applying indirect stress to the suspected fracture site. Compress the rib anteroposteriorly if a fracture is suspected at a lateral location. Compress the rib medially if a posterior or anterior fracture is suspected** (Figure 60-1). **Pain occurring at the suspected fracture site during application of indirect stress is clinical evidence of a fracture or separation and should be documented on the chart.**

✔ Obtain any history of chronic pulmonary problems or heavy smoking.

✔ **Unless the patient is elderly or has pulmonary disease, have him try out a rib belt while he is waiting for x-ray films.**

✔ **Send the patient for posteroanterior and lateral chest radiographs to rule out a pneumothorax, hemothorax, and pulmonary contusion. Additional oblique rib films for radiologic documentation of a fracture are optional and often**

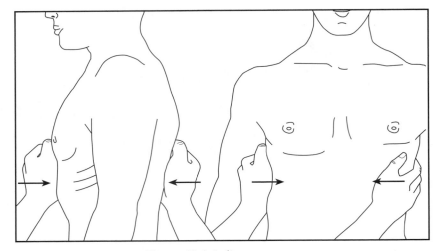

Figure 60-1 Indirect stress test.

Figure 60-2 Proper placement of elastic and Velcro rib belt.

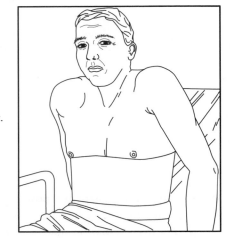

unproductive, especially with anterior cartilage injuries, but these films may be indicated when there is a suspicion of multiple rib fractures, especially in the elderly patient.

✔ If there is no suspicion of underlying injury and there is clinical or radiologic evidence of a rib fracture or chondral separation, **provide a potent oral analgesic such as ibuprofen (Motrin), naproxen (Anaprox), acetaminophen plus hydrocodone (Lorcet), or acetaminophen plus oxycodone (Percocet).**

✔ **Instruct the patient regarding the intermittent use of an elastic and Velcro rib belt if it reduces pain.** Place the bottom of the belt at the inferior tip of the xiphoid process, tightening it around the chest enough to obtain maximum pain relief. The rib belt may be worn almost continuously for the first 1 to 4 days, but it should be removed as comfort allows thereafter (Figure 60-2).

✔ Instruct the patient regarding the importance of deep breathing and coughing (without the rib belt but using a pillow splint) to help prevent pneumonia. Tell him to take enough pain medicine to allow coughing and deep breathing.

✔ Provide the patient with appropriate documentation for missing work, and refer him for follow-up care in 48 hours. Tell him to expect gradually decreasing discomfort for about 2 weeks, and forbid strenuous activity for approximately 8 weeks.

✔ Severe worsening of chest pain, shortness of breath, fever, or purulent sputum may signal pulmonary complications and should prompt a return visit. A greater incidence of complications can be expected in patients with displaced rib fractures.

✔ **When patients are elderly, suffer pulmonary or cardiac compromise, or have multiple fractures or other injuries that might compromise respiratory dynamics, consider hospitalization for observation, pain control, and respiratory therapy.** Blood gases and pulmonary function tests can aid in the evaluation of breathing.

✔ When there is no clinical or radiologic evidence of a fracture, treat the pain as any other contusion would be treated, using an appropriate analgesic.

What Not To Do:

✘ Do not confuse simple rib fractures with massive blunt trauma to the chest. The evaluation and management are quite different.

✘ Do not tape ribs or use continuous strapping. This will lead to an atelectatic lung prone to pneumonia.

✘ Do not assume there is no fracture just because the x-ray films are normal. Rib fractures are often not apparent on x-ray films, especially when they occur in the cartilaginous portion of the rib. The patient deserves the disability period and analgesics commensurate with the real injury.

DISCUSSION

Most fractures and separations are treated with immobilization, but ribs are a special problem because patients have to continue breathing. In the presence of severe pain, consider the use of an intercostal nerve block or injection of the fracture hematoma with 0.5% bupivacaine (Marcaine). Because of the risks of pneumothorax or hemothorax, in most cases this procedure should be reserved for secondary management when initial treatment has proven ineffective.

SUGGESTED READINGS

Lazcano A, Dougherty J, Kruger M: Use of rib belts in acute rib fractures, *Am J Emerg Med* 7:97-100, 1989.

Quick G: A randomized clinical trial of rib belts for simple fractures, *Am J Emerg Med* 8:277-281, 1990.

61

Tear Gas Exposure (Lacrimators)

Presentation

The patient may have been sprayed with tear gas (e.g., Mace) during a riot being dispersed by the police, or he may have accidentally sprayed himself with his own can. He complains of burning of the eyes, nose, mouth, and skin; tearing and inability to open his eyes because of the severe stinging; sneezing; coughing; runny nose; and perhaps a metallic taste, with a burning sensation of the tongue, nausea, vomiting, and abdominal pains. These signs and symptoms last for 15 to 30 minutes after exposure. Redness and edema may be noted for 1 to 2 days after exposure to these aerosol agents.

What To Do:

✔ **Segregate victims so that others are not contaminated. Medical personnel should don gowns, gloves, and masks before helping victims remove contaminated clothing, place the clothing in sealed plastic bags, and then shower with soap and water to remove the tear gas from their skin. Exposed eyes should be irrigated with copious amounts of tepid water for at least 15 minutes.**

✔ **If eye pain lasts longer than 15 to 20 minutes, examine the eyes with fluorescein dye, looking for corneal erosions,** which may be produced by tear gas.

✔ **Look for signs of and warn the patient about allergic reactions to tear gas, including bronchospasm and contact dermatitis.**

What Not To Do:

✗ Do not rush or allow others to rush to the aid of the patient who has been exposed to tear gas; rushing heedlessly can result in contamination and incapacitation of those attempting to help the patient.

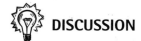 **DISCUSSION**

Agents commonly used as tear gas include CN (Mace), which is sprayed in a weak water solution; CS, which is burned and produces symptoms as long as the victim remains in the smoke; and CR, which is more potent and longer lasting. Another agent used in personal-protection spray canisters is capsicum powder, the active ingredient in hot peppers; exposure to this agent is handled in the same fashion.

62

Upper Respiratory Tract Infection (Common Cold)

Presentation

Most patients with colds do not visit a physician unless they are unusually ill (e.g., the duration of the cold is prolonged, lasting more than a few days, or the cold is progressing into bronchitis, sinusitis, or serous otitis, with new symptoms). The patient may request a note excusing her from work or a prescription for antibiotics, which "seemed to help" the last time she had a cold.

The common denominator of upper respiratory tract infections is inflammation of the respiratory mucosa. The nasal mucosa is usually red, swollen, and wet with reactive mucus. The pharynx (see Chapter 34) is inflamed directly or by drainage of mucus from the nose, and swallowing may be painful. Pharyngitis secondary to nasal drainage is typically worst when the patient wakes in the morning, and signs and symptoms may be localized to the side that is dependent during sleep.

Occlusion of the ostia of the paranasal sinuses (see Chapter 36) permits buildup of mucus and pressure, leading to pain and predisposing to bacterial superinfection. Occlusion of the orifices of the eustachian tubes in the posterior pharynx permits imbalance of middle ear pressure and serous otitis (see Chapter 35). The larynx can be inflamed directly or secondary to mucous drainage or forceful coughing, lowering the pitch and volume of the voice or causing hoarseness. The trachea can also be inflamed, producing coughing, and the bronchi can develop a bacterial superinfection or bronchospasm with wheezing. In addition to all these illnesses of the upper respiratory tract mucosa, there can be reactive lymphadenopathy of the anterior cervical chain, diffuse myalgias, and side effects of self-medication.

What To Do:

✔ Perform a complete history and physical examination, documenting which of the aforementioned signs and symptoms are present; ruling out some other, underlying ailment; and noting any sign of bacterial superinfection of the ears, sinuses, pharynx, tonsils, epiglottis, bronchi, or lungs, which might require antibiotics or other therapy.

✔ **Explain the course of the viral illness and the inadvisability of indiscriminate use of antibiotics.** Tailor drug treatment to the patient's specific complaint as follows:

✔ **For fever, headache, and myalgia, prescribe acetaminophen 650 mg q4h or ibuprofen 600 mg q6h.**

✔ **To decongest the nose, ostia of sinuses, and eustachian tubes, start with topical sympathomimetics (0.5% phenylephrine nose drops q4h, but only for 3 days) and add systemic sympathomimetics (pseudoephedrine 60 mg q6h or phenylpropanolamine 25 mg q4h). An alternative to sympathomimetics is ipratropium (Atrovent) nasal spray, twice in each nostril 3 to 4 times daily.** There is no rebound congestion after extended use.

✔ To dry out the nose, or if the symptoms are probably caused by an allergy, try antihistamines (e.g., chlorpheniramine 4 mg q6h). Topical ipratropium also dries the nasal mucosa.

✔ **To suppress coughing, prescribe dextromethorphan or codeine 10 to 20 mg q6h. To avoid sedation and narcotic use, prescribe benzonatate (Tessalon) 100 to 200 mg q8h, which provides airway anesthesia.**

✔ **For bronchitis or suspected bronchospasm, treat the cough using inhaled bronchodilators such as albuterol two puffs q1-8h prn and inhaled steroids such as beclomethasone four puffs q12h.**

✔ Arrange for follow-up if symptoms persist or worsen or if new problems develop.

What Not To Do:

✘ Do not get bullied into inappropriately prescribing antibiotics. Most colds are self-limiting illnesses, and many treatments may appear to work by coincidence alone. Do not prescribe antibiotics simply because the insistent patient will probably be successful in obtaining them elsewhere anyway. This is not justification for poor medical practice.

✘ Do not undertake expensive diagnostic testing in uncomplicated cases.

DISCUSSION

Colds are produced by more than 100 different adenoviruses and rhinoviruses, and influenzavirus, coxsackievirus, and measles can also present as upper respiratory tract infections. Especially during the winter months, when colds are epidemic, keeping abreast of what is "going around" will help you intelligently advise patients regarding incubation periods, contagiousness, expected symptoms, and duration of symptoms and will also make it easier to pick an unusual syndrome out of the background.

Some of the medications recommended earlier are available in various combinations over the counter. Bacterial superinfections require antibiotics. *Mycoplasma pneumoniae* can present with headache, cough, myalgias, and perhaps bullous myringitis and may respond to erythromycin. Coughing can precede wheezing as an early sign of asthma, and response to

167

Continued

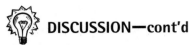 **DISCUSSION—cont'd**

beta-agonists helps make the diagnosis. Antibiotics have not proved to be very useful for treating acute bronchitis, and vitamin C therapy as prophylaxis for colds has not done well in controlled trials either.

Patients' satisfaction has been shown to be related more to their perception of the amount of time the physician spends explaining the illness and treatment than to whether they received a prescription for an antibiotic.

SUGGESTED READINGS

Clemens CJ, Taylor JA, Almquist JR, et al: Is an antihistamine-decongestant combination effective in temporarily relieving symptoms of the common cold in preschool children? *J Pediatr* 130:463-466, 1997.

Gonzales R, Steiner JF, Sande MA: Antibiotic prescribing for adults with colds, upper respiratory infections, and bronchitis by ambulatory care physicians, *JAMA* 278:901-904, 1997.

Hamm RM, Hicks RJ, Bemben DA: Antibiotics and respiratory infections: are patients more satisfied when expectations are met? *J Fam Pract* 43:56-62, 1996.

part 6

Gastrointestinal Emergencies

63 Anal Fissure

Presentation

The patient complains of painful defecation and perhaps constipation. The pain occurs with and immediately after defecation, and the patient is relatively comfortable between bowel movements. Bleeding with defecation may occur but is usually slight, only staining the toilet tissue. Mucus discharge may increase perineal moisture and cause itching. Examination of anus reveals a radial tear or ulceration of the posterior midline 95% of the time (the fissure is anterior in 10% of women but only 1% of men). If the condition becomes chronic, distal edema may produce a "sentinel pile."

What To Do:

✔ **Provide topical anesthesia with lidocaine jelly or viscous lidocaine to perform a reasonably comfortable rectal examination. An injection of lidocaine into the anal sphincter may be necessary** to produce adequate pain relief. **If this is done, take advantage of this local anesthesia to dilate the sphincter using a gentle two-finger digital examination.** This dilation will help break the cycle of pain and spasm.

✔ **Advise the patient to use psyllium seed supplements** (e.g., Metamucil) to soften stools **and to use a glycerin suppository twice daily** to maintain lubrication of the anal canal.

✔ **Topical nitroglycerin ointment (2%) may be applied bid to reduce spasm.**

✔ Instruct the patient to use warm, soothing sitz baths after each painful bowel movement.

✔ **Prescribe analgesics if needed, but remember that narcotics are constipating.**

✔ Inform the patient that an acute superficial fissure will take about 1 month to heal. He should follow-up if symptoms continue.

What Not To Do:

✗ Do not assume that a lesion located outside the anteroposterior midline sagittal plane of the anus is an anal fissure. Other possibilities include ulcerative colitis, squamous cell carcinoma, leukemia, tuberculosis, syphilis, herpes, and trauma from instrumentation and anal intercourse.

✗ Do not confuse a "sentinel pile" with a hemorrhoidal vein.

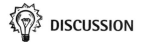

DISCUSSION

Anal fissures are more common in men and probably begin by the tearing of the mucosa during defecation, due to a tight or abnormally shaped external sphincter. This starts a vicious cycle of pain causing spasm in the anal sphincter, which causes increased friction during defecation, leading to further tearing and pain. The cycle can be broken with analgesia, lubrication, relaxation of spasm, or all three. If the fissure is large, it may become ulcerated and infected, not heal spontaneously, and require surgical excision.

Pruritus ani has multiple etiologies. Infections such as pinworms, *Candida albicans*, *Tinea cruris*, and erythrasma can cause anal itching. Mechanical trauma from overly vigorous cleansing of the perianal area may also cause pruritus and may be aggravated by diarrhea and the presence of external or prolapsed hemorrhoids or multiple skin tags, which make cleansing more difficult. Another cause of pruritus ani is allergic or contact dermatitis from agents such as soaps, perfumes in toilet tissue and feminine hygiene sprays, as well as spicy foods, tomatoes, citrus fruits and colas, coffee, and chocolate. Other causes of pruritus ani include chronic anorectal disease and cancer. If a specific cause of anal pruritus can be determined, then treat it accordingly. If the etiology is obscure, the patient can be treated with hydrocortisone cream to reduce itching and inflammation, followed by zinc oxide as a barrier cream. The patient should be instructed to gently cleanse the anal area with a cotton ball and a perineal cleansing lotion after each bowel movement and to obtain follow-up care. A systemic antipruritic agent such as hydroxyzine (Vistaril) 50 mg qid may be prescribed.

SUGGESTED READINGS

Brenner BE, Simon RR: Anorectal emergencies, *Ann Emerg Med* 12:367-376, 1983.

Lieberman DA: Common anorectal disorders, *Ann Intern Med* 101:837-846, 1984.

Lund JN, Scholefield JH: A randomized, prospective, double-blind, placebo-controlled trial of glyceryl trinitrate ointment in treatment of anal fissure, *Lancet* 349:11-14, 1997.

chapter

64 Diarrhea

Presentation

Complaints may range from acute, copious diarrhea that produces shock to concern because an occasional stool is not well formed. Typically, there is crampy pain throughout the abdomen, especially before a diarrhea stool, and some irritation of the anus. Tenesmus (the frequent urge to defecate) can exist without diarrhea.

What To Do:

✔ **Ask specifically about the frequency of stools, the volume** (much liquid implies a defect in absorption in the small bowel, while tenesmus producing little more than mucus implies inflammation of the rectosigmoid wall), **the character** (color, odor, blood, or mucus), **and the consistency** (like water or just loose stool). **Ask about travel, medications (including antibiotics), prior similar symptoms, and nocturnal symptoms (rare with functional disease).**

✔ Perform orthostatic vital signs and urinalysis and weigh pediatric patients. Any symptoms, fall in pressure, or pulse rise of more than 20 beats per minute after standing for a minute suggests hypovolemia. A urine specific gravity of 1.020 or greater also suggests hypovolemia, and ketones of 2+ or greater suggest starvation ketosis.

✔ **Perform a rectal examination and obtain a sample of stool for occult blood testing and for Wright's or Gram's stain.** If the rectal ampulla is empty, you can still swab the mucosa and may get an even better specimen for stool culture. A spontaneous specimen is also good. **If the patient has recently been on antibiotics, test the stool for *Clostridium difficile* toxin.**

✔ **If the patient has a fever or the stool is positive for occult blood or there are any white cells in a 400× field, assume the problem is invasive or inflammatory (*Campylobacter* organisms, salmonellae, shigellae, entamebae, ulcerative colitis, and so on). Send a stool culture, prescribe ciprofloxacin 500 mg bid ×3 days, and schedule follow-up.** Ask the patient to bring a fresh stool sample in a specimen cup at follow-up in case it needs to be examined for ova and parasites.

✔ **If there are no white blood cells on microscopic examination of the stool and the stool is negative for occult blood, assume the diarrhea is due to a virus or toxin. Afebrile patients with limited diarrhea require no treatment other than fluid and electrolyte replacement.** These patients will not benefit from antibiotics and require follow-up only if they have continued diarrhea, abdominal pain, or fever.

✔ **Patients who feel sick and appear to be dehydrated will benefit from rapid re-hydration with IV 0.9% NaCl or lactated Ringer's solution, 1–2 L over an hour for an adult with normal cardiovascular and renal function.** Children may be re-hydrated with an initial infusion of 20 ml/kg.

✔ **Both classes of diarrhea are best treated with absorbent bulk laxatives, such as bran or ground psyllium seeds** (Metamucil 1 tbsp in a glass of water up to qid).

✔ **To adsorb toxins and provide some binding effect, add Amphogel, Diasorb, or Kaopectate, 1 tbsp qid, or bismuth subsalicylate (Pepto-Bismol) 2 tbsp each half-hour until symptoms subside, or to a total of eight doses** (this does contain salicylates, and bismuth will turn stools black).

✔ **For travelers without signs of invasive or inflammatory diarrhea, give a single dose of ciprofloxacin (Cipro) 500 mg or ofloxacin (Floxin) 400 mg PO to reduce the duration and severity of symptoms.** If symptoms persist or the diarrhea is severe or associated with high fever or bloody stools, prescribe ciprofloxacin 500 mg bid or ofloxacin 300 mg bid for 3 days. Trimethoprim plus sulfamethoxazole (Bactrim) can be used for children.

✔ **With infants and small children, oral rehydration therapy should be the main treatment.** Antimicrobial drugs should be given only for dysentery (bloody diarrhea) and suspected cholera. Have the parents give an oral rehydration mixture with the goal of replacing the fluid lost. **For every 1 cup of diarrhea lost, give a cup of the following recipe:**
½ **to 1 cup precooked baby rice cereal**
2 cups water
¼ **tsp salt**
Mix the rice cereal, water, and salt together until the mixture thickens but is not too thick to drink. Be sure the ingredients are well mixed. A pinch of the artificial sweetener aspartame (Equal) can be added to make it more palatable. Have the parents give the mixture by spoon often and have them offer the child as much as she will accept (every minute if she will accept it). Even if the child is vomiting, the mixture can be offered in small amounts (½–1 tsp) every few minutes. Banana or other nonsweetened mashed fruit can help provide potassium. **Alternatively, one can give commercial rehydration fluids such as Rehydralate, Ricelyte, or Pedialyte, which are sold in drugstores.**

✔ **During or after diarrhea, children should be given frequent small meals** (six or more times a day) and actively encouraged to eat. Parents should use well-cooked staple starches that can be easily digested such as rice, corn, potatoes, or noodles in a soft mashed form. Infants should be given a thick porridge or semiliquid pulp. Milk products and cereals are usually well tolerated.

✔ **Patients with severe dehydration that cannot be reversed orally may require large amounts of IV fluids and occasionally must be admitted to the hospital.**

What Not To Do:

✘ Do not omit the rectal examination, which may disclose a fecal impaction or abscess.

✘ Do not stop or reduce breast feeding when a baby has diarrhea. Infants with diarrhea should be breastfed as often and for as long as they want.

✘ Do not give or recommend sugary drinks such as Gatorade, sweetened commercial fruit drinks, cola drinks, or apple juice, which may cause an osmotic diarrhea and a net loss of fluid.

✘ Do not give additional aspirin-containing drugs to patients taking bismuth subsalicylate (Pepto-Bismol).

✘ Do not routinely use narcotics to paralyze peristalsis. Lomotil, Imodium, paregoric, and so on will reduce cramps and frequency of diarrhea, but they may slow elimination of toxins and organisms, may have little effect on the symptoms of electrolyte imbalance, and may even potentiate bowel perforation in invasive conditions such as salmonella, amebic dysentery, and ulcerative colitis.

 DISCUSSION

Most cases of mild-to-moderate diarrhea (defined as five or fewer unformed stools a day without fever, blood, or significant cramps, pain, nausea, or vomiting) can be handled without an investigation of the etiology.

When bran or psyllium is prescribed, patients may remind you that they have diarrhea, not constipation, but because these agents absorb water in the gut lumen, they can relieve both problems and obviate the rebound constipation often produced by the narcotic and binding agents also used to treat diarrhea.

The three most common causes of diffuse colonic inflammation and thus fecal leukocyte exudate are shigellae, salmonellae, and *Campylobacter* organisms. Fecal leukocytes can also be a sign of ulcerative colitis.

Most bacterial diarrheas do not require treatment with antibiotics, which can produce a carrier state. The presumptive ciprofloxacin strategy described here will suit most patients whose signs and symptoms justify using antibiotics but may have to be modified in follow-up based on the patient's course and stool culture results.

Infants can become severely dehydrated in short order with viral diarrhea. Older patients medicated for pain or psychosis can develop a fecal impaction, which can also present as diarrhea. Irritable bowel syndrome, food allergy, lactose intolerance, and parasite infestation can produce relapsing diarrhea, but the pattern may only become apparent on follow-up.

SUGGESTED READINGS

Cohen MB, Mezoff AG, Laney DW, et al: Use of a single solution for oral rehydration and maintenance therapy of infants with diarrhea and mild to moderate dehydration, *Pediatrics* 95:639-645, 1995.

Margolis PA, Litteer T, Hare N, et al: Effects of unrestricted diet on mild infantile diarrhea, *Am J Dis Child* 144:162-164, 1990.

Reid SR, Bonadino WA: Outpatient rapid intravenous rehydration to correct dehydration and resolve vomiting in children with acute gastroenteritis, *Ann Emerg Med* 28:318-323, 1996. (editorial, pages 353-354).

Salam I et al: Randomized trial of single-dose ciprofloxacin for traveller's diarrhea, *Lancet* 344:1537, 1994.

Sigel D, Cohen PT, Neighbor M, et al: Predictive value of stool examination in acute diarrhea, *Arch Pathol Lab Med* 111:715-718, 1987.

65

Enterobiasis (Threadworm, Pinworm)

Presentation

The patient complains of severe perianal itching, which is worse at night, and may contribute to insomnia or superinfection of the excoriated perianal skin. Often, an entire family is affected.

What To Do:

✔ **Examine the anus to rule out other causes of itching,** such as rectal prolapse, fecal leakage, hemorrhoids, lice (pediculosis), fungal infections (tinea or candidiasis), or bacterial infections (erythrasma).

✔ **Look for pinworms directly** (especially if the patient comes in at night) by pressing the sticky side of cellophane tape wrapped around a tongue blade to the perianal skin. Examine the tape under the low power of the microscope for female worms, approximately 1 cm long, 0.5 mm in diameter, with pointed tails (Figure 65–1). (Use shiny rather than "invisible" tape, because the latter's rough surface makes microscopy difficult.)

✔ **If you see pinworms or still suspect them, administer an oral dose of pyrantel pamoate 11 mg/kg (maximum 1 g) to all family members (over the counter Antiminth oral suspension, 50 mg/ml, Reese's Pinworm Medicine).** Two prescription medications are mebendazole (Vermox) 100 mg chewable tablet once PO (not for infants) and albendazole (Albenza) 400 mg in adults or 10 mg/kg in children. All three of these medications may be repeated in 2 weeks, and none are considered completely safe during pregnancy.

✔ Explain to all concerned that this is not a dangerous infection and should be eradicated from the whole family after one treatment (which may be repeated in 2 or more weeks if there are recurrences).

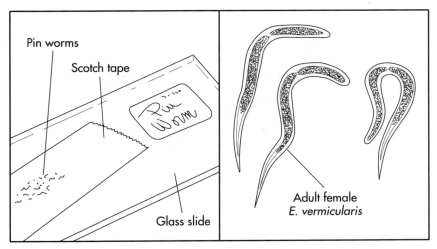

Figure 65-1 Pinworm examples.

💡 DISCUSSION

Pinworms mostly live in the colon, and females migrate down to the perianal skin to lay eggs at night. Eggs on contaminated fingers reenter via the mouth but remain viable for several days on surfaces around the house. Perhaps 10% of the US population harbors pinworms, especially children.

66

Esophageal Food Bolus Obstruction (Steakhouse Syndrome)

Presentation

The patient develops symptoms either immediately after swallowing a large mouthful of food (usually inadequately chewed meat), or as the result of intoxication, wearing dentures, or being too embarrassed to spit out a large piece of gristle. The patient often develops substernal chest pain that may mimic the pain of a myocardial infarction. This discomfort increases with swallowing and is followed by retained salivary secretions, which unlike infarction leads to drooling. The patient usually arrives with a receptacle under her mouth into which she is repeatedly spitting. At times these secretions will cause paroxysms of coughing, gagging, or choking.

What To Do:

✔ Complete a history and physical examination. If an esophageal perforation is suspected because of severe pain and diaphoresis, take PA and lateral x-rays of the neck and chest, looking for subcutaneous emphysema, pneumomediastinum, pneumothorax, and pleural effusion.

✔ **If the patient is troubled by drooling and spitting of saliva, offer to insert a small nasogastric tube to the point of obstruction and attach it to low intermittent suction.** This insertion will assist the patient in handling excess secretions and reduce the risk of aspiration.

✔ If the history and physical findings are ambiguous, but there remains a question of esophageal obstruction, give 5 ml of dilute barium PO and x-ray the chest to locate the foreign body. **When the history and physical findings are classic for a meat impaction in the esophagus, there is no need to perform a barium swallow,** which may later obscure the view for a consulting endoscopist.

✔ **Give 1 mg (1 unit) of glucagon IV to decrease lower esophageal sphincter pressure (infuse slowly to prevent nausea and vomiting).** This decrease in pressure will sometimes allow for passage of a food bolus. **If there is no response, repeat after 30 minutes.**

✔ One means of passing a lower esophageal meat impaction of less than 6 hours into the stomach if glucagon has failed is to **have the patient sit up and drink 100 ml of a carbonated beverage or EZ gas** (sodium bicarbonate, citric acid, simethicone) **followed by 240 ml of water.**

✔ If the food does not pass spontaneously and there is no access to a gastroenterologist with an endoscope, prepare the patient for manual extraction. Start an IV line for drug administration and anesthetize the pharynx with 20% benzocaine (Hurricane) spray, viscous lidocaine 2%, or lidocaine 10% oral spray. Place the patient on her side and slowly administer diazepam intravenously until the patient is very drowsy. Take a gastric Ewald lavage tube, cut off the end until there are no side ports, and round off the new tip with scissors. Push the Ewald tube through the patient's mouth until the obstruction is reached. Take a large aspiration syringe, have an assistant apply suction to the free end of the Ewald tube, and slowly withdraw it. If suction is maintained, the bolus will come up with the tubing.

✔ If the patient is unable to tolerate this procedure or if foreign body removal was unsuccessful, consult with an endoscopist for an early removal with a flexible fiberoptic esophagoscope.

✔ **When removal of the food bolus has been successful, early medical follow-up should be provided for a comprehensive evaluation of the esophagus.** Patients who have experienced a prolonged obstruction or do not have complete resolution of all their symptoms should be admitted to the hospital for further observation and management.

What Not To Do:

✔ Do not ignore a patient's claims of a foreign body stuck in the esophagus. The patient is usually right.

✔ Do not try to force the food bolus down with the Ewald tube or any other catheter or dilator. This may cause an esophageal tear or perforation.

✔ Do not use oral enzymes such as papain, trypsin, or chymotrypsin. This treatment is slow, ineffective, and may possibly carry a risk of enzyme-induced esophageal perforation.

✔ Do not attempt to remove a hard, sharp, esophageal foreign body using any of the above techniques. These techniques very likely will cause an esophageal injury.

✔ Do not give glucagon to patients with pheochromocytoma or insulinoma.

✔ Do not use barium-impregnated cotton balls to detect esophageal foreign bodies. If a foreign body is present, they will obscure the view for the endoscopist.

 DISCUSSION

Patients who experience a food bolus obstruction of the esophagus are usually over 60 years of age and often have an underlying structural lesion. One of the more common lesions is a benign stricture secondary to reflux esophagitis. Another abnormality, the classic Schatzki's

Continued

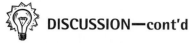 **DISCUSSION—cont'd**

ring (distal esophageal mucosal ring), especially above a hiatal hernia, may present with the "steakhouse syndrome" in which obstruction occurs and is relieved spontaneously. Other associated problems include postoperative narrowing, neoplasms, and cervical webs, as well as motility disorders, neurologic disease, and collagen vascular disease.

Chicken bones are the foreign bodies that most often cause esophageal perforation in adults. Meat impacted in the proximal two thirds of the esophagus is unlikely to pass and should be removed as soon as possible. Meat impacted in the lower third frequently does pass spontaneously, and the patient can safely wait, under medical observation, up to 12 hours before extraction. Even if a meat bolus does pass spontaneously, endoscopy must still be done later to assess the almost certain (80% to 90%) underlying pathology. Additional modes of therapy include the use of sublingual nitroglycerin or nifedipine to relax the lower esophageal sphincter, but they are not usually as effective as IV glucagon, which itself is of questionable efficacy.

SUGGESTED READINGS

Blair SR, Graeber GM, Cruzzavala JL, et al: Current management of esophageal impactions, *Chest* 104:1205-1209, 1993.

Kozarek RA, Sanowski RA: Esophageal food impaction: description of a new method for bolus removal, *Dig Dis Sci* 25:100-103, 1980.

Rice BT, Spiegel PK, Dombrowski PJ: Acute esophageal food impaction treated by gas-forming agents, *Radiology* 146:299-301, 1983.

Tibbling L, Bjorkhoel A, Jansson, et al: Effect of spasmolytic drugs on esophageal foreign bodies, *Dysphagia* 10:126-127, 1995.

67

Food Poisoning—
Staphylococcal

Presentation

The patient seeks medical care 1 to 6 hours after eating, because of severe nausea, vomiting, and abdominal cramps that progress later into diarrhea. He may appear very ill: pale, diaphoretic, tachycardic, orthostatic, perhaps complaining of paresthesias, or feeling as if he is "going to die." Others may have similar symptoms from eating the same food. The physical examination, however, is reassuring. There is minimal abdominal tenderness, localized, if at all, to the epigastrium or to the rectus abdominis muscle (which is strained by the vomiting).

What To Do:

✔ Completely examine the patient, and perform any tests needed to rule out myocardial infarction, perforated ulcer, dissecting aneurysm, or any of the catastrophes that can present in a similar fashion.

✔ In the meantime, **rapidly infuse 0.9% NaCl or Ringer's lactate solution IV and observe the patient,** doing repeated vital sign checks and physical examinations. In younger patients, who have the renal and cardiovascular reserve to handle rapid hydration, 1 to 2 L infused over an hour often provides dramatic improvement of all symptoms.

✔ If the patient is improving and beginning to tolerate oral fluids, discharge him with instructions to advance his diet over the next 24 hours, starting with an oral rehydration solution such as the following recipe from the World Health Organization:
¾ tsp of table salt
1 tsp of baking soda
1 cup of orange juice
4 tbsp of sugar
4 cups of water

✔ He should expect to be eating and feeling well in another 1 or 2 days.

✔ **If symptoms resolve more slowly, discharge the patient with a single dose of an antiemetic or antispasmodic such as a prochlorperazine (Compazine) 25 mg suppository or a dicyclomine (Bentyl) 20 mg tablet.**

181

✔ If hypotension or other significant signs or symptoms persist, if the patient cannot tolerate parenteral rehydration, or if he cannot resume oral intake, he may have to be admitted to the hospital for further evaluation and treatment.

What Not To Do:

✔ Do not immediately resort to medications (e.g., Compazine, Tigan) for nausea and vomiting. They may interfere with elimination of toxins and do not help correct the fluid and electrolyte imbalances responsible for many of the symptoms.

✔ Do not immediately resort to medications (e.g., Lomotil, Imodium) for cramping and diarrhea for the same reasons.

✔ Do not skimp on IV fluids.

✔ Do not pursue expensive laboratory investigations on straightforward cases.

✔ Do not presume food poisoning without a good history for it.

DISCUSSION

Many of the symptoms accompanying any gastroenteritis seem to be related to electrolyte disturbances and dehydration, which can be substantial even in the absence of copious vomiting and diarrhea. These symptoms can be resistant to oral rehydration, because the gut is unable to absorb and allows liter after liter of fluid to pool in its lumen. Lactated Ringer's solution is the choice for IV rehydration, because it approximates normal serum electrolytes and can be infused rapidly. Lactated Ringer's approximately replaces the electrolytes lost in diarrhea, although normal saline has more of the chloride lost by vomiting.

The most common food poisoning seen in most emergency departments is caused by the heat-stable toxin of staphylococci, which is introduced into food from infections in handlers and grows when the food sits warm. Chemical toxins have a similar presentation, but the onset of symptoms may be more immediate. Other bacterial food poisonings usually present with onset of symptoms later than 1 to 6 hours after eating, less nausea and vomiting, more cramping and diarrhea, and longer courses. A clearly implicated food source may give a clue to the etiology: shellfish suggesting *Vibrio parahaemolyticus;* rice suggesting *Bacillus cereus;* meat or eggs suggesting staphylococci, *Campylobacter* organisms, clostridia, salmonellae, shigellae, enteropathic *Escherichia coli,* or *Yersinia* species.

Whenever someone suffers any gastrointestinal upset, it is natural, if not instinctive, to implicate the last food eaten. Caution patients (especially if they are planning to sue the food supplier) that the diagnosis of food poisoning cannot be established without a group outbreak or a sample of tainted food for analysis.

68 Foreign Body, Rectal

Presentation

An object is generally inserted by the patient or a partner for sexual stimulation; it then causes pain or bleeding or becomes irretrievable. There may be rectal or lower abdominal pain, obstipation, or acute urinary retention. Sometimes the patient will not volunteer that any object has been inserted or will give outlandish explanations such as having sat or fallen onto the object. When interviewed privately, however, the patient will usually give an accurate account of the foreign body.

What To Do:

✔ Try to determine how long the foreign body has been lodged and if any attempts at removal have been made. Ask specifically about any assault or rape and respond accordingly. Give special consideration to the psychiatric patient.

✔ **Perform an abdominal and rectal examination but defer the rectal examination if the foreign body is known to be dangerously sharp.** If there are signs of peritoneal inflammation (i.e., rebound tenderness or pain with movement), suspect a perforation of the bowel, start appropriate IV lines, draw blood for laboratory analysis, obtain flat and upright abdominal x-rays to look for free air, notify surgical consultants, and administer IV antibiotics.

✔ **If there are no signs of perforation, flat and upright abdominal films may still be obtained to help define the nature, size, and number of foreign objects (as well as to reveal unsuspected free air).**

✔ **When there is no suspicion of a bowel perforation, sedate the patient with IV benzodiazepines and narcotics to help in the removal of the foreign body.** Place the patient on his side in the Sims' position. **If anal discomfort persists, instill lidocaine jelly for mucosal anesthesia or locally infiltrate 1% lidocaine with epinephrine into the anal sphincter.** The method of removal must be individualized depending on the size, shape, consistency, and fragility of the object.

✔ When the object can be reached by the examining finger and is of a nature that will allow it to be grasped, a lax anal sphincter may allow slow insertion of as much of a gloved hand as possible to grab the object and gradually extricate it. Perforate fruit with the fingertips to obtain a more effective grasp.

✔ **If unable to pull out the foreign body by hand, the following are techniques that can be used to get a purchase on the object and break the vacuum behind it:**
- **Slide a large Foley catheter with a 30 cc balloon past the object, inflate the balloon, and apply traction to the catheter. (This can be used in conjunction with any of the other techniques.) Two catheters may occasionally be needed, and air can be instilled through the lumen of the catheter** (Figure 68-1).
- **Under direct visualization with an anoscope or vaginal speculum, attempt to grasp the object with a tenaculum, sponge forcep, Kelly clamp, or tonsil snare** (Figure 68-2).
- An open object, like a jar or bottle, can be filled with wet plaster, into which a tongue blade can be inserted like a popsicle stick. When the plaster hardens, traction can be applied to the tongue blade (Figure 68-3).
- Forceps or soup spoons can be used to "deliver" a round object (Figure 68-4).

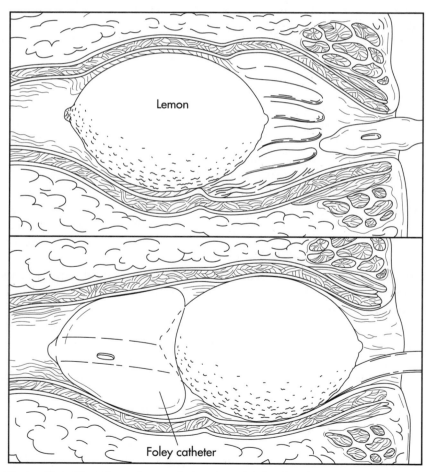

Figure 68-1 The Foley catheter technique is used to break a vacuum behind an object.

✔ **With an object that is too high to reach, the patient can be admitted and sedated for removal the next day.**

✔ When the object cannot be removed due to patient discomfort or sphincter tightness, removal must be accomplished in the OR under spinal or general anesthesia.

✔ When blood is present in the rectum or the object is capable of doing harm to the bowel, sigmoidoscopy should be performed after removal of the foreign body. When pain persists or there is any lingering suspicion of a bowel perforation, keep the patient for a 24-hour observation.

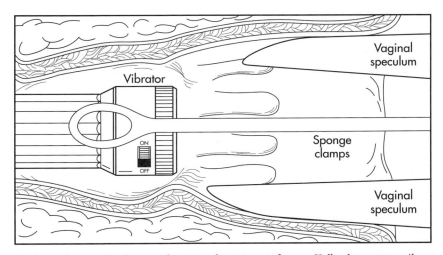

Figure 68-2 Grasp the object with a tenaculum, sponge forceps, Kelly clamp, or tonsil snare.

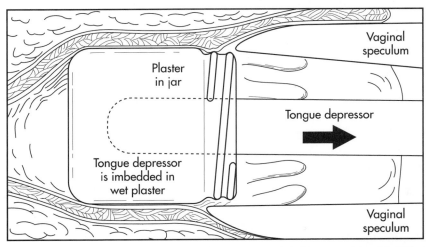

Figure 68-3 Fill jars or bottles with plaster and insert tongue blade like a popsicle stick. When plaster hardens, traction can be applied.

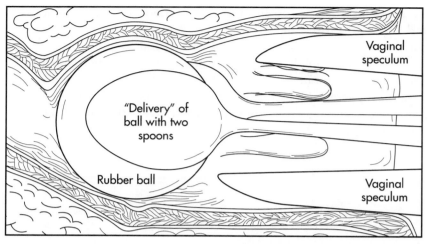

Figure 68-4 Round objects can be removed with forceps or soup spoons.

What Not To Do:

✗ Do not pressure the patient into giving you an accurate story. He may be embarrassed and intimidation will not help.

✗ Do not push the object higher into the colon while attempting to remove it.

✗ Do not blindly grab for an object with a tenaculum or other such device. This can itself lead to a perforation.

✗ Do not attempt to remove sharp, jagged objects such as broken glass via the rectum. These should only be removed under anesthesia in surgery.

✗ Do not send home a patient who is having continued pain. Admit him and observe for peritoneal signs, increased pain, fever, and a rising white blood cell count.

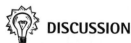 **DISCUSSION**

Most rectal foreign bodies (i.e., vibrators, dildos, broom handles, bottles, lightbulbs, balls, fruits, and vegetables) can be removed safely in the emergency department. Some practitioners quite reasonably forego x-rays before manipulation if the patient is free of pain and fever and if the object is benign. The famous gerbil is urban folklore. Consider recommending sexual or psychological counseling.

SUGGESTED READINGS

Couch CH, Tan EGC, Watt AG: Rectal foreign bodies, *Med J Aust* 144:512-515, 1986.

69

Foreign Body, Swallowed

Presentation

Parents bring in a young child shortly after she has swallowed a coin, safety pin, or toy. The child may be asymptomatic or have recurrent or transient symptoms of vomiting, drooling, dysphagia, pain, or a foreign body sensation. Disturbed or retarded adults may be brought from mental health facilities to the hospital on repeated occasions, at times accumulating a sizable load of ingested material.

What To Do:

✔ Ask about symptoms and examine the patient, looking for signs of airway obstruction (coughing, wheezing), bowel obstruction, or perforation (vomiting, melena, abdominal pain, abnormal bowel sounds).

✔ **Obtain PA and lateral x-ray views of the throat and chest to at least the mid-abdomen to determine if indeed anything was ingested or if the foreign body has become lodged or produced an obstruction.** A barium swallow may occasionally be necessary to locate a nonopaque foreign body in the esophagus.

✔ **A foreign body with sharp edges or a blunt foreign body lodged in the esophagus for more than a day should be removed endoscopically,** because it is likely to cause a perforation and is still accessible.

✔ **When a coin or other smooth object has been lodged in the upper esophagus of a healthy child for less than 24 hours, it can often be removed using a simple Foley catheter technique.** When available, it should be performed under fluoroscopy, although it can be done as a blind procedure. With the patient mildly sedated (e.g., midazolam [Versed] 0.5 mg/kg per rectum, intranasally or PO, with a half-hour allowed for absorption), position with the head down (Trendelenburg) and prone to minimize the risk of aspiration. Restrain uncooperative patients. Have a functioning laryngoscope, forceps, and airway equipment at hand. Test the balloon of an 8 to 12 Fr Foley catheter to ensure that it inflates symmetrically. Lubricate the catheter with water-soluble jelly and insert it through the nose into the esophagus to a point distal to the foreign body. Inflate the balloon with 5 ml of air and apply gentle traction on the catheter until the foreign body reaches the base of the tongue. Terminate the procedure if you encounter any resistance. While encouraging the patient to cough or spit out the foreign body, further traction will cause involuntary gagging and expectoration. Immediately deflate the balloon and remove the catheter. If a first attempt at removal fails, make a second and third try and then consult an endoscopist. When removal is successful, discharge the patient after a period of observation (Figure 69-1).

✔ Esophageal bougienage is another safe, effective, and inexpensive method to advance coins or smooth objects from the distal esophagus into the stomach without sedation. Wrap the patient in a bed sheet with arms at the side and an assistant holding her upright. Advance a well lubricated, blunt, round-tipped Hurst-type esophageal dilator through the mouth and esophagus into the stomach, then remove it. Obtain a postprocedure radiograph of the chest and upper abdomen to document the location of the

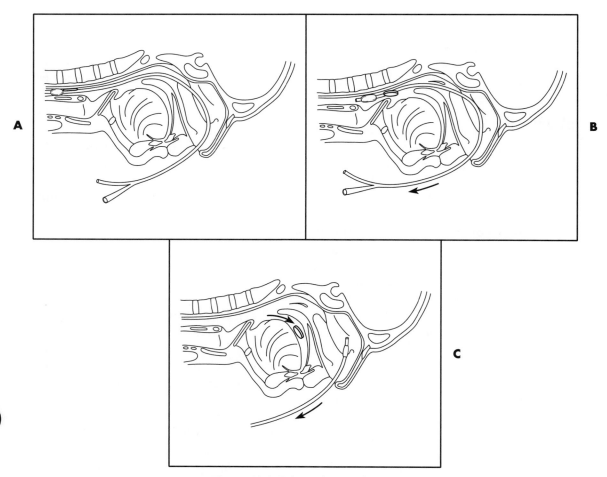

Figure 69-1 Foley catheter technique.

foreign body. Esophageal bougienage should be limited to witnessed ingestions of a single coin lodged for less than 24 hours with no previous history of esophageal foreign body, disease, or surgery and no respiratory compromise. Dilator size should be 28 Fr for ages 1 to 2, 32 Fr for ages 2 to 3, 36 Fr for ages 3 to 4, 38 Fr for ages 4 to 5, and 40 Fr over 5 years of age.

✔ **When a foreign body has passed into the stomach and there are no symptoms that demand immediate removal, discharge the patient with instructions to return for reevaluation in 7 days** (or sooner if she develops nausea, vomiting, abdominal pain, rectal pain, or rectal bleeding). Pediatricians have a saying that objects larger than 2 inches will not pass the second portion of the duodenum in a child under 2 years old. **Having parents sift through stools is often unproductive** (one missed stool negates days of hard work). **It may be helpful to give a bulk laxative to help decrease the intestinal transit time.**

What Not To Do:

✘ Do not use ipecac for foreign body ingestions. Emesis is effective for emptying the stomach of liquid but not for removing foreign bodies from the esophagus or stomach.

✘ Do not forcefully remove an esophageal foreign body, especially if it is causing pain. This removal may lead to injury or perforation.

✘ Do not automatically assume that an ingested foreign body should be surgically removed. The vast majority of potentially injurious foreign bodies pass through the alimentary tract without mishap. Operate only when the patient is actually being harmed by the swallowed foreign body or when there is evidence that it is not moving down the alimentary tract.

✘ Do not miss additional coins after removing one from the proximal esophagus. Take a repeat x-ray film after removal of one coin.

✘ Do not ignore the potential hazards of button battery ingestions (see below).

 DISCUSSION

Children swallow coins more than any other foreign body. Although the large majority of coins swallowed by healthy children pass through the gastrointestinal tract without difficulty, the most common complication is failure of the swallowed coin to traverse the esophagus completely.

The narrowest and least distensible strait in the gastrointestinal tract is usually the cricopharyngeus muscle at the level of the thyroid cartilage. Next narrowest is usually the pylorus, followed by the lower esophageal sphincter and the ileocecal valve. Thus anything that passes the throat will probably pass through the anus as well. In general, foreign bodies below the diaphragm should be left alone. A swallowed foreign body can irritate or perforate the GI tract anywhere but does not require treatment until complications occur.

189

Continued

DISCUSSION—cont'd

A significant portion of children with esophageal foreign bodies are asymptomatic; therefore any child suspected of ingesting a foreign body requires an x-ray to document whether or not it is present, and if so where it is located. Children with distal esophageal coins may be safely observed up to 24 hours before an invasive removal procedure, since most will spontaneously pass the coins. Even safety pins and razor blades usually pass without incident.

Large button batteries (the size of quarters) have become stuck in the esophagus, eroded through the esophageal wall, and produced a fatal exsanguination, but the smaller variety and batteries that passed into the gut have not been such a danger. Any button battery lodged in the esophagus should be considered a true emergency and removed immediately by an endoscopist. A button battery found in the stomach should be allowed to pass spontaneously. Smaller batteries need only weekly x-ray follow-up; the larger ones should be checked every 48 hours. Failure to pass the pylorus within 2 to 4 days is an indication for endoscopic removal. A metal detector can be used instead of repeated x-rays.

SUGGESTED READINGS

Binder L, Anderson WA: Pediatric gastrointestinal foreign body ingestions, *Ann Emerg Med* 13:112-117, 1984.

Connors GP: A literature-based comparison of three methods of pediatric esophageal coin removal, *Pediatric Emergency Care* 13:154-157, 1997.

Connors GP, Chamberlain JM, Ochsenschlager DW: Symptoms and spontaneous passage of esophageal coins, *Arch Pediatr Adolesc Med* 149:36-39, 1995.

Dokler ML, Bradshaw J, Mollitt DL, et al: Selective management of pediatric esophageal foreign bodies, *Am Surg* 61:132-134, 1995.

Ginaldi S: Removal of esophageal foreign bodies using a Foley catheter in adults, *Am J Emerg Med* 3:64-66, 1985.

Gracia C, Frey CF, Bodai BI: Diagnosis and management of ingested foreign bodies: a ten-year experience, *Ann Emerg Med* 13:30-34, 1984.

Hodge D, Tecklinburg F, Fleisher G: Coin ingestion: does every child need a radiograph? *Ann Emerg Med* 14:443-446, 1985.

Emslander HC, Bonadio W, Klatzo M: Efficacy of esophageal bougienage by emergency physicians in pediatric coin ingestion, *Ann Emerg Med* 27:726-729, 1996.

Schunk JE, Harrison M, Corneli HM, et al: Fluoroscopic Foley catheter removal of esophageal foreign bodies in children: experience with 415 episodes, *Pediatrics* 94:709-714, 1994.

70

Gas Pain and Constipation

Presentation

Sharp, crampy, migratory, and bloating abdominal pains may double the patient over, but last only a few seconds and are relieved by bowel movement and passing flatus. These pains may be related to loud bowel sounds *(borborygmi)* but not to position or eating and are not accompanied by other symptoms, such as nausea, vomiting, diarrhea, anorexia, or urinary urgency. Pain may be worse after meals and rarely are patients awakened with nocturnal symptoms. The physical examination is also benign, with no tenderness, masses, organomegaly, or other abnormalities, and the patient does not appear ill between the episodes of abdominal pain. Bowel sounds may become loud during each episode of cramps.

What To Do:

✔ Take a thorough history and try to determine the time of onset of symptoms and whether their severity is increasing or decreasing. Ask if there was a similar episode in the past. Perform a complete physical examination, including rectal and/or pelvic examination, and a repeat abdominal examination after an interval.

✔ If the presentation is not clear, consider using diagnostic tests like urinalysis (to help rule out renal colic or urinary tract infection); hemoglobin and hematocrit (to demonstrate an underlying anemia); differential white blood cell count (a clue to infection or inflammation); abdominal x-rays (to show free peritoneal air, bowel obstruction, or fecal impaction); ultrasonography (for pyloric stenosis, malrotation and intussusception in children, or appendicitis and gallbladder disorders).

✔ **If constipation is part of the problem, disimpact the rectum by pulling out hard stool *(scybala)* and follow with one oil retention enema,** which can be both diagnostic and therapeutic. **For dry, obstipated feces, repeated tap water enemas should be administered once or twice daily until clear before cathartics are used.**

✔ Instruct the patient to relieve symptoms with ambulation and local heat, and to return if symptoms do not resolve over the next 12 to 24 hours.

✔ Instruct the patient to drink 6 to 10 glasses of water a day.

✔ **Suggest adding bulk fiber, 10 g per day, in the form of bran, psyllium (Meta-mucil), methylcellulose (Citrucel), or calcium polycarbophil (FiberCon tablets) for prophylaxis. The last two products are made from synthetic fiber and produce less gas.** When possible, medications that may be constipating should be discontinued or replaced.

✔ **In addition, sorbitol solution or lactulose (Cephulac, Chronulac) can be safely prescribed 15 to 30 ml qd or bid 3 times a week. Additionally, bisacodyl (Dulcolax) 5 mg or senna (Senokot) two tablets can be given at bedtime and are available over the counter.**

✔ If the problem is chronic or recurrent or associated with alternating constipation and diarrhea, suspect irritable colon, inflammatory bowel disease, or diverticulitis, and arrange for a more comprehensive evaluation. If there is weight loss, anemia, occult blood in the stool, abdominal distension or mass, or a family history of colon cancer, refer the patient for colonoscopy.

✔ For infant colic (defined as crying for a minimum of 3 hours daily 3 days per week for the previous 3 weeks, without weight loss, vomiting, or diarrhea) instruct the parents to administer 2 ml of 12% sucrose in distilled water with each episode for a one- to two-day trial. If this is not successful, a higher concentration of sucrose may be more effective.

What Not To Do:

✘ Do not discharge the patient without 1 to 2 hours of observation, and two abdominal examinations. Many abdominal catastrophes may appear improved for short periods, only to worsen in an hour or two.

✘ Do not add fiber supplements without an adequate intake of fluids. Otherwise, they may actually exacerbate symptoms.

✘ Avoid long-term use of cathartic laxatives in otherwise healthy and active elderly patients because of the potential for adverse effects, including malabsorption, dehydration, electrolyte imbalances, and fecal incontinence.

DISCUSSION

While a patient may swallow excessive air in response to anxiety, an increased rate of "empty" swallowing may also accompany a number of gastrointestinal abnormalities including hiatal hernia and chronic cholecystitis. Heartburn increases salivation and therefore the frequency of swallowing. In addition to air swallowing, intraluminal gas-producing bacteria provide the other major mechanism for causing excess intestinal gas. A patient may be helped by reducing or eliminating her intake of foods that contain nonabsorbable carbohydrates such as beans, broccoli, cauliflower, and cabbage. Alternatively, she can be instructed to take Beano food enzyme tablets with these healthful foods.

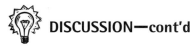 **DISCUSSION—cont'd**

Patients who have had at least 12 months of straining, lumpy, or hard stools, feeling of incomplete bowel evacuation at least a quarter of the time, or less than two bowel movements in a week fit the criteria for functional constipation due to poor transit time. If a patient has prolonged defecation or she occasionally needs manual disimpaction, she may have rectal outlet delay, due to anal fissure, rectal surgery, trauma, or megacolon. Rectosigmoid outlet delay is treated with glycerin suppositories on a regular schedule or mineral oil enemas daily or every other day half an hour after eating.

Constipation is one of the most common causes of pediatric abdominal pain. After a digital rectal examination, a glycerin suppository in infants or a single cleansing enema in children may provide rapid symptomatic relief. Be aware that constipation in infants is defined by stool consistency, not frequency, and that breastfed infants may normally have periods of 7 to 10 days without stools.

Colic attacks usually start when an infant is 7 to 10 days old and increase in frequency for the next 1 to 2 months. They tend to be worse in the evening, and subside by the age of 3 months. They do not just happen suddenly one night when the infant is 6 to 8 weeks old. In that situation, look for some other acute problem such as intussusception, corneal abrasion, incarcerated hernia, or digital hair tourniquet.

Common conditions associated with constipation in the elderly include dietary habits, hypercalcemia, hypokalemia, hypomagnesemia, mechanical obstruction, diabetes, hypothyroidism, Parkinson's disease, stroke, depression, and many medications, including anticholinergics, opiate analgesics, calcium channel blockers, calcium or aluminum containing antacids, antihistamines, and NSAIDs.

71

Hemorrhoids (Piles)

Presentation

Patients with external hemorrhoids generally complain of a painful anal lump that is discovered to be purple and covered with anal skin. It may have been precipitated by straining during defecation, heavy lifting, or pregnancy, but in most cases there was no definite preceding event. The external hemorrhoidal swelling is caused by thrombosis of the vein, is very tender to palpation, and usually does not bleed unless there is erosion of the overlying skin.

Patients with internal hemorrhoids usually seek help because of painless (or nearly painless) bright red bleeding at the time of defecation. Patients usually notice intermittent spotting on toilet tissue or episodic streaking of stool with blood. A prolapsed internal hemorrhoid appears as a protrusion of painless, moist red mass covered with rectal mucosa at the anal verge. Prolapsed internal hemorrhoids may become strangulated and thrombosed, and thus painful. Itching is not a common symptom of hemorrhoids.

What To Do:

✔ If the problem is rectal bleeding, it should be approached as any other gastrointestinal bleeding. The amount of bleeding should be quantified with orthostatic vital signs and a hematocrit; the rectum should then be examined with an anoscope. **For nonthreatening rectal bleeding from hemorrhoids, the initial management should include a high fiber diet, stool softeners, and bulk laxatives,** and the patient should be instructed to spend less time sitting on the commode. Prolapsed or strangulated hemorrhoids warrant surgical consultation and possible hospital admission. **All patients with rectal hemorrhage should be referred for a thorough gastroenterologic evaluation,** which might include proctosigmoidoscopy, barium enema, or colonoscopy. Young patients in whom hemorrhoids are the obvious source of bleeding may not require more than a digital rectal examination and anoscopy.

✔ **If the problem is pain, the rectum should be examined using a topical anesthetic (lidocaine jelly) as a lubricant. First, look for thrombosed external hemorrhoids and prolapsed internal hemorrhoids.** Have the patient perform a Valsalva maneuver as you provide traction on the skin of the buttocks, to evert the anus. **Examine the posterior mucosa for anal fissures.** After the topical anesthesia has taken effect, complete the digital rectal examination, looking for internal hemorrhoids and evidence of rectal abscesses or other masses.

✔ **If topical mucosal anesthetic does not give enough relief to permit examination, follow with subcutaneous injection of 5 to 10 ml of 1% lidocaine with epinephrine or bupivacaine for extended pain relief.**

✔ **If topical anesthetics on the rectal mucosa help control the pain, provide for more of the same, perhaps also with some added corticosteroid for antiinflammatory effect (Anusol-HC cream).** Suppositories are convenient but may not deliver the medication to where it is needed, so prescribe cream or foam (Proctofoam-HC, applied externally rather than internally).

✔ **Instruct the patient to treat lesser pain and itching with witch hazel compresses; a medium potency steroid cream; and ice packs followed by warm sitz baths.** Zinc oxide paste or petroleum jelly may ease defecation and soothe itching. **Prevent constipation by using bulk laxatives (i.e., bran, psyllium, polycarbophil, see Chapter 70) and stool softeners (docusate [Colace] 50 to 100 mg qd) and arrange follow-up.** Inform the patient that hemorrhoids may recur and require surgical removal.

✔ **Small ulcerated external hemorrhoids usually do not require any treatment for hemostasis.** Bulk laxatives and gentle cleansing are generally all that is required.

✔ **If a thrombosed external hemorrhoid is still moderately to severely painful after topical anesthesia, apply an ice pack for 15 minutes and then, using the smallest needle available, inject around it with a local anesthetic to allow for examination and excision. The thrombus may be enucleated via an elliptical incision over the anal mucosa. Locular clots can be broken up by inserting a straight hemostat into the wound and spreading the tips, thereby allowing the clots to be expressed.** Pain relief from this simple surgical technique can be dramatic, but excision is not effective unless the entire thrombosed lesion is completely removed. Apply a compression dressing and tape the buttocks together for 12 hours to minimize bleeding. The patient can then begin the nonsurgical treatment described above. Schedule a follow-up examination in 2 days. Narcotics may be prescribed for a day but should be switched to NSAIDs as soon as the risk of bleeding has lessened so they do not cause constipation (Figure 71-1).

What Not To Do:

✘ Do not labor to reduce prolapsed hemorrhoids unless they are part of a large rectal prolapse with some strangulation. Everything may prolapse again when the patient stands or strains.

✘ Do not traumatize the patient when doing an examination.

✘ Do not miss infectious and neoplastic processes that can resemble or coexist with hemorrhoids.

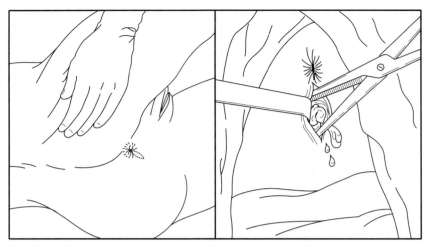

Figure 71-1 Thrombosed hemorrhoid excision.

✘ Do not excise a thrombosed hemorrhoid when the patient has a bleeding abnormality, is taking an anticoagulant or daily aspirin, or has increased portal venous pressure.

✘ Do not have the patient sit on a doughnut–shaped cushion. This may actually increase venous congestion.

 DISCUSSION

Three quarters of Americans have hemorrhoids at some time in their lives. Predisposing factors include heredity, portal hypertension, low fiber diet, obesity, straining to defecate, and pregnancy.

Internal hemorrhoids are classified into four groups. First-degree internal hemorrhoids do not protrude, cannot be palpated by digital examination, and require anoscopy for diagnosis. Second-degree hemorrhoids protrude with defecation but reduce spontaneously. Third-degree hemorrhoids protrude and require manual reduction. Fourth-degree hemorrhoids are irreducibly prolapsed.

Elastic banding techniques can be 80% to 90% curative for second-, third-, and fourth-degree internal hemorrhoids but can increase prolapse of first-degree hemorrhoids. Patients with bleeding diatheses, prolapse, or both internal and external hemorrhoids are best treated by surgical resection.

The diagnosis of "hemorrhoids" may cover a variety of minor ailments of the anus, which may or may not be related to the hemorrhoidal veins. Anal and perianal itching can be caused by dermatologic conditions such as psoriasis and allergic dermatitis. Infections of anal and perianal area include candidiasis, erythrasma, and pinworm (see Chapter 65). Perianal itching can also be the result of precancerous and cancerous lesions, so punch biopsy is indicated when pruritus ani is chronic.

72

Innocuous Ingestions

Presentation

Frightened parents call or arrive in the emergency department (ED) with a 2-year-old child who has just swallowed some household product such as laundry bleach.

What To Do:

✔ Establish exactly what was ingested (have them locate the container or bring in a sample if possible), how much, how long ago, as well as any symptoms and treatment so far.

✔ If there is any question about the substance, its toxicity, or its treatment, call the regional poison control center. In fact, it is a good policy to call the regional poison center even if you are completely comfortable managing the case, so they can record the ingestion for epidemiologic purposes.

✔ If there is any question of this being a toxic ingestion, follow the instructions of the regional poison center.

✔ Reassure the parents and child, and instruct them to call or return to the ED if there are any problems. Teach parents how to keep all poisons beyond the reach of children and how to call the regional poison center first for any future ingestions.

What Not To Do:

✘ Do not totally believe what is told about the nature of the ingestion. Often some of the information immediately available is wrong. Suspect the worst.

✘ Do not depend on product labels to give you accurate information on toxicity. Some lethal poisons carry warnings no more serious than "use as directed," or "for external use only."

✘ Do not follow the instructions on the package regarding what to do if a product is ingested. These are often inaccurate or out-of-date.

✘ Do not give ipecac for emesis of liquids that are corrosive or toxic only when aspirated, such as hydrocarbons.

✘ Do not improvise treatment of a patient referred by the regional poison center. They probably have special information and a treatment plan to share, if they have not called already.

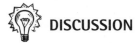

DISCUSSION

Fortunately, most products designed to be played with by children are also designed to be nontoxic when ingested. This includes chalk, crayons, ink, paste, paint, and Play-Doh. Many drugs, such as birth control pills and thyroid hormone, are relatively nontoxic, as are most laundry bleaches, the mercury in thermometers, and many plants. On the other hand, some apparently innocuous household products are surprisingly toxic, including camphorated oil, cigarettes, dishwasher soap, oil of wintergreen, and vitamins with iron. Because both the ingredients of common products and the treatment of ingestions continue to change, broad statements and lists are not reliable. The best strategy is always to call the regional poison center (see Appendix F).

73

Singultus (Hiccups)

Presentation

Recurring, unpredictable, clonic contractions of the diaphragm produce sharp inhalations. Hiccups are usually precipitated by some combination of laughing, talking, eating, and drinking but may also occur spontaneously. Most cases also resolve spontaneously and do not come to a physician's office unless prolonged or severe.

What To Do:

✔ **Stimulate the patient's soft palate by rubbing it with a swab, catheter tip, or finger, just short of stimulating a gag reflex, and continue this for a few minutes. Alternatively, stimulate the same general area by depositing a tablespoon of granulated sugar at the base of the tongue, in the area of the lingual tonsils, and letting it dissolve.** Such maneuvers (or their placebo effect) may abolish simple cases of hiccups.

✔ If hiccups continue, look for an underlying cause, and ask about precipitating factors or previous episodes. Persistence of hiccups during sleep suggests an organic cause; conversely, if a patient is unable to sleep or if the hiccups stop during sleep and recur promptly on awakening, this suggests a psychogenic or idiopathic etiology.

✔ Look in the ears (foreign bodies against the tympanic membrane can cause hiccups). Examine the neck, chest, and abdomen, perhaps including upright chest x-rays, to look for neoplastic or infectious processes irritating the phrenic nerve or diaphragm. Pericarditis and aberrant cardiac pacemaker electrode placement are potential sources of persistent hiccups, as well as acute and chronic alcohol intoxication and gastroesophageal reflux. Perform a neurologic examination, looking for evidence of partial continuous seizures or brainstem lesions. Early multiple sclerosis is thought to be one of the most frequent neurologic causes of intractable hiccups in young adults.

✔ Routine laboratory evaluation may include a CBC with differential (looking for infection or neoplasm) and electrolytes (hyponatremia can cause persistent hiccups).

✔ **If hiccups persist, try chlorpromazine (Thorazine) 25 to 50 mg PO tid or qid. (The same dose may be given IM.) Alternatively, haloperidol (Haldol) 2 to 5 mg IM followed by 1 to 4 mg PO tid for 2 days may be equally effective** with less potential for side effects. **Another approach is to use metoclopramide (Reglan)**

10 mg IV or IM followed by a maintenance regimen of 10 to 20 mg PO qid for 10 days. A final choice is nifedipine (Procardia) 10 to 20 mg PO tid or qid.

✔ Arrange for follow-up and additional evaluation. Although unlikely, there are potentially serious complications such as dehydration and weight loss resulting from the inability to tolerate fluids and food.

 DISCUSSION

Hiccups are a common malady and fortunately usually transient and benign. The common denominator among various hiccup cures seems to be stimulation of the glossopharyngeal nerve, but as for every self-limiting disease, there are always many effective cures.

"... hold your breath, and if after you have done so for some time the hiccup is no better, then gargle with a little water, and if it still continues, tickle your nose with something and sneeze, and if you sneeze once or twice, even the most violent hiccup is sure to go."
—Eriximachus the physician to Aristophanes, in Plato's *Symposium*.

SUGGESTED READINGS

Friedman NL: Hiccups: a treatment review, *Pharmacotherapy* 16:986-995, 1996.

Kolodzik PW, Eilers MA: Hiccups (singultus): review and approach to management, *Ann Emerg Med* 20:565-573, 1991.

Launois S, Bizec JL, Whitelaw WA, et al: Hiccup in adults: an overview, *Eur Resp J* 6:563-575, 1993.

Nathan MD, Leshner RT, Keller AP: Intractable hiccups (singultus), *Laryngoscope* 90:1612-1618, 1980.

Wagner MS, Stapczynski JS: Persistent hiccups, *Ann Emerg Med* 11:24-26, 1982.

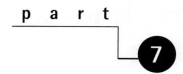

part

7

Urologic Emergencies

74 Blunt Scrotal Trauma

Presentation

Blunt injuries to the scrotum usually occur in patients less than 50 years of age as a result of an athletic injury, a straddle injury, an automobile or industrial accident, or an assault. Patients present with various degrees of pain, ecchymosis, and swelling (Figure 74-1).

What To Do:

✔ Get a clear history of the exact mechanism of the trauma and the point of maximum impact. **Determine if there was any bloody penile discharge or hematuria** and whether or not the patient has any preexisting genital pathology such as prior genitourinary surgery, infection, or mass.

✔ Gently examine the external genitalia with the understanding that intense pain may result in a suboptimal examination. **If scrotal swelling is not too severe, try to palpate and assess the intrascrotal anatomy.**

✔ **Obtain a urinalysis. If blood is present in the urine (or at the urethral meatus) do a digital examination of the prostate** (elevation of the prostate implies injury of the membranous urethra) and obtain urologic consultation. **There is a high risk of urethral injury in straddle injuries.**

✔ **When pain or swelling prevents demonstration of normal intrascrotal anatomy, obtain an ultrasound study or testicular scan to help determine the need for operative intervention.**

✔ With serious perineal injury, obtain x-rays of the pelvis.

✔ **When urologic intervention is not required, provide analgesia, bed rest, scrotal support, a cold pack, and urologic follow-up** (Figure 74-2).

What Not To Do:

✘ Do not miss testicular torsion, which can be associated with minor-to-moderate blunt trauma.

✘ Do not miss the rare traumatic testicular dislocation that results in an "empty scrotum." The testis is found superficially beneath the abdominal wall in about 80% of such cases. Immediate urology consultation is required.

✘ Do not discharge a patient until he can demonstrate the ability to urinate.

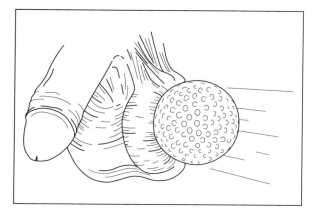

Figure 74-1 Blunt injury to the scrotum.

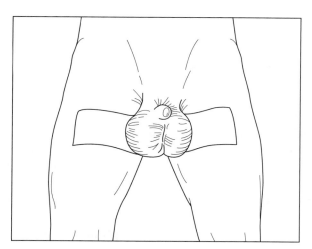

Figure 74-2 Scrotal support.

 DISCUSSION

The majority of blunt testicular injuries result in either contusions or ruptures. If Doppler or testicular scan studies demonstrate a serious injury, then early exploration, evacuation of hematoma, and repair of testicular rupture tend to result in an earlier return to normal activity, less infection, and less testicular atrophy.

c h a p t e r

75

Colorful Urine

Presentation

The patient may complain of or be frightened about the color of his urine; color may be one component of some urinary complaint, or the color may be noted incidentally on urinalysis.

What To Do:

✔ **Ask about symptoms of urinary urgency, frequency, and crampy pains (suggesting stones), as well as any food colorings, OTC or prescription medications, or diagnostic dyes recently ingested.** Ascertain the circumstances surrounding the notice of the color: Did the color only appear after the urine contacted the container or the water in the toilet bowl? Did the urine have to sit in the sun for hours before the color appeared?

✔ **Obtain a fresh urine sample for analysis. Persistent foam suggests protein, or yellowfoam, bilirubin,** which should also show up on a dipstick test. **A positive dipstick for blood implies the presence of red cells, free hemoglobin, or myoglobin,** which can be double-checked by examining the urinary sediment for red cells and the serum for hemoglobinemia. In patients with normal renal function, hemoglobinuria can be distinguished from myoglobinuria by drawing a blood sample, spinning it down, and looking at the serum. Free hemoglobin produces a pink serum that will test positive with the dipstick. Myoglobin is cleared more efficiently by the kidneys, usually leaving a clear serum that tests negative with the dipstick.

✔ **If the urine is red and acidic but does not contain hemoglobin, myoglobin, or red blood cells, suspect an indicator dye such as phenolphthalein** (the former laxative in Ex-Lax) in which case the red should disappear when the urine is alkalinized with a few drops of KOH. People with a particular metabolic defect produce red urine whenever they eat beets. Blackberries can turn acidic urine red, while rhubarb, anthraquinone laxatives, and some diagnostic dyes will redden urine only when it is alkaline.

✔ **Orange urine may be produced by phenazopyridine (Pyridium) or ethoxazene (Serenium),** both of which are used as urinary tract anesthetics to diminish dysuria. Rifampin will also turn urine orange.

✔ **Blue or green urine may be caused by a blue dye such as methylene blue,** a component in several medications (Trac Tabs, Urised, Uroblue) used to reduce symptoms of cystitis. A blue pigment may also be produced by *Pseudomonas* infection.

✔ **Brown or black urine** (not due to myoglobin or bilirubin) **may be caused by L-dopa, melanin, phenacetin, or phenol poisoning.** Metabolites of the antihypertensive methyldopa (Aldomet) may turn black on contact with bleach (which is often present in toilet bowls). Contamination with povidone-iodine (Betadine) solution or douche can turn urine brown. Melanin and melanogen, found in the urine of patients with melanoma, will darken standing urine from the air-exposed surface downward.

What Not To Do:

✘ Do not allow the patient to alter his urine factitiously. Have someone observe urine collection and inspect the specimen at once.

✘ Do not let a urine dipstick sit too long in the sample (allowing chemical indicators to diffuse out) or hold the dipstick vertically (allowing chemicals to drip from one pad to another and interfere with reagents).

✘ Do not be misled by dye in urine interfering with dipstick indicators. Pyridium can make a dipstick appear falsely positive for bilirubin, while contamination with hypochlorite bleach can cause a false positive test for hemoglobin. Also the urobilinogen dipstick test is not adequate for diagnosing porphyria.

 DISCUSSION

Porphyrins or eosin dyes fluoresce under ultraviolet light. Eosin turns urine pink or red but fluoresces green. Automobile radiator antifreeze contains fluorescein, to help locate leaks with ultraviolet light. Because this dye is excreted in the urine, green fluorescence can be a clue to ethylene glycol poisoning.

76 Epididymitis

Presentation

An adult male complains of dull-to-severe unilateral scrotal pain developing over a period of hours to a day and radiating to the ipsilateral lower abdomen or flank. There may be a history of recent urethritis, prostatitis, or prostatectomy (allowing ingress of bacteria), strain from lifting a heavy object, or sexual activity with a full bladder (allowing reflux of urine). There may be fever or urinary urgency or frequency. Nausea is unusual.

The epididymis is tender, swollen, warm, and difficult to separate from the firm, nontender testicle. Increasing inflammation can extend up the spermatic cord and fill the entire scrotum, making examinations more difficult, as well as produce frank prostatitis or cystitis. The rectal examination therefore may reveal a very tender, boggy prostate.

What To Do:

✔ **Ascertain that the testicle is normal in position and perfusion, with a normal cremasteric reflex.** Doppler ultrasound or a testicular perfusion scan, which is better, may help pick up a decrease in arterial flow from spermatic cord to testicle as seen in testicular torsion.

✔ Palpate and auscultate the scrotum to rule out a hernia. Gently palpate the prostate once, looking for prostatitis. In older men, percuss for dullness above the pubic symphysis to evaluate urinary retention and bladder distension. Culture urine and any urethral discharge to identify a bacterial organism.

✔ When a mass is present, consider the diagnosis of a hydrocele, testicular tumor, or abscess, best evaluated with ultrasound.

✔ On rare occasions for severe pain, infiltrate the spermatic cord above the inflammation with local anesthetic for better palpation and diagnosis (e.g., 1% lidocaine without epinephrine). Lesser pain may respond to antiinflammatory analgesics (Motrin to Percodan).

✔ **Prescribe antibiotics for likely organisms. In men under 35, ceftriaxone (Rocephin) 250 mg IM in the emergency department and a prescription for doxycycline (Vibramycin) 100 mg bid for 10 days should eradicate _Neisseria gonorrhoeae_ and _Chlamydia trachomatis._** An alternative treatment is ofloxacin (Floxin) 300 mg bid × 10 days. **In men over 35, ciprofloxacin (Cipro) 500 mg bid, ofloxacin (Floxin) 200 mg bid, or trovafloxacin (Trovan) 200 mg qd for 10 to 14 days may be better for gram-negative bacteria.**

✔ **Arrange for 2 to 3 days of strict bed rest, with the scrotum elevated, using an athletic supporter when up, warm tub baths, and urologic follow-up within several days. Prior to 72 hours, ice compresses may be helpful.**

What Not To Do:

✘ Do not miss testicular torsion. It is far better to have the urologist explore the scrotum and find epididymitis than to delay and lose a testicle to ischemia (which can happen in only 4 to 6 hours). When torsion is strongly suspected, do not delay the management of the case by waiting for the results of ancillary tests.

 DISCUSSION

A significant number of pediatric patients with epididymitis will have a urologic abnormality. Testicular torsion is more likely in children and adolescents and has a more sudden onset, although it can be recurrent and is often related to exertion or direct trauma, and is more often associated with nausea and vomiting. If the spermatic cord is twisted, the testicle may be high, the epididymis may be in a position other than its normal posterior position, and there will most likely be no cremasteric reflex. A testicular scan can help differentiate torsion from the sometimes similar presentation of acute epididymitis. When torsion is highly suspected, try a therapeutic and diagnostic detorsion by externally rotating the testicle (move the anterior aspect from medial to lateral) at least 180 degrees with the patient standing or supine. Continue rotating one to three turns until the pain is promptly relieved.

SUGGESTED READINGS

Caldamone AA, Valvo JR, Altebarmakian VK, et al: Acute scrotal swelling in children, *J Ped Surg* 19:581–584, 1984.

Knight PJ, Vassy LE: The diagnosis and treatment of the acute scrotum in children and adolescents, *Ann Surg* 200:664–673, 1984.

77

Genital Herpes Simplex

Presentation

The patient may be distraught with severe genital pain or just concerned about paresthesias and subtle genital lesions, desirous of pain relief during a recurrence, or suffering complications such as superinfection or urinary retention. Often, there are associated systemic symptoms such as fever, myalgias, and headache.

Instead of the classic grouped vesicles on an erythematous base, herpes in the genitals usually appears as groupings of 2 to 3 mm ulcers, representing the bases of abraded vesicles (Figure 77-1). Resolving lesions are also less likely to crust on the genitals. Lesions can be tender, and should be examined with gloves on, because they shed infectious viral particles. Inguinal lymph nodes may be painful but are usually bilateral and not confluent.

What To Do:

✔ If necessary for the diagnosis, perform a Tzanck prep, by scraping the base of the vesicle (this hurts!), spreading the cells on a slide, drying, and staining with Wright's or Giemsa stain. The presence of multinucleate giant cells with nuclear molding confirms the diagnosis of herpes. Alternatively, use this sample for herpes virus culture, if available, and if there is any doubt about the diagnosis.

✔ Send a serologic test for syphilis and culture any cervical or urethral discharge in search of other infections requiring different therapy.

✔ **For the immunocompetent patient, prescribe acyclovir (Zovirax) 400 mg tid for 10 days. Alternative treatment regimens include famciclovir (Famvir) 250 mg tid for 5 to 10 days, and valacyclovir (Valtrex) 1000 mg bid for 10 days. For recurrent infections, prescribe acyclovir 400 mg tid, famciclovir 125 mg bid, or valacyclovir 500 mg bid for 5 days.**

✔ **Prescribe antiinflammatory analgesics (Motrin to Percodan) for pain. Try sitz baths for comfort.**

✔ Warn the patient of the following:
1) Lesions and pain can be expected to last 2 weeks during the initial attack (usually less in recurrences).

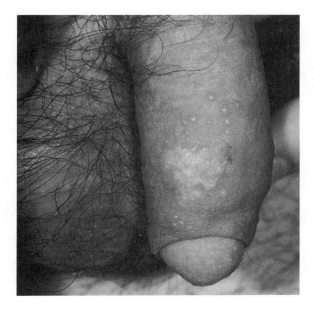

Figure 77-1 Herpes simplex of the penis. *(From Habif TP: Clinical dermatology: a color guide to diagnosis and therapy, ed 3, St Louis, 1996, Mosby.)*

2) Although acyclovir reduces shedding, the patient should assume he is contagious whenever there are open lesions (and can potentially transmit the virus at other times as well).
3) He should be careful about touching lesions and washing hands, because other skin can be inoculated.
4) Recurrences can be triggered by any sort of local or systemic stress and will not be helped by topical acyclovir.

What Not To Do:

✗ Do not confuse these lesions with the painless, raised, genital ulcer of syphilis, or the erosive lesions of Stevens-Johnson syndrome, which will also involve at least one other mucous membrane such as oral mucosa, pharynx, larynx, lips, or conjunctiva.

 DISCUSSION

Currently there is no role for topical acyclovir in the treatment of genital herpes. Oral prophylaxis has been shown to be effective.

SUGGESTED READINGS

Benedetti J, Corel L, Ashley R: Recurrence rates in genital herpes after symptomatic first-episode infection, *Ann Intern Med* 121:847-854, 1994.

chapter

78

Gonorrhea (GC, Clap)

Presentation

A young man may present with symptoms of urethritis (dysuria, a purulent discharge), or perhaps prostatitis (low back pain) or epididymitis (scrotal pain). A young woman may have cervicitis or pelvic infection (low abdominal pain and tenderness, dysuria, and vaginal, cervical, or urethral discharge). Both sexes may present with gonococcal proctitis (rectal pain, rectal discharge, tenesmus) or pharyngitis. Either sex may be asymptomatic after contact with a partner known to be infected with gonorrhea.

What To Do:

✔ Obtain a sexual history and look for rash, arthritis, tenosynovitis, perihepatitis, or pain on moving the cervix. These are signs of disseminated infection, which may require a longer course of treatment or hospital admission.

✔ **Gram stain any discharge or exudate and examine it for gram-negative diplococci ingested by polymorphonuclear leukocytes,** which corroborate the diagnosis of gonorrhea (their absence does not rule out the possibility).

✔ Culture the throat, urethra, cervix, anus—wherever the patient is symptomatic or exposed, according to the history. To avoid killing the organism, use a special transport medium or plate immediately on room-temperature Thayer-Martin medium; incubate soon after collection.

✔ With female patients, send a urine or blood test to rule out pregnancy.

✔ Send blood for syphilis serology and be sure someone will review and act on the results. Incubating primary syphilis with negative serology should be eradicated by the regimens below, but established secondary or tertiary syphilis with positive serology will require a longer course of antibiotics.

✔ **Gonorrhea can be treated with one dose of ceftriaxone (Rocephin) 125 mg IM; for oral treatment, cefixime (Suprax) 400 mg; or in the nonpregnant patient, ciprofloxacin (Cipro) 500 mg or ofloxacin (Floxin) 400 mg one PO.**

✔ **Treat all cases of gonococcal urethritis or pelvic infection for chlamydia, which is a likely copathogen. Cover both possibilities by adding doxycycline (Vibramycin) 100 mg or ofloxacin (Floxin) 300 mg bid for 7 days, or azithromycin (Zithromax) 1000 mg PO once.** If the patient is pregnant, as an alternative to azithromycin, use erythromycin ethyl succinate (EES) 800 mg qid × 7 days or erythro-mycin base, not estolate, 500 mg qid × 7 days.

✔ Instruct the patient to avoid sexual contact for 5 days, arrange for a follow-up reexami-nation and reculture to ensure eradication, and report the infection, if required by law.

✔ **Treat sexual partners of patients exposed to gonorrhea with the same antibi-otic regimens (cultures may be omitted).**

✔ Instruct the patient on the correct use of the condom to prevent reinfection.

What Not To Do:

✘ Do not pretend to rule out venereal disease on the basis of a "negative" sexual history. Simply taking cultures during the physical examination is often preferable to badgering a patient about intimate details she would rather not reveal.

✘ Do not be misled by extracellular gram-negative diplococci, which can be among the normal flora of the pharynx or vagina. Do not send culture or serology tests unless some-one will see and act on the results.

✘ Do not fail to suspect and treat gonococcal in sexually active women with the mild and nonspecific symptoms of primary gonorrhea.

DISCUSSION

Disseminated gonorrhea with arthritis and dermatitis presents with fever, chills, polyarticu-lar arthritis, a characteristic petechial or tender papular rash of the distal extremities, and tenosynovitis of extensor tendons of the hands, wrists, or ankle tendons. This represents a more serious infection requiring a more comprehensive evaluation, extended parenteral an-tibiotic therapy, and hospitalization of all but the mildest cases.

The Centers for Disease Control and Prevention update treatment recommendations every few years, incorporating changes in antibiotics and sensitivity.

79

Phimosis and Paraphimosis

Presentation

Phimosis is the inability to retract the foreskin over the glans and is usually due to a contracted preputial opening (Figure 79-1). Patients with phimosis may seek acute medical care when they develop signs and symptoms of infection, such as pain and swelling of the foreskin and a purulent discharge. Paraphimosis occurs when the foreskin cannot be replaced in its normal position after it is retracted behind the glans. The tight ring of preputial skin, which is caught behind the glans, creates a venous tourniquet effect and leads to edematous swelling of the glans (Figure 79-2).

What To Do:

✔ **For paraphimosis, squeeze the glans firmly for at least 10 minutes to reduce the edematous swelling. Wrap the shaft and swollen glans with a gauze pad followed by a 2-inch elastic bandage that will produce constant, gentle compression. After 10 to 15 minutes, remove the bandage, push the glans proximally, and slide the prepuce back over the glans** (Figure 79-3).

✔ If manual reduction fails, anesthetize the dorsal foreskin and carefully incise the constricting tissue with a vertical incision.

✔ **If the phimosis patient has secondary urinary obstruction, catheterize the urethra with a small gauge catheter.** If you cannot find the urethral meatus, try using a nasal speculum to widen the opening or anesthetize the dorsal foreskin and carefully incise the constricting tissue with a vertical incision (dorsal slit) to allow retraction.

✔ **Treating phimosis usually involves the management of acute infection. Frequent hot compresses or soaks are needed along with antibiotics.** Topical antibiotics like bacitracin may be adequate when poor hygiene leads to infection in the pediatric patient. Sexually transmitted diseases should be suspected and treated appropriately in adolescents and adults. Candidal infections, with their typical white cheesy exudate, can be treated with a single dose of fluconazole (Diflucan) 200 mg PO.

✔ Instruct parents in the technique and importance of proper cleaning of their son's prepuce. Have them place him in a tub of warm water to alleviate dysuria.

✔ In both paraphimosis and phimosis, follow-up care should be provided. When swelling and inflammation subside, circumcision should be considered.

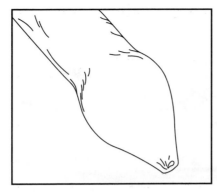

Figure 79-1 Phimosis.

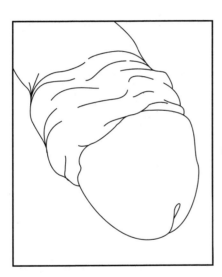

Figure 79-2 Paraphimosis.

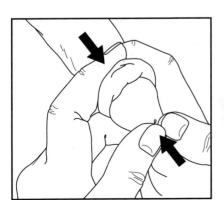

Figure 79-3 Manual reduction of paraphimosis by counter-pressure between thumbs and fingers.

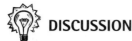 **DISCUSSION**

Poor hygiene and chronic inflammation are the usual causes of stenosing fibrosis of the preputial opening. It can be normal for boys up to 5 years of age not to be able to retract the foreskin completely. In the case of a neglected paraphimosis, arterial occlusion may supervene, and gangrene of the glans develops. When phimosis results in acute urinary retention, the tip of a hemostat can be inserted into the scarred end of the foreskin and gently opened, allowing the patient to void satisfactorily until urologic consultation can be obtained. One common cause of paraphimosis is retracting the foreskin to clean the glans and insert a Foley catheter, then forgetting to reduce the foreskin afterwards.

80

Prostatitis

Presentation

A man complains of fever, chills, and perineal or low back pain and may have urinary urgency and frequency, as well as signs of obstruction to urinary flow, ranging from a weak stream to urinary retention. On gentle examination, the prostate is swollen and tender. The infection may spread from or into the contiguous urogenital tract (epididymis, bladder, urethra) or the bloodstream.

What To Do:

✔ **Perform a rectal examination and, only once, gently palpate the prostate to see if it is tender, swollen, edematous, warm, fluctuant, or boggy.**

✔ Evaluate and treat for possible associated urinary retention (see Chapter 82). In severe cases, a suprapubic catheter may be preferable to a Foley catheter for bladder decompression and urinary drainage because it avoids trauma to the prostate and resulting pain and hematogenous spread of infection.

✔ Culture the urine to help identify the organism responsible (although there is no guarantee that the bacteria in the prostate will be in the urine).

✔ **For patients 35 years and younger, treat for gonorrhea and other urethritis** (see Chapters 78 and 81) **with ceftriaxone (Rocephin) 125 mg IM to 1000 mg IV and azithromycin (Zithromax) 1000 mg PO or doxycycline (Vibramycin) 100 mg PO bid for 7 days.**

✔ **For men over 35 years old, begin empirical treatment with ciprofloxacin (Cipro) 400 mg IV, then 500 mg PO bid, or prescribe ofloxacin (Floxin) 400 mg bid or the less expensive trimethoprim plus sulfamethoxazole (Bactrim DS) bid for 10 to 14 days.**

✔ For pain and fever, prescribe NSAIDs. **If the patient needs narcotics, add stool softeners to prevent constipation.**

✔ Arrange for urologic follow-up.

What Not To Do:

✗ Do not massage or repeatedly palpate the prostate. Rough treatment is unlikely to help drain the infection or produce the responsible organism in the urine but is likely to extend or worsen a bacterial prostatitis or precipitate bacteremia or septic shock.

DISCUSSION

Blood in the ejaculate may be a sign of inflammation in the prostate and epididymis or, especially in younger males, may simply be a self-limiting sequela of vigorous sexual activity.

81 Urethritis (Drip)

Presentation

A male complains of dysuria, a burning discomfort along the urethra, or a urethral discharge. A copious, thick, yellow-green discharge that stains underwear is characteristic of gonorrhea, whereas a thin, white, scant discharge with milder symptoms is characteristic of chlamydia. Urethritis in a female may be asymptomatic or indistinguishable from cystitis or vaginitis or may be manifest as UTI symptoms with a low concentration of bacteria on urine culture or tenderness localized to the distal periurethral area of the anterior vaginal wall. In addition to increased vaginal discharge, women may have intermenstrual bleeding, especially postcoital spotting and cervical friability.

What To Do:

✔ **Gram stain any urethral discharge, looking for gram-negative diplococci inside white cells, which imply gonococcal infection** (see Chapter 78).

✔ Order a serologic test for established syphilis. Further antibiotic treatment is required if the RPR or VDRL is positive.

✔ **Examine the urine sediment for swimming protozoa, implying infection with *Trichomonas vaginalis*, best treated with metronidazole (Flagyl) 500 mg bid × 7 days, or 2 g PO once.**

✔ **If there is no sign of gonorrhea or *Trichomonas* organisms causing the urethritis, assume the infection is caused by chlamydia or *Ureaplasma* organisms, best treated with doxycycline 100 mg bid for 7 days, or azithromycin 1000 mg PO once.** Alternatively, prescribe ofloxacin (Floxin) 300 mg bid for 7 days. (If the patient is pregnant, use erythromycin ethyl succinate (EES) 800 mg qid × 7 days or erythromycin base, not estolate, 500 mg qid × 7 days).

✔ Ask about sexual partners who should also be treated.

✔ Instruct the patient on the correct use of the condom to prevent reinfection.

What Not To Do:

✘ Do not send off a serologic test for syphilis without following up on the results.

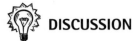

DISCUSSION

Cultures and fluorescent antibody tests to diagnose chlamydia are expensive and insensitive, so presumptive treatment remains the best strategy. Many gonorrhea victims develop a rebound urethritis, probably with chlamydia, following single-dose antibiotic treatment.

Nongonococcal urethritis is the most common sexually treated disease among US men. Complications include acute epididymitis, Reiter's syndrome, and persistent or recurrent urethritis. More important, failure to identify and treat nongonococcal urethritis places female sexual partners at risk for mucopurulent cervicitis, pelvic inflammatory disease (PID), ectopic pregnancy, and tubal infertility. Sexually-transmitted infections that produce cervical inflammation in women and urethritis in men may facilitate transmission of human immunodeficiency virus (HIV).

Although more expensive, a single dose of azithromycin ensures compliance compared to 7 days of doxycycline. Although most patients probably take doxycycline long enough to eradicate uncomplicated chlamydial infections, some may develop persistent or recurrent urethritis from stopping early.

SUGGESTED READINGS

Augenbraun M, Bachmann L, Wallace T, et al: Compliance with doxycycline therapy in sexually transmitted disease clinics, *Sex Transm Dis* 25: 1-4, 1998.

Stamm WE, Hicks CB, Martin DH, et al: Azithromycin for empirical treatment of the nongonococcal urethritis syndrome in men, *J Am Med Assoc* 274:545-549, 1995.

82

Urinary Retention

Presentation

The patient, usually male, may complain of increasing dull low abdominal discomfort and the urge to urinate, without having been able to urinate for many hours. Elderly and debilitated patients may be asymptomatic or have vague discomfort with urinary frequency but small volumes, overflow, or stress incontinence. A firm, distended bladder can be palpated between the symphysis pubis and umbilicus. Rectal examination may reveal an enlarged or tender prostate or suspected tumor.

What To Do:

✔ **Delaying only long enough for good aseptic technique, pass a Foley catheter into the bladder** and collect the urine in a closed bag. Reassuring the patient and having him breathe through his mouth may help relax the external sphincter of the bladder and facilitate the passage of the catheter.

✔ **If passage remains difficult in a male patient, distend the urethra with lubricant such as K-Y jelly or lidocaine jelly 2% in a catheter-tipped syringe (Uroject, Uro-Jet) and try a 16, 18, or 20 Fr Foley catheter. Leave the lidocaine jelly in place 5 to 20 minutes to obtain good mucosal anesthesia** (Figure 82-1).

✔ **If the problem is negotiating the curve around a large prostate, use a Coudé catheter.**

✔ If the bladder still cannot drain, obtain urologic consultation for stylets, sounds, filiforms, and followers, or consider a percutaneous suprapubic catheterization.

✔ Check renal and urinary function with a urinalysis, a urine culture, and serum BUN, and creatinine determinations. Examine the patient to ascertain the cause of obstruction.

✔ If there is an infection of the bladder, give antibiotics (see Chapter 83).

✔ If the volume drained is modest (1 to 1.5 L) and the patient stable and ambulatory, attach the Foley catheter to a leg bag and discharge him for follow-up (and probably catheter removal) the next day.

✔ If the volume drained is small (100 to 200 ml), remove the catheter and search for alternate etiologies of the abdominal mass and urinary urgency.

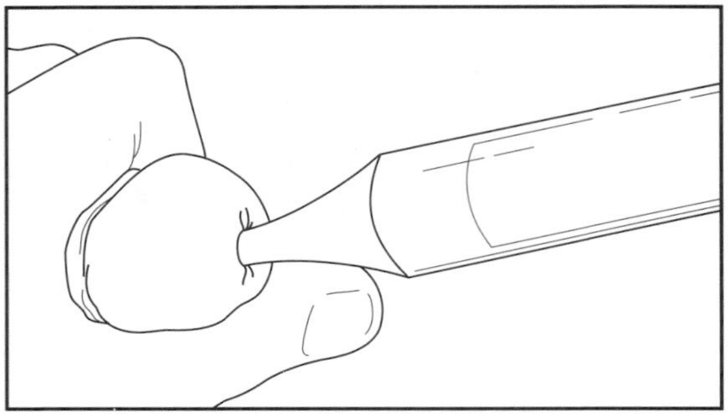

Figure 82-1 Lidocaine jelly administrator.

What Not To Do:

✘ Do not use stylets or sounds unless you have experience instrumenting the urethra—these devices can cause considerable trauma.

✘ Do not remove the catheter right away if the bladder was significantly distended. Bladder tone will take several hours to return, and the bladder may become distended again.

✘ Do not clamp the catheter to slow decompression of the bladder, even if the volume drained is greater than 2 L.

✘ Do not use bethanechol (Urecholine) unless it is clear that there is no obstruction, inadequate (parasympathetic) bladder tone is the only cause of the distension, and there is no possibility of gastrointestinal disease.

✘ Do not routinely treat the bacteria cultured from a distended bladder—they may only represent colonization, which will resolve with drainage.

DISCUSSION

Urinary retention may be caused by stones lodged in the urethra or urethral strictures (often from gonorrhea); prostatitis, prostatic carcinoma, or benign prostatic hypertrophy; and tumor or clot in the bladder. Any drug with anticholinergic effects or alpha adrenergic effects, such as antihistamines, ephedrine sulfate, and phenylpropanolamine, can precipitate urinary retention. Neurologic etiologies include cord lesions and multiple sclerosis. Patients with genital herpes may develop urinary retention from nerve involvement. Urinary retention has also been reported following vigorous anal intercourse. The urethral catheterization outlined is appropriate initial treatment for all these conditions.

Sometimes hematuria develops midway through bladder decompression, probably representing loss of tamponade of vessels injured as the bladder distended. This should be watched until the bleeding stops (usually spontaneously) to be sure that there is no great blood loss, no other urologic pathology responsible, and no clot obstruction.

83

Urinary Tract Infection, Lower (Cystitis)

Presentation

The patient (usually female) complains of urinary frequency and urgency, internal dysuria, and suprapubic pain. The onset of symptoms is generally abrupt, often causing her to seek care within 24 hours. There may have been some antecedent trauma (sexual intercourse) to inoculate the bladder, and there may be blood in the urine (hemorrhagic cystitis). Usually, there is no labial irritation, external dysuria, or vaginal discharge (which would suggest vaginitis); and no fever, chills, nausea, flank pain, or costovertebral angle tenderness (which would suggest an upper urinary tract infection [UTI]).

What To Do:

✔ Examine a clean-catch urine specimen. Instruct the patient to wipe the introitus from front to back and begin urinating into the toilet before filling the sample cup. In women of childbearing age, send a urine pregnancy test: this will influence choice of antibiotic and follow-up. Use a dipstick test for leukocyte esterase, send for a urinalysis, or Gram stain a sample of urine. Epithelial cells on the microscopic examination are evidence of contamination from the vagina. The presence of any white cells or bacteria in a clean sample confirms the infection. A positive nitrite on dipstick is helpful, but a negative test does not rule out infection because many bacteria do not produce nitrites. Menses or vaginal discharge make a clean catch difficult. One technique is to insert a tampon before giving the sample. A better technique is urinary catheterization.

✔ **If the clinical picture is clearly of an uncomplicated lower urinary tract infection in a nonpregnant patient, give trimethoprim 160 mg plus sulfamethoxazole 800 mg (Bactrim DS or Septra DS) one tablet bid for 3 days or a 3-day regimen of a quinolone such as ciprofloxacin (Cipro) 250 mg bid, norfloxacin (Noroxin) 400 mg bid, or ofloxacin (Floxin) 200 mg bid.** Single-dose treatment with two TMP/SMX DS tablets is also effective in the young healthy female, but does have a higher early recurrence rate. **In pregnancy, give a single dose of 200 mg of** nitrofurantoin (Macrodantin). Amoxicillin or cephalosporins are alternatives in pregnancy, but not quinolones (or sulfas in the last trimester).

✔ Instruct the patient to drink plenty of liquids (such as cranberry juice).

✔ If the dysuria is severe, also prescribe phenazopyridine (Pyridium) 200 mg tid for 2 days only, to act as a surface anesthetic in the bladder. Warn the patient that it will stain her urine (and perhaps clothes) orange.

✔ Extend therapy to 7 days and obtain cultures when treating a patient who is unreliable, diabetic, symptomatic more than 5 days, older than 50 years of age, or younger than 16 years of age. Also, extend treatment and obtain cultures on all male patients and those with an indwelling urinary catheter, renal disease, obstructive urinary tract lesions, recurrent infection, or other significant medical problems.

✔ If there are no bacteria or few white cells, no hematuria or suprapubic pain, gradual onset over 7 to 10 days, and a new sexual partner, the dysuria may be caused by a chlamydial or ureaplasmal urethritis (see Chapter 81). Perform a pelvic examination and obtain samples for culture and microscopic examination. Ask the patient about the use of spermicides or douches, which may irritate the periurethral tissue and cause dysuria.

✔ When there is a history of previous episodes of lower UTI symptoms with negative urinalysis, cultures, and work ups for sexually transmitted diseases, consider a paraurethral gland infection as the cause of this female urethral syndrome. This is usually associated with tenderness at either side of the distal third of the urethra, adjacent to the urethral meatus. Treat presumed chlamydia with doxycycline or erythromycin for 2 to 4 weeks. Older women or young women after an initial treatment failure should be given a quinolone for at least a month. Hot sitz baths may provide comfort.

✔ If there is external dysuria, vaginal discharge, odor, itching, and no frequency or urgency, then evaluate for vaginitis (see Chapter 93) with a pelvic examination.

✔ Arrange for follow-up in 2 days if the symptoms have not completely resolved. If necessary, urine culture and a longer course of antibiotics can be undertaken then. Arrange follow-up for all children because a UTI may be the first evidence of underlying urinary tract pathology.

What Not To Do:

✘ Do not forget to check for pregnancy.

✘ Do not undertake expensive urine cultures for every lower UTI of recent onset in nonpregnant, normal healthy women with no history of recent UTI or antibiotic use.

✘ Do not use the single-dose or 3-day regimens for a possible upper UTI or pyelonephritis (see Chapter 84).

✘ Do not rely on gross inspection of the urine sample. Cloudiness is usually caused by crystals, and odors can result from diet or medication.

✘ Do not require a follow-up visit or culture after therapy unless symptoms persist or recur.

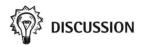 **DISCUSSION**

Lower UTI or cystitis is a superficial bacterial infection of the bladder or urethra. The majority of these infections involve *Escherichia coli, Staphylococcus saprophyticus,* or enterococci.

The urine dipstick is a reasonable screening measure that can direct therapy if results are positive. Under the microscope in a clean sediment (free of epithelial cells), one white cell per 400× field suggests a significant pyuria, although clinicians accustomed to imperfect samples usually set a threshold of 3 to 5 WBCs per field. In addition, *Trichomonas* organisms may be appreciated swimming in the urinary sediment, indicating a different etiology for urinary symptoms or associated vaginitis. In a straightforward lower UTI, urine culture may be reserved for cases that fail to resolve with single-dose or 3-day therapy. In complicated or doubtful cases or with recurrences, a urine culture before initial treatment may be helpful.

Risk factors for UTI in women include pregnancy, sexual activity, use of diaphragms or spermicides, failure to void postcoitally, and history of prior UTI. Healthy women may be expected to suffer a few episodes of lower UTI in a lifetime without indicating any major structural problem, but recurrences at short intervals suggest inadequate treatment or underlying abnormalities.

Young men, however, have longer urethras and far fewer lower UTIs, and probably should be evaluated urologically after just one episode unless they have a risk factor such as an uncircumcised foreskin, HIV infection, or homosexual activity, and respond successfully to initial treatment. In sexually active men, consider urethritis or prostatitis as the etiology. In men over 50 years of age, there is a rapid increase in UTI due to prostate hypertrophy, obstruction, and instrumentation.

SUGGESTED READINGS

Stamm WE, Hooton TM: Management of urinary tract infections in adults, *N Engl J Med* 329:1328-1334, 1993.
Valenstein PN, Koepke JA: Unnecessary microscopy in routine urinalysis, *Am J Clin Pathol* 82:444-448, 1984.

84

Urinary Tract Infection, Upper (Pyelonephritis)

Presentation

The patient has some combination of urinary frequency, urgency, dysuria, malaise, flank pain, nausea, vomiting, fever, and chills that have been progressive over several days. On physical examination, the patient is febrile, ill-appearing, and tachycardic. There is tenderness elicited by percussing the costovertebral angle over the kidneys and mild-to-moderate lateral abdominal and suprapubic tenderness. The urinalysis may help establish the diagnosis with pyuria, bacteriuria, and tubular casts of white cells.

What To Do:

✔ Examine the urine using a Gram's stain for the presence of gram-positive cocci (presumptively enterococci) or the more usual gram-negative rods, and send for culture and sensitivity.

✔ If the patient appears toxic, with a high fever or white count, nausea or vomiting (preventing adequate oral medication and hydration), or if the patient is pregnant or there is any sign of urinary obstruction or developing sepsis, she should be admitted to the hospital for IV antibiotics.

✔ **For stable, otherwise healthy patients, start with a first dose of IV antibiotics in the emergency department (ampicillin 1000 mg plus gentamicin 80 mg, ceftriaxone 1000 to 2000 mg, ofloxacin 200 to 400 mg, or ciprofloxacin 200 to 400 mg), then discharge home on oral hydration and 2 weeks of oral antibiotics (trimethoprim 160 mg plus sulfamethoxazole 800 mg bid, ciprofloxacin 500 mg bid, norfloxacin 400 mg bid, or ofloxacin 400 mg bid × 14 days).**

✔ Instruct the patient to return for reevaluation in 24 to 48 hours and sooner if symptoms worsen. Most patients improve on this regimen, but the others will require hospital admission if they do not improve in 2 days.

What Not To Do:

✗ Do not routinely obtain blood cultures, which are of little value in uncomplicated cases.

✗ Do not forget a pregnancy test in women of childbearing age, and do not give amino-glycosides or fluoroquinolones in pregnancy.

✗ Do not lose the patient to follow-up. Although lower urinary tract infections (UTIs) often resolve without treatment, upper UTIs inadequately treated can lead to renal damage or sepsis.

✗ Do not miss a diagnosis of pyelonephritis in the absence of fever when other signs and symptoms are present.

✗ Do not miss an infection above a ureteral stone or obstruction. Crampy, colicky pain or hematuria with the symptoms above calls for sonography or an excretory urogram (IVP). Antibiotics and hydration alone may not cure an infected obstruction.

DISCUSSION

Although oral antibiotics are usually sufficient treatment for upper UTIs, there is a significant incidence of renal damage and sepsis as sequelae, mandating good follow-up or admission when necessary. By the same token, lower UTIs can ascend into upper UTIs, or it can be difficult to decide the level of a given UTI, in which case it should be treated as an upper UTI.

Studies have shown that a 14-day course of oral therapy is highly effective for the woman with clinical evidence of pyelonephritis without sepsis, nausea, or vomiting. Quinolones such as ofloxacin (Floxin), ciprofloxacin (Cipro), and norfloxacin (Noroxin) are highly effective and probably the drugs of choice in this setting, except for pregnant women, for whom they are contraindicated. Trimethoprim-sulfamethoxazole (Bactrim, Septra) could also be used, although resistance of 5% to 15% of pathogens may be a more important factor in the selection of therapy for pyelonephritis than for cystitis.

SUGGESTED READINGS

Pinson AG, Philbrick JT, Lindbeck GH, et al: ED management of acute pyelonephritis in women: a cohort study, *Am J Emerg Med* 12:271-278, 1994.

Pinson AG, Philbrick JT, Lindbeck GH, et al: Fever in the clinical diagnosis of acute pyelonephritis, *Am J Emerg Med* 15:148-151, 1997.

Thanassi M: Utility of urine and blood cultures in pyelonephritis, *Acad Emerg Med* 4:797-800, 1997.

Gynecologic Emergencies

85 Bartholin Abscess

Presentation

A woman complains of vulvar pain and swelling that has developed over the past 2 to 3 days, making walking and sitting very uncomfortable. On physical examination in the lithotomy position, there is a unilateral (occasionally bilateral), tender, fluctuant, erythematous swelling at 5 or 7 o'clock within the posterior labium minus (Figure 85-1).

What To Do:

✔ **If the swelling is mild without fluctuance (bartholinitis) or if the abscess is not pointing, the patient can be placed on antibiotics like ciprofloxacin (Cipro) 500 mg plus azithromycin (Zithromax) 1000 mg PO once, or ceftri-axone (Rocephin) 125 mg IM once plus doxycycline (Vibramycin) 100 mg PO bid for 7 days,** and instructed to take warm sitz baths. Early follow-up should be provided.

✔ **When the abscess is pointing, an incision should be made over the medial bulging mucosal surface with a #15 scalpel blade and the pus evacuated.**

✔ **After drainage, a Word catheter should be inserted through the incision. Inflate the tip of the catheter with sterile water to hold it in place and prevent premature closure of the opening** (Figure 85-2).

✔ **After drainage, the patient should be placed on antibiotics as above and instructed to take sitz baths.**

✔ Provide for a follow-up examination within 48 hours.

What Not To Do:

✘ Do not mistake a nontender Bartholin duct cyst, which does not require immediate treatment, for an inflamed abscess.

✘ Do not mistake a more posterior perirectal abscess for a Bartholin abscess. The perirectal abscess requires a different treatment approach.

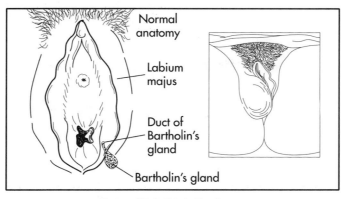

Figure 85-1 Bartholin abscess.

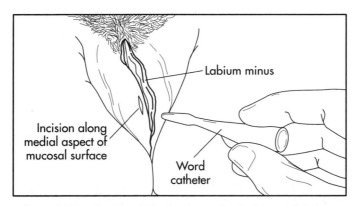

Figure 85-2 Insertion of Word catheter after incision and drainage.

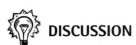 **DISCUSSION**

The most common organisms involved in the development of a Bartholin abscess are gonococci, streptococci, *Escherichia coli*, Proteus, and Chlamydia, and often more than one organism is present. Bilateral infections are more commonly characteristic of gonorrhea.

The Word catheter is an inflatable latex balloon on the tip of a 1-inch single-barreled catheter designed to retain itself in the abscess cavity for 4 to 6 weeks to help ensure the development of a wide marsupialized opening for continued drainage. It seldom stays in place that long. Iodoform or plain ribbon gauze can be inserted into the incised abscess as a substitute. If a wide opening persists, recurrent infections are not likely to occur, but they are common if the stoma closes.

86

Contact
Vulvovaginitis

Presentation

Patients complain of vulvar itching and swelling. Occasionally there will be tenderness, pain, burning, and dysuria severe enough to cause urinary retention. The vulvovaginal area is inflamed, erythematous, and edematous. In more severe cases there may be vesiculation and ulceration, and in cases where there is a chronic contact dermatitis there may be lichenification, scaling, and skin thickening.

What To Do:

✔ **Try to identify an offending agent and have the patient stop using it. Most reactions are caused by agents that the patient unknowingly applies or uses for hygienic or therapeutic purposes.** Chemically scented douches, soaps, bubble baths, deodorants, and perfumes, as well as dyed or scented toilet paper, dyed underwear, scented tampons or pads, and feminine hygiene products are the most common causative agents. Less commonly, plant allergens such as poison oak or poison ivy may be inadvertently applied and trigger the reaction.

✔ Rule out an alternate cause of vulvar puritus such as pinworms (see Chapter 65) or *Trichomonas* organisms (see Chapter 93). *Candida albicans* may also be the cause of pruritus, but it may present as an overgrowth when contact vulvovaginitis is the primary problem.

✔ **Instruct the patient in the use of cool baths and wet compresses using boric acid or Burow's solution (Domboro).**

✔ **Prescribe liberal amounts of topical corticosteroids like fluocinolone (Synalar cream 0.025%) or triamcinolone (Aristocort A 0.025% cream) bid to qid (dispense 15 g).**

✔ In more severe cases, also prescribe oral steroids in a tapering dose-pack schedule like prednisone (Sterapred DS or Sterapred DS 12 day) or methylprednisolone (Medrol Dosepack 8 mg) for 6 days of systemic therapy.

What Not To Do:

✗ Do not have the patient use hot baths or compresses. This will usually exacerbate the burning and pruritus.

✗ Do not prescribe antihistamines. They are relatively ineffective in treating contact vulvitis and may increase discomfort by drying the vaginal mucosa.

 DISCUSSION

The major problem with managing contact vulvovaginitis is identifying the primary irritant or allergen. In many cases, more than one substance is involved or potentially involved and may be totally unsuspected by the patient (such as the use of scented toilet paper). For this reason, a thorough investigative history is very important.

87

Dysmenorrhea (Menstrual Cramps)

Presentation

A young woman complains of crampy, labor-like pains that began before the visible bleeding of her menstrual period. The pain is focused in the lower abdomen, low back, suprapubic area, or thighs, and may be associated with nausea, vomiting, increased defecation, headache, muscular cramps, and passage of clots. The pain is most severe on the first day of the menses, and may last from several hours to several days. Often, this is a recurrent problem, dating back to the first year after menarche. Rectal, vaginal, and pelvic examination disclose no abnormalities.

What To Do:

✔ Ask about the duration of symptoms and onset of similar episodes (onset of dysmenorrhea after menarche suggests other pelvic pathology). Ask about appetite, diarrhea, dysuria, dyspareunia, and other symptoms suggestive of other pelvic pathology.

✔ Perform a thorough abdominal and speculum and bimanual pelvic examination, looking for signs of infection, pregnancy, or uterine or adnexal disease.

✔ **Confirm that the patient is not pregnant with a urine pregnancy test (or serum beta hCG if available).**

✔ **For uncomplicated dysmenorrhea, try NSAIDs such as ibuprofen (Motrin) 600 to 800 mg, or naproxen (Naprosyn) 500 mg PO initially, tapering to maintenance doses (half the loading dose q6h).**

✔ Arrange for work up of endometriosis or other underlying causes, and suggest aspirin or oral contraceptives for prophylaxis.

What Not To Do:

✘ Do not treat acute dysmenorrhea with aspirin alone. Aspirin begun 3 days before the period, 650 mg qid, is effective prophylaxis, but it is not as good after the onset of symptoms.

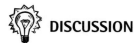 **DISCUSSION**

Menstrual cramps affect more than half of all menstruating women, with 10% to 15% suffering enough pain to miss work, school, or home activities. It is most common during the late teens and twenties. Overproduction of prostaglandins E and F in menstrual blood appears to stimulate uterine contractions, and thus many of the symptoms of dysmenorrhea.

88

Foreign Body, Vaginal

Presentation

This usually is a problem of children, who may insert a foreign body and not tell their parents, or may be the victims of child abuse. The patient is finally brought to the emergency department with a foul-smelling purulent discharge with or without vaginal bleeding. Vaginal foreign bodies in the adult may be a result of a psychiatric disorder or unusual sexual practices. Occasionally a tampon or pessary is forgotten or lost and causes discomfort and a vaginal discharge.

What To Do:

✔ **Visualize the foreign body using a nasal speculum in the pediatric patient or a vaginal speculum in the adult. Consider using conscious sedation in a child or frightened adult.**

✔ **Pediatric patients may be placed in the knee-chest position and, while performing a rectal examination, the foreign body may be expelled from the vagina by pushing it with the examining finger in the rectum.**

✔ **Friable foreign bodies such as wads of toilet paper may be flushed out using warm water, an infant feeding tube, and a standard syringe.**

✔ **Lost or forgotten tampons can be removed with vaginal forceps** that are first pierced through the finger of a latex glove, so that when the malodorous foreign body is extracted, the glove can immediately be pulled over it to reduce the odor before it is discarded in a sealed plastic bag. **The vagina should then be swabbed with a Betadine solution.**

✔ In difficult cases, or when large or sharp objects are involved, young and adult patients may require general anesthesia to allow removal under direct vision. When general anesthesia is not required, conscious sedation should be considered.

✔ The patient should empty her bladder and lie in stirrups in the lithotomy position. **Insert a Foley catheter to break any suction between the foreign body and the vaginal mucosa. Most objects can then be grasped with ring forceps, a tenaculum, or the plaster and tongue blade method** (see Chapter 68).

✔ Reserve x-rays for radio-opaque foreign bodies concealed in the bladder or urethra. Objects in the vagina are usually apparent on examination.

What Not To Do:

✘ Do not ignore a vaginal discharge in a pediatric patient or assume it is the result of a benign vaginitis. Perform a bimanual or rectoabdominal examination to palpate a hard object and then do a gentle speculum examination to look for a foreign body or signs of vaginal trauma.

✘ Do not forget to ask about possible sexual abuse and consult with protective services if it cannot be ruled out.

 DISCUSSION

Vaginal foreign body removal is generally not a problem, but when large objects make removal more difficult, use the additional techniques described for rectal foreign bodies (see Chapter 68).

89

Genital Warts
(Condylomata acuminata)

Presentation

Patients complain of perineal itching, burning, pain, and tenderness or they may be asymptomatic, especially with cervical and vaginal involvement, but noticed distinctive fleshy warts of the external genitalia or anus. Lesions are pedunculated or broad based with pink to gray soft excrescences, occurring in clusters or individually.

What To Do:

✔ External warts seldom require biopsy for diagnosis. The differential diagnosis of anogenital warts includes molluscum cantagiosum, verruca vulgaris (common nongenital wart), secondary syphilis (condyloma lata), hypertrophic vulvar dystrophies, and vulvar intraepithelial and invasive neoplasias. Consider atypical, pigmented, intravaginal, cervical, and persistent warts for referral for gynecologic evaluation. Recognition of cervical lesions may require colposcopy.

✔ **Prescribe imiquimod (Aldara) cream 5%, 12 single-use packets. Have the patient apply a thin layer of cream to external genital and perianal warts, rubbed in until the cream is no longer visible, with hand washing before and after cream application. This should be repeated 3 times per week, prior to normal sleeping hours, and left on the skin for 6 to 10 hours before being washed off. This should continue until there is total clearing of the warts or for a maximum of 16 weeks.**

✔ **An alternative for self-treatment is to prescribe podofilox 0.5% solution (Condylox) 3.5 ml. Patients may apply podofilox with a cotton swab to warts twice daily for 3 days, followed by 4 days of no treatment.** The patient should be careful to avoid surrounding normal tissue. **This cycle may be repeated as necessary for a total of 4 cycles.** Total wart area treated should not exceed ten square centimeters, and total volume of podofilox should not exceed 0.5 ml per day. If possible, apply the initial treatment to demonstrate the proper application technique and identify which warts should be treated.

✔ **Alternatively, apply 25% podophyllin in tincture of benzoin (Podocon–25) 15 ml using the above application technique** and with the same dosage restrictions. **Have the patient thoroughly wash off in 1 to 4 hours.** This may be repeated weekly if necessary, but if warts persist after six applications the patient should be referred for alternative therapy.

✔ If the patient is pregnant, has severe involvement, or has profuse anal or rectal warts, she should be referred for cryotherapy, application of trichloroacetic acid, ablation with carbon dioxide laser, electrocautery, or surgical extirpation.

✔ **If the patient's male partner also has visible lesions, he can be treated using the same regimens.**

✔ Counsel both about the unpredictable natural history of the disease and the possible increased risk of lower genital tract malignancy. Infected women should have an annual Pap smear.

What Not To Do:

✘ Do not use podofilox or podophyllin during pregnancy. There have been a few cases of toxicity reported when large amounts of podophyllin have been used.

✘ Do not mistake "pearly penile papules" for warts. These dome–shaped or hairlike projections around the corona of the glans penis are normal variants in up to 10% of men.

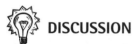

DISCUSSION

Genital warts are a result of infection with human papillomavirus (HPV). The virus is currently considered a leading candidate as a causative agent in squamous carcinomas of both the female and male genital tracts. The sexual transmission of HPV is well documented, with the highest prevalence in young, sexually active adolescents and adults. HPV types 6 and 11 are the most prevalent types associated with condyloma acuminata and are not considered to have the malignant potential of types 16, 18, and others. HPV frequently coexists with other sexually transmitted diseases. HPV lesions are difficult to eradicate, with a very high recurrence rate, and there is still no definitive therapy.

90

"Morning After" Contraception

Presentation

A woman had unprotected sexual intercourse in the last 24 hours and wants to prevent an unplanned pregnancy. This may be part of the prophylactic treatment of a rape victim.

What To Do:

✔ **Obtain a serum pregnancy test. If the test is already positive, the following measures will not be sufficient and will harm the fetus.**

✔ **Prescribe a contraceptive in large doses for a short time to prevent implantation. Expect some nausea. Examples include one of the following:**
- Emergency Contraceptive Kit (Preven Kit) contains four pills of levonorgestrel and ethinyl estradiol, along with a patient information book and urine pregnancy test
- Norgestrel and ethinyl estradiol (Ovral) PO two now and two in 12 hours
- Four pills now and four in 12 hours of lower dose contraceptives like Levlen, Lo/Ovral, Nordette, Tri-Levlen, or Triphasil
- Diethylstilbestrol 25 mg PO bid for 5 days
- Conjugated estrogen (Premarin) 30 mg PO qd for 5 days
- Conjugated estrogen (Premarin) 50 mg IV (slow push) qd for 2 days

✔ **Ask about exposure to sexually transmitted diseases, which might require separate testing and prophylaxis.**

✔ **Arrange for follow-up if this treatment fails to prevent pregnancy.**

What Not To Do:

✘ Do not use this emergency rescue technique as a substitute for condoms, which also help prevent sexually transmitted infections.

SUGGESTED READINGS

Association of Reproductive Health Professionals hotline (800) 584-9911.

Ovral as a morning after contraceptive, *Med Letter Drugs Ther* 31:93, 1989.

Trussell J, Ellertson C, Rodriguez G: The Yuzpe regimen of emergency contraception: how long after the morning after? *Obstet Gynecol* 88:150-154, 1966.

91 Pelvic Inflammatory Disease

Presentation

A woman 15 to 30 years of age, possibly with a new sex partner, complains of lower abdominal pain. There may be associated vaginal discharge, malodor, dysuria, dyspareunia, menorrhagia, or intermenstrual bleeding. Patients with more severe infections may develop fever, chills, malaise, nausea, and vomiting. Women with severe pelvic pain tend to walk slightly bent over, holding their lower abdomen, and shuffling their feet. Abdominal examination reveals lower quadrant tenderness, sometimes with rebound, and occasionally there will be right upper quadrant tenderness due to gonococcal perihepatitis (Fitz-Hugh–Curtis syndrome). Pelvic examination demonstrates bilateral adnexal tenderness as well a uterine fundal and cervical motion tenderness. Many women with pelvic inflammatory disease (PID) exhibit subtle or mild symptoms with absence of fever, cervical motion tenderness, adnexal tenderness, and leukocytosis.

What To Do:

✔ **Always perform a pelvic examination on women with lower abdominal complaints or lower abdominal tenderness.** The examination should be thorough, yet performed as gently and briefly as possible to avoid exacerbating a very painful condition. **When pain is intolerable, provide IV narcotic analgesia.**

✔ **Obtain endocervical cultures for *Neisseria gonorrhoeae* and *Chlamydia trachomatis.***

✔ **Obtain blood for syphilis serology and recommend HIV testing.**

✔ **Obtain urine for urinalysis and blood or urine for pregnancy testing.**

✔ Consider obtaining a leukocyte count, sedimentation rate, and C-reactive protein. These are indicators of clinical severity, but normal results do not rule out PID.

✔ **Determine pH of any vaginal discharge and make wet mount examinations and Gram's stains of endocervical secretions,** looking for *Candida* organisms, *Trichomonas* organisms, clue cells, and any gram-negative diplococci inside polymorphonuclear neutrophils (almost diagnostic of gonorrhea).

✔ **Perform pelvic ultrasound if there is a suspected mass, severe pain, or a positive pregnancy test.**

✔ Because no laboratory tests are diagnostic for PID, and the clinical diagnosis is also non-specific, **assume a diagnosis when there are lower abdominal pain with tenderness on examination, bilateral adnexal tenderness, and cervical motion tenderness plus one of the following: temperature ≥38° C (100.4° F), leukocytosis 10,500 WBC/mm³, inflammatory mass on pelvic examination or ultrasound, elevated C-reactive protein, erythrocyte sedimentation rate ≥15 mm/h, or evidence of gonorrhea or chlamydia in the endocervix** (by positive antigen test, Gram's stain, or mucopurulent cervicitis). **Subtle findings may only include a history of abnormal uterine bleeding, dyspareunia, vaginal discharge, or cervical purulence. When in doubt, always treat.**

✔ **Remove any intrauterine device (IUD).**

✔ **Treat suspected cases while awaiting diagnostic confirmation.**

✔ Hospitalize adolescents with salpingitis and all patients with pelvic or tubo-ovarian abscess, pregnancy, fever 38.5° C, nausea and vomiting that preclude oral antibiotics, current use of an IUD, septicemia or other serious disease, high risk of poor compliance, failed follow-up, and failure on 48 hours of the outpatient therapy below. Inpatient treatment consists of IV antibiotics continued for at least 48 hours after the patient demonstrates significant clinical improvement.

✔ **Treat mild-to-moderate cases as outpatients with one dose of ceftriaxone (Rocephin) 250 mg IM, followed by a prescription for doxycycline (Vibramycin) 100 mg bid for 14 days.** For more severe cases with a high probability of resistant anaerobic infection, add metronidazole (Flagyl) 500 mg PO bid for 14 days. A completely oral alternative is ofloxacin (Floxin) 400 mg bid × 14 days plus metronidazole 500 mg bid, also for 14 days, or trovafloxacin (Trovan) alone, 200 mg qd for 14 days.

✔ Provide for follow-up examination in 2 to 3 days.

✔ **Provide analgesics as needed.**

✔ Instruct the patient to abstain from sexual intercourse for at least 2 weeks.

✔ Unless sexual acquisition can be excluded with certainty, treat the partner for presumptive gonorrhea and chlamydia with ceftriaxone (Rocephin) 125 mg IM once or ciprofloxacin (Cipro) 500 mg PO once plus doxycycline (Vibramycin) 100 mg PO bid × 7 days or azithromycin (Zithromax) 1000 mg PO once.

✔ Counsel the patient about the sexually transmitted nature of PID and its risks for infertility (15% to 30% per episode) and ectopic pregnancy, which is increased sixfold to tenfold. Barrier methods of contraception (condoms and diaphragms) reduce the risk. Vaginal spermicides are also bactericidal.

What Not To Do:

✗ Do not use ofloxacin or trovafloxacin in pregnant women or patients under 18 years of age.

✗ Do not miss the more unilateral disorders like ectopic pregnancy, appendicitis, ovarian cyst or torsion, and diverticulitis. Early consultation by both general surgeon and obstetrician/gynecologist is sometimes necessary.

✘ Do not diagnose PID in a patient with a positive pregnancy test without ruling out ectopic pregnancy, usually with a sonogram.

✘ Do not ignore pelvic symptoms if the patient has gonococcal perihepatic inflammation.

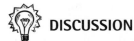 **DISCUSSION**

PID is defined as salpingitis, often accompanied by endometritis or secondary pelvic peritonitis, which results from an ascending genital infection. Prompt diagnosis and early, presumptive treatment are crucial to maintaining fertility. There is an increased risk for PID in sexually active adolescents compared with women over 20 years of age. There is also increased risk with multiple sex partners, use of an IUD, previous history of PID, and vaginal douching. The incubation period for PID varies from 1 to 2 days to weeks or months.

Infection with *N. gonorrhoeae* and *C. trachomatis* is more common within the first 1 or 2 weeks after the onset of menstruation. One half of women with a sexually transmitted microorganism will also harbor a concomitant organism from the vaginal flora. *Haemophilus influenzae*, enteric gram-negative rods, and group B streptococci are also involved.

Laparoscopy is indicated in severe cases, if diagnosis is uncertain, or if there is inadequate response to initial antibiotic therapy. A diagnosis of PID in children or young adolescents should prompt an evaluation for possible child abuse.

92

Vaginal Bleeding

Presentation

A menstruating woman complains of greater-than-usual bleeding, which is either off of her usual schedule (metrorrhagia), lasts longer than a typical period, or is heavier than usual (menorrhagia), perhaps with crampy pains and passage of clots.

What To Do:

✔ Obtain orthostatic pulse and blood pressure measurements, a complete blood count, and pregnancy test (urine or serum beta hCG). Although less reliable than hemoglobin and hematocrit, try to quantify the amount of bleeding by the presence of clots and the number of saturated pads used.

✔ If there is significant bleeding, demonstrated by pallor, lightheadedness, tachycardia, orthostatic pressure changes, a pulse increase of more than 20 per minute on standing, or a hematocrit below 30%, start an IV line of lactated Ringer's solution and have blood ready to transfuse on short notice.

✔ **Obtain a menstrual, sexual, and reproductive history.** Are her periods usually irregular, occasionally this heavy? **Does she take oral contraceptive pills, and has she missed enough to produce estrogen-withdrawal bleeding?** Is an IUD in place and contributing to cramps, bleeding, and infection? Was her last period missed or light, or is this period late, suggesting an anovulatory cycle, a spontaneous abortion, or an ectopic pregnancy? Ask about bruising, petechiae, or other signs suggestive of a coagulopathy. Ask about use of anticoagulants like aspirin or Coumadin. Ask about any history of thyroid, renal, or hepatic disease.

✔ **Perform a speculum and bimanual vaginal examination,** looking particularly for signs of pregnancy, such as a soft, blue cervix, enlarged uterus, or passage of fetal parts with the blood. **Ascertain that the blood is coming from the cervical os, and not from a laceration, polyp, cervical lesion, or other vaginal or uterine pathology or infection.** Feel for adnexal masses, as well as pelvic fluid or tenderness. Spread any questionable products of conception on gauze or suspend in saline to differentiate from organized clot. **Press ring forceps against the cervix to see whether they enter the uterus indicating that the internal os is open** (indicating an inevitable, complete, or

243

incomplete abortion) or closed (not pregnant or a threatened abortion, the fetus having roughly even odds of survival, and is generally treated with bedrest alone).

✔ **If the hCG is elevated, obtain a transvaginal or abdominal ultrasound.** For an intrauterine pregnancy, the sonogram will help assess the age and viability of the fetus. An ectopic gestational sac may be seen. A sonogram showing an empty uterus, despite a positive pregnancy test, is consistent with either an ectopic pregnancy or a recent complete abortion.

✔ **With incomplete abortions, deliver any products of conception that protrude from the cervical os using steady gentle traction with sponge forceps while massaging the uterus. If bleeding continues, start an IV infusion of oxytocin (Pitocin) 20 mU/min to diminish the rate of hemorrhage.** Obtain gynecologic consultation. **After all spontaneous abortions, test the mother's Rh status and, if negative, administer Rh immunoglobulin (RhoGAM) 50 μg IM if the uterus was less than 12 weeks size, 300 μg IM if larger.**

✔ **The stable patient with a threatened abortion may be sent home unless there is severe pain or hemorrhage.** Bedrest has not been shown to improve the outcome for a threatened abortion but is still usually part of the regimen.

✔ **When the patient is hemodynamically stable and any anatomic lesions, systemic disease, infection, and pregnancy have been ruled out, begin treatment for dysfunctional uterine bleeding. Patients with moderate hemorrhage can be started on oral contraceptive pills like Ortho-Novum 1/50 or Norinyl 1 + 50, administered at a dose of two to four pills a day for 3 to 5 days until the bleeding stops, and then decreased to one pill a day until the month's pack is completed.** For more severe hemorrhage, conjugated estrogen (Premarin) 25 mg can be given intravenously every 4 to 6 hours until the bleeding slows, to a maximum of four doses. Add prochlorperazine (Compazine) to control nausea. Begin a high dose combination of estrogen and synthetic progestin (Provera 5 mg qid) at the same time, later reduced to qd for 21 days, and stopped to allow a controlled withdrawal bleed.

✔ **Simple menorrhagia and mild dysfunctional uterine bleeding can be treated with standard regimens of oral contraceptives plus NSAIDs given on the first day of the menstrual period.**

✔ **If the cause of the uterine bleeding was missed oral contraceptive pills, the patient may resume the pills but should use additional contraception for the first cycle to prevent pregnancy.** If the cause is a new IUD, the patient may elect to have it removed and use another contraceptive technique.

✔ In most cases, the patient should be referred for follow-up to a gynecologist for definitive diagnosis, adjustment of medications, or further treatment. She may be evaluated via hysteroscopy, ultrasound, and endometrial biopsy. A dilation and curettage may stop bleeding from polyps, submucous leiomyomas, and retained products of conception.

What Not To Do:

✘ Do not leap to a diagnosis of dysfunctional uterine bleeding without ruling out pregnancy.

✘ Do not rule out pregnancy or venereal infection on the basis of a negative sexual history—confirm with physical examination and laboratory tests.

✘ Do not give aspirin for menorrhagia. It is not effective and may increase bleeding.

 DISCUSSION

The patient's age should direct you to the most likely etiology of her vaginal bleeding. In prepubertal girls, look for anatomic lesions, rectal fissures, trauma, or foreign bodies, and consider abuse. In postmenarchal adolescents and women of reproductive age, consider pregnancy-related problems first, then dysfunctional uterine bleeding (anovulatory cycles), infection with sexually transmitted diseases, anatomic lesions (fibroids, cervical polyps), and systemic illnesses (hypothyroidism, bleeding disorders). In perimenopausal and postmenopausal women, strongly consider the possibility of malignant disease and then evaluate for anovulatory dysfunctional uterine bleeding, liver disease, anticoagulation therapy, and bleeding disorders.

Dysfunctional uterine bleeding is a diagnosis of exclusion. It is usually hormonal in etiology and can be the result of abnormal endogenous hormone production or the result of problems with the administration of prescribed synthetic sex hormones like oral contraceptive pills. During an anovulatory cycle, there is no progesterone, which results in a chaotic estrogen-stimulated endometrial proliferation. The uterine lining therefore hypertrophies and sloughs erratically, resulting in excessive or irregular uterine bleeding. This occurs most commonly around the time of menarche in girls and menopause in women. Other causes include a severely restricted diet, prolonged exercise, and significant emotional stress. Breakthrough bleeding is a form of estrogen withdrawal while taking low estrogen dose oral contraceptives. Changing to a higher dose pill will generally eliminate this problem. Also consider drug interactions with certain anticonvulsants and antibiotics.

The essential steps in the emergency evaluation of vaginal bleeding are fluid resuscitation of shock, if present, and recognition of any anatomic lesion, infection, or pregnancy, and its complications of spontaneous abortion or ectopic pregnancy. Treatment of the more chronic and less severe dysfunctional uterine bleeding usually consists of iron replacement and optional use of oral contraceptives to decrease menstrual irregularity (metrorrhagia) and volume (menorrhagia).

Progesterone 100 mg IM or medroxyprogesterone (Provera) 10 mg PO qd × 10 days can also be given to stop dysfunctional uterine bleeding by creating a pharmacologic curettage. Warn the patient that after the initial reduction of bleeding, there will be an increase in hemorrhage when the uterine lining is sloughed.

SUGGESTED READINGS

Falcone T, Desjardins C, Bourque J, et al: Dysfunctional uterine bleeding in adolescents, *J Reprod Med* 39:761-764, 1994.

93 Vaginitis

Presentation

A woman complains of itching and irritation of the labia and vagina, vaginal discharge or odor, external dysuria, vague low abdominal discomfort, or dyspareunia. (Suprapubic discomfort, internal dysuria, and urinary urgency and frequency suggest cystitis.) Abdominal examination is benign, but examination of the introitus may reveal erythema of the vulva and edema of the labia (especially with *Candida* organisms). Speculum examination may disclose a diffusely red, inflamed vaginal mucosa with vaginal discharge. A thin, homogenous, gray-to-white discharge adhering to the vaginal wall is characteristic of bacterial vaginosis (previously called anaerobic or *Gardnerella vaginalis* overgrowth). Profuse, frothy, greenish discharge is characteristic of *Trichomonas* organisms. Vulvar pruritus and a thick white discharge resembling cottage cheese are due to *Candida* organisms. Bimanual examination should show a nontender cervix and uterus, without adnexal tenderness or masses or pain on cervical motion.

What To Do:

✔ Take a brief sexual history. Ask if partners are experiencing related symptoms.

✔ **Perform speculum and bimanual pelvic examination. Collect urine for possible culture and pregnancy tests that may influence treatment. Swab the cervix or urethra to culture for *Neisseria gonorrhoeae* and swab the endocervix to test for Chlamydia. Touch pH indicator paper** (Hydrion pH papers, ColorpHast pH Test Strips) **to the vaginal mucus. A pH >4.5 suggests bacterial vaginosis or *Trichomonas* organisms, but this is only useful if there is no blood or semen to buffer vaginal secretions.**

✔ **Dab a drop of vaginal mucus on a slide, add a drop of 0.9% NaCl and a cover slip, and examine under 400× magnification for swimming protozoa (*Trichomonas vaginalis*), epithelial cells covered by adherent bacilli ("clue cells" of bacterial vaginosis), or pseudohyphae and spores ("spaghetti and meatballs" appearance of *Candida albicans*)** (Figure 93-1).

✔ If epithelial cells obscure the view of yeast, add a drop of 10% KOH, smell whether this liberates the odor of stale fish (characteristic of *Gardnerella* organisms [bacterial vaginosis], *Trichomonas* organisms, and semen), and look again under the microscope.

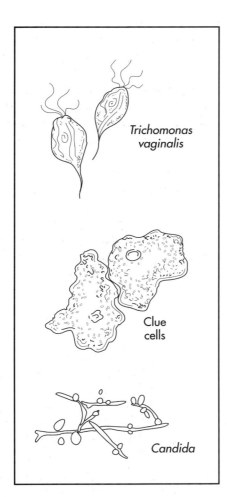

Figure 93-1 Test vaginal mucus on a slide with saline.

✔ **Gram stain a second specimen. This is an even more sensitive method for detecting *Candida* organisms and clue cells (Figure 93-2), as well as a means to assess the general vaginal flora,** which is normally mixed with occasional predominance of gram-positive rods. Many white cells and an overabundance of pleomorphic gram-negative rods suggest *Gardnerella* organisms infection. **Gram-negative diplococci inside white cells suggest gonorrhea.**

✔ **If *Trichomonas vaginalis* is the etiology, discuss with the patient the options of metronidazole (Flagyl) 500 mg bid × 7 days, or 2000 mg once.** The latter has practically as good a cure rate, obviously better compliance, and shortens the time the patient must abstain from alcohol—24 hours after the last dose because of metronidazole's disulfiram-like activity. **A 1500 mg single dose of metronidazole has been shown to be as effective as the recommended 2000 mg dose** and may reduce the frequency of side effects. **Sexual partners must receive the same treatment,** and

247

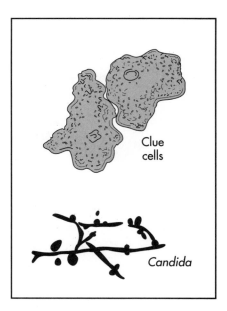

Figure 93-2 Gram's stain is an even more sensitive method of testing for *Candida* organisms and clue cells.

advise the patient and her partner to refrain from intercourse or to use a condom until cure has been confirmed at follow-up. In the first trimester of pregnancy, substitute intravaginal clotrimazole 100 mg vaginal suppository qhs × 14 days, which is less effective, but safer than metronidazole vaginal gel. **Metronidazole is contraindicated in the first trimester of pregnancy and controversial thereafter.** Treatment of asymptomatic pregnant patients can be delayed until after delivery.

✔ **If *Candida albicans* is the etiology, recommend miconazole (Monistat) or clotrimazole (Gyne-Lotrimin) 200 mg vaginal suppositories to be inserted qhs × 3 days. These treatments are available without prescription.** Prescription alternatives for recurrences that are active against fungi other than *Candida* organisms are butoconazole (Femstat) and terconazole (Terazol) one 5-gram applicator of cream qhs for 3 days and 7 days, respectively. Use of cream also allows its soothing application on irritated mucosa. **For convenience, prescription clotrimazole (Mycelex-G) 500 mg vaginal tablet only needs to be used once, but may be less effective. A single oral dose of fluconazole (Diflucan) 150 mg PO is at least as effective as intravaginal treatment of vulvovaginal candidiasis, and many patients seem to prefer it.** Fluconazole may be repeated up to once a month for recurrent infection. Gastrointestinal side effects are fairly common, and serious side effects can occur. In pregnancy, halve the dose and double the course of topical clotrimazole. Sex partners need not be treated unless they have balanitis.

✔ **If the diagnosis is bacterial vaginosis, the strongest treatment is metronidazole (Flagyl) 500 mg bid or clindamycin (Cleocin) 300 mg bid × 7 days.** For intravaginal treatment, use metronidazole 0.75% vaginal gel (MetroGel-Vaginal) one applicator intravaginally bid for 5 days or clindamycin 2% vaginal cream (Cleocin), one 5-gram applicator intravaginally qhs for 7 days. **Intravaginal treatment is more expensive** but carries fewer gastrointestinal side effects than the oral form, and some patients prefer using intravaginal products for treating this vaginosis. Metronidazole cannot be used during the first trimester of pregnancy, but clindamycin can. Sex partners need not be treated unless they have balanitis.

✔ To prevent rebound *Candida albicans* after antibiotics reduce the normal vaginal flora, or for treatment of mild vaginitis, consider douching with 1% acetic acid (half-strength vinegar) to maintain a normal low pH vaginal ecology.

✔ **Remember that any given patient may harbor more than one infection.**

✔ **Arrange for follow-up and instruct the patient in prevention of vaginitis.** She should avoid routine douching, perfumed soaps and feminine hygiene sprays, and tight, poorly ventilated clothing.

What Not To Do:

✘ Do not prescribe sulfa creams for nonspecific vaginitis. The treatments above are more effective.

✘ Do not miss underlying pelvic inflammatory disease, pregnancy, or diabetes, all of which can potentiate vaginitis.

✘ Do not miss candidiasis because the vaginal secretions appear essentially normal in consistency, color, volume, and odor. Nonpregnant patients may not develop thrush patches, curds, or caseous discharge.

✘ Do not treat sexual partners of patients with bacterial vaginosis or *Candida albicans* unless they show signs of infection or have been causing recurrent infections.

 DISCUSSION

Both *Candida albicans* and *Gardnerella vaginalis* (previously known as *Haemophilus vaginalis* or *Corynebacterium vaginale* and now referred to as bacterial vaginosis), are part of the normal vaginal flora. A number of anaerobes share the blame in bacterial vaginosis. An alternate therapy uses active-culture yogurt douches to repopulate the vagina with lactobacilli.

Candida albicans is more common in the summer, under tight or nonporous clothing (jeans, synthetic underwear, wet bathing suits), and in users of contraceptives (which alter vaginal mucus), as well as in diabetes mellitus, steroid-induced immunosuppression, HIV infection, and use of broad-spectrum antibiotics.

Trichomonas organisms can be passed back and forth between sexual partners, a cycle that can be broken by treating both partners. *Trichomonas* organisms sometimes produce vague, mild abdominal symptoms.

Ask patients with vulvar pruritus, erythema, and edema, but with otherwise nondiagnostic saline, KOH, and Gram stain microscopy, about the use of hygiene sprays or douches, bubble baths, or scented toilet tissue. Contact vulvovaginitis may result from an allergic or chemical reaction to any one of these or similar products and can be treated by removing the offending substance and prescribing a short course of a topical or systemic corticosteroid (see Chapter 86).

SUGGESTED READINGS

Abbott J: Clinical and microscopic diagnosis of vaginal yeast infection: a prospective analysis, *Ann Emerg Med* 25:587-591, 1995.

Ferris DG, Litaker MS, Woodward L, et al: Treatment of bacterial vaginosis: a comparison of oral metronidazole, metronidazole vaginal gel, and clindamycin vaginal cream, *J Fam Pract* 41:443-449, 1995.

Martin DH, Mroczkowski TF, Dalu ZA, et al: A controlled trial of a single dose of azithromycin for the treatment of chlamydial urethritis and cervicitis, *N Engl J Med* 327:921-925, 1992.

Schwebke JR, Hillier SL, Sobel JD, et al: Validity of the vaginal Gram stain for the diagnosis of bacterial vaginosis, *Obstet Gynecol* 88:573-576, 1996.

Spence MR, Hartwell TS, Davies MC, et al: The minimum single oral metronidazole dose for treating trichomoniasis: a randomized, blinded study, *Obstet Gynecol* 85:699-703, 1997.

Swedberg J, Steiner JF, Deiss F, et al: Comparison of a single-dose vs one-week course of metronidazole for symptomatic bacterial vaginosis, *J Am Med Assoc* 254:1046-1049, 1985.

part

9

Musculoskeletal Emergencies

94

Acromioclavicular (Shoulder) Separation

Presentation

After a direct blow or a fall onto the superior surface of the lateral aspect of the shoulder, with the arm abducted, the patient complains of shoulder pain increased by moderate motion of the arm. The acromioclavicular (AC) joint is tender to palpation (it is superficial and easily palpated). There may be no deformity, or there may be a step-off between the acromion process of the scapula and the distal end of the clavicle, or the distal clavicle may be displaced superiorly and no longer connected to the acromion (roughly corresponding to first-, second-, or third-degree disruption of the AC joint. The patient may come in right away because it hurts even without movement (first- or second-degree tear), or she may come in days later without pain, having noted that the injured shoulder hangs lower or the clavicle rides higher (third degree) (Figure 94–1).

What To Do:

✔ **Provide analgesia as needed, ice compresses for acute injuries, and a sling.**

✔ Palpate the entire shoulder girdle, including the head of the humerus. There should only be tenderness over the AC joint. Gentle passive rotation of the humerus should not cause more pain, but there may be pain on pulling the humerus down towards the feet, distracting the AC joint. Strength may be decreased because of pain, but other bones, joints, range of motion, sensation, and circulation should be documented as being intact.

✔ **X-ray the shoulder** to be sure there is no associated fracture of the lateral clavicle or fracture or dislocation of the humerus. An anteroposterior view of the uninjured shoulder can help determine if the AC joint is widened. **Weight-bearing stress views are uncomfortable and unnecessary.**

✔ **Grade I injuries with a tender but stable AC joint and less than 3 mm widening require only sling immobilization for 10 to 14 days. Grade II injuries, with 3 to 5 mm of subluxation, are treated the same.**

✔ **Grade III injuries, with 5 mm or half the diameter of the clavicle displaced, are a consequence of disruption of the AC and the coracoclavicular ligaments, and call for orthopedic referral in 1 to 2 days. Higher grades, with marked dis-**

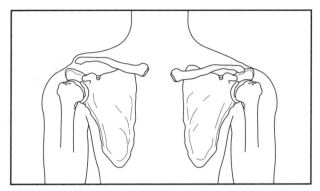

Figure 94-1 Step-off deformity of Grade III injury. *(From Knoop KJ, Stack LB, Storrow AB:* Atlas of Emergency Medicine, *New York, 1997, McGraw-Hill.) (Courtesy of Frank Birinyi, MD.)*

placement of the distal clavicle posteriorly, superiorly, or inferiorly, require immediate orthopedic consultation.

✔ **Prescribe NSAIDs and narcotic analgesics as needed, along with ice compresses for 20 minutes 3 to 4 times daily for 3 days.**

✔ Arrange for reevaluation by an orthopedic surgeon and for physical therapy to begin shoulder range-of-motion exercises within a week.

What Not To Do:

✘ Do not confuse the deformity of a displaced AC ligament tear with a dislocated shoulder, which is accompanied by loss of the normal deltoid convexity and inability to rotate the shoulder internally and externally at the side.

✘ Do not bother with weight-bearing x-ray views to differentiate separations based on the widening of the distance between the clavicle and scapula. These views are painful and inaccurate.

✘ Do not try to tape or strap the clavicle and scapula back into position. Patients have suffered ischemic necrosis of the skin from overzealous strapping.

✘ Do not allow the patient to wear a sling and immobilize the shoulder for more than a week without at least beginning pendulum exercises. The shoulder capsule will contract and restrict the range of motion.

DISCUSSION

Nearly all patients with grade I and 90% of those with grade II injuries recover fully after 10 to 14 days of simple sling immobilization. The patient should avoid heavy lifting for 8 to 12 weeks and be referred to an orthopedic surgeon for any problems with pain or diminished range of motion.

Continued

DISCUSSION—cont'd

A partial tear of the ligaments between acromion and clavicle produces pain but no widening of the joint (first-degree separation). A second-degree AC separation shows up on x-ray as a widened joint but is otherwise the same on examination and treatment. In a third-degree or complete separation, the ligament from the coracoid process to the clavicle is probably also torn, allowing the collarbone to be pulled superior by the sternocleidomastoid muscle, but often relieving the pain of the stretched AC joint. Long-term shoulder joint stability and strength after a grade III tear remain almost normal, but patients may desire surgical repair to regain the appearance of the normal shoulder or the last few percent of function for athletics.

95 Ankle Sprain

Presentation

Patients usually describe stepping off a curb or into a hole. Sports-related injuries often occur after jumping and landing on another player's foot, which causes an inversion of the ankle. The sensation of a "pop" or "snap" at the time of injury with immediate loss of function suggests disruption of a ligament. Severe swelling in the first hour suggests bleeding from the torn ends. The body's response to the injury begins with inflammation, which produces swelling, warmth, pain, and stiffness that build to a maximum about 1 day after the injury.

Patients usually either arrive immediately after the injury or 1 to 2 days later, complaining of pain, swelling, and partial or complete inability to walk. Patients are usually tender around the lateral malleolus, particularly anteriorly, because the anterior talofibular ligament is the first to tear when the ankle is inverted.

What To Do:

✔ **Get a detailed description of the mechanism of injury, and ask if the patient could bear weight immediately after the injury.** Ask if there have been previous injuries of the ankle. (Patients with a previous ankle injury have an increased risk of recurrence.)

✔ Document the degree and location of swelling and discoloration. Check the sensation and circulation distal to the injury (a slight decrease relative to the uninjured foot might be attributed to the swelling).

✔ **Palpate sites of potential injury: the fibula up to the knee, the base of the fifth metatarsal on the lateral foot, the tarsal navicular bone anteriorly, the deltoid ligament medially, and finally, the anterior talofibular ligament in front of the lateral malleolus. Note if there is tenderness along the posterior distal six centimeters of the lateral malleolus, the posterior medial malleolus, or the tip of either malleolus.** Start palpating gently and away from the injury to overcome the tendency to flinch at the first touch. Save the most likely site of injury for last, because the pain may inhibit any further examination.

✔ **If there is not too much pain, check joint stability with the anterior drawer test** (Figure 95-1) and the talar tilt test. Grasp the tibia with one hand and the heel with the other hand and push the leg posterior while holding the foot still. Anterior

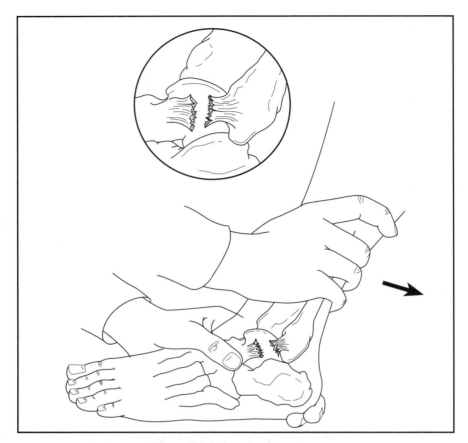

Figure 95-1 Anterior drawer test.

displacement of the talus can be felt or seen as a dimple over the anterolateral ankle compared to the uninjured side. A positive anterior drawer indicates a torn anterior talofibular ligament. The talar tilt test is also performed with the foot in the neutral position. Gently invert the ankle and compare the range of movement and the mushiness of the end point with the uninjured side. An intact calcaneofibular ligament should prevent inversion. Often these tests cannot be accomplished because the ankle is too painful, in which case the tests may be deferred for up to 1 week.

✔ **If there is significant medial ankle injury or severe lateral injury, perform a squeeze test to determine if there is a tear of the syndesmosis between the distal tibia and fibula.** With the knee flexed at 90 degrees, place your hand over the mid portion of the lower leg with your thumb on the fibula and your fingers on the medial tibia. Squeeze the fibula and tibia together. Pain during this test signifies syndesmotic injury, predicts a prolonged recovery, and calls for an orthopedic referral.

✔ **Elevate the foot** (preferably above the level of the heart), **apply an ice pack for 20 minutes, and compress the ankle with a splint or elastic bandage.**

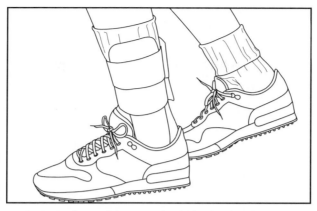

Figure 95-2 Grade I and II sprains should be fitted with a stirrup splint.

✔ **Optional x-rays of the ankle or foot may be ordered to rule out a fracture, but radiographs are not necessary (and likely to be negative) unless there was either: (1) inability to bear weight both immediately and in the initial physical examination, or (2) bony tenderness to palpation of the ankle in the posterior distal six centimeters of the lateral malleolus or the posterior distal medial malleolus, or bony tenderness of the foot at the tarsal navicular or the base of the fifth metatarsal bone.** The use of these decision rules must remain secondary to the judgment and common sense of the clinician. **Be liberal in imaging patients with other distracting painful injuries, altered sensorium, intoxication, paraplegia, or bone disease.** Weight bearing is defined as the ability to transfer weight twice onto each leg, a total of four steps, regardless of limping. Assess ability to bear weight after determining bony tenderness and do not coerce the patient.

✔ **Instruct the patient to elevate and rest the ankle as much as possible and apply ice for three or four periods of 15 to 20 minutes a day for 3 days, insulating the skin from the ice with a towel to prevent frostbite.**

✔ **Patients with mild-to-moderate sprains (grades I to II) should be fitted with a stirrup-type splint** (Figure 95-2) **that prevents inversion and eversion of the ankle, given crutches and instructions how to ambulate with crutches, and prescribed NSAIDs like ibuprofen 200 to 800 mg q6h.** For follow-up, instruct the patient to walk using a stirrup splint as soon as it is tolerable and for the next 4 to 6 weeks and to use crutches for the shortest time possible. These sprains can be referred to a primary care specialist for follow-up in 2 weeks.

✔ Patients with moderate-to-severe sprains (grades II to III) should be placed in a soft, bulky compression dressing. If there is instability or fracture, incorporate a plaster sugar-tong splint (see Figure 95-3) that extends almost the entire length of the tibia and fibula just below the knee. Narcotic analgesics like hydrocodone may be needed for pain relief. Moderate-to-severe sprains, recurrent sprains, sprains with instability or syndesmotic injury, and most injuries with associated fractures should be given an orthope-

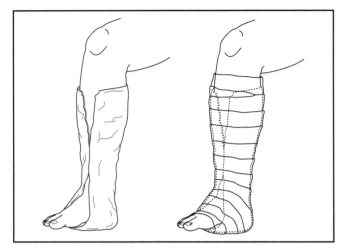

Figure 95-3 Severe sprains and fractures should be treated with a "sugar-tong" splint or Jones dressing.

dic referral within 1 week. Obtain orthopedic consultation in cases of delayed recovery, diagnostic uncertainty, and treatment involving competitive athletes.

✔ Tender or swollen ankle sprains in children with open growth plates are considered to be nondisplaced physeal (Salter I) fractures, even with negative x-rays, and are usually immobilized for 3 to 4 weeks.

✔ **Patients not receiving x-rays at the initial visit should be instructed to seek follow-up if their symptoms have not improved after 1 week.**

What Not To Do:

✘ Do not have the patient apply heat during the recovery phase. It is unnecessary and increases the swelling.

✘ Do not overlook fractures of the anterior process of the calcaneus, tarsal navicular, talar dome or the rest of the talus, or os trigonum, all visible on the ankle x-rays.

✘ Do not completely rule out a fracture based upon a negative x-ray.

 DISCUSSION

Blunt ankle trauma is one of the most common injuries seen in emergency departments and ankle sprains are the most common sports-related orthopedic injury, but less than 15% have clinically significant fractures. The old tradition of radiographic examination of all ankle injuries is no longer required, and the Ottawa decision rules described here have led to reductions of negative x-rays, unnecessary radiation, and waiting times and costs, all without missed fractures or patient dissatisfaction.

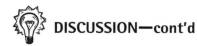

DISCUSSION—cont'd

Mild or grade I sprains usually involve partial tearing of ligament fibers and minimal swelling, with no joint instability. Moderate or grade II sprains are characterized by some pain, edema, ecchymosis, and point tenderness over the involved structures, resulting in partial loss of joint motion. Some ligament fibers may be completely torn, but overall stability of the joint remains intact. Severe or grade III sprains exhibit gross instability with complete tearing of all ligament fibers, marked swelling, and severe pain.

Medial ligament injuries usually result from an eversion stress. Because the deltoid ligament is so strong, it is rarely injured in isolation but rather in association with lateral malleolus fracture.

A minor sprain usually keeps an athlete out of competition for 2 weeks, and a moderate sprain usually keeps an athlete out of competition for 5 weeks. Taping, lace-up braces, and air stirrup orthoses can all be helpful in the rehabilitation of ankle injuries.

SUGGESTED READINGS

Anis AH, Steill IG, Stewart, et al: Cost-effectiveness analysis of the Ottawa ankle rules, *Ann Emerg Med* 26:422-428, 1995.

Auleley GR, Ravaud P, Giraudeau B, et al: Implementation of the Ottawa ankle rules in France: a multicenter randomized controlled trial, *JAMA* 277:1935-1939, 1997.

Chande VT: Decision rules for roentgenography of children with acute ankle injuries, *Arch Pediatr Adolesc Med* 149:255-258, 1995.

Eiff MP, Smith AT, Smith GE: Early mobilization versus immobilization in the treatment of lateral ankle sprains, *Am J Sports Med* 22:83-88, 1994.

Halvorson G, Iserson KV: Comparison of four ankle splint designs, *Ann Emerg Med* 16:1249-1252, 1987.

Lucchesi GM, Jackson RE, Peacock WF, et al: Sensitivity of the Ottawa rules, *Ann Emerg Med* 26:1-5, 1995.

Stiell IG, Greenberg GH, McKnight RD, et al: Decision rules for the use of radiography in acute ankle injuries: refinement and prospective validation, *JAMA* 269:1127-1132, 1993.

Stiell IG, McKnight RD, Greenberg GH, et al: Implementation of the Ottawa ankle rules, *JAMA* 271:827-832, 1994.

vanDijk CN, Lim LS, Bossuyt PM, et al: Physical examination is sufficient for the diagnosis of sprained ankles, *J Bone Joint Surg Br* 78:958-962, 1996.

Boutonnière Finger

Presentation

After jamming the tip of a partially extended finger (resulting in hyperflexion of the proximal interphalangeal [PIP] joint) or with direct trauma over the joint, the patient develops a painful, swollen PIP joint. Tenderness is greatest over the dorsum of the base of the middle phalanx, and there is diminished extensor tendon strength with pain when the middle phalanx is extended against resistance. The classic boutonnière deformity is rarely present in the acute stage of injury.

What To Do:

✔ Obtain a detailed history of the mechanism of injury.

✔ **Perform a complete examination,** palpating for point tenderness of the dorsum of the joint, the collateral ligaments, and the volar plate. Test for joint stability in all directions, test sensation, and check for injuries proximal and distal to the PIP joint.

✔ **Check for a possible tear of the central slip of the extensor digitorum communis tendon. With the patient's PIP joint flexed at 90 degrees over a straight edge (such as a counter top), apply resistance to active extension over the middle phalanx.** If the central slip is disrupted, the patient will not be able to apply pressure against the resistance. It is possible for the patient to extend the injured finger using the lateral bands of the extensor tendon, causing the distal phalanx to hyperextend (Figure 96-1, *A, B,* and *C*).

✔ **Test for collateral ligament stability with varus and valgus stress** (Figure 96-1, *D*).

✔ **If avulsion of the central slip of the extensor tendon is suspected, splint the PIP joint in extension.** The splint should leave the distal interphalangeal (DIP) and metacarpophalangeal joints completely mobile or the collateral ligaments will contract. Active DIP flexion should be encouraged. This action pulls the PIP extensor hood mechanism distally thereby further approximating the two ends of the ruptured central slip. The PIP joint should remain constantly splinted for 8 to 10 weeks and then occasionally splinted for another 8 to 10 weeks whenever the patient engages in any activity likely to cause reinjury (Figure 96-2).

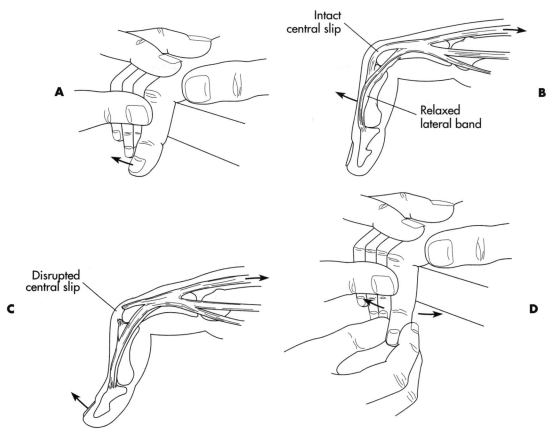

Figure 96-1 Extension against resistance tests for a central slip avulsion **(A, B, C).** Varus and valgus stress at the PIP joint tests for collateral ligament instability **(D).**

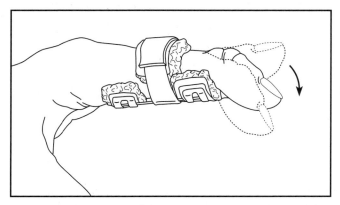

Figure 96-2 Suspected avulsion of the central slip of the extensor tendon necessitates splinting the PIP joint in extension, while allowing the DIP joint to go through a full range-of-motion. *(From Ruiz E, Cicero JJ:* Emergency management of skeletal injuries, *St Louis, 1995, Mosby.)*

✔ **Provide standard NSAIDs along with initial cold compresses and elevation.**

✔ **Recommend orthopedic referral in 1 week.**

What Not To Do:

✘ Do not overlook associated injuries that may cause joint instability. Such injuries may require immediate orthopedic consultation.

DISCUSSION

Volar dislocation of the PIP joint is uncommon but may cause rupture of the central slip mechanism. Although the acute manifestations may be limited to swelling and tenderness over the PIP joint, with time the lateral bands will slip and volar collapse will ensue, allowing the joint to herniate dorsally through the defect in the tendon—like a button through a buttonhole. Eventually, a position of flexion at the PIP joint and hyperextension at the DIP joint becomes fixed, producing the classic buttonhole or boutonnière deformity.

Early diagnosis is clearly the key to prevention, and because the acute injury may suggest nothing more than a contusion or sprain, any injury around the PIP joint should be viewed with suspicion.

A boutonnière finger, like a mallet finger, requires complete and prolonged immobilization. Unfortunately, many people do not seek help for a central slip avulsion until a deformity has developed, and at that point surgery may be required to correct the retinacular structures and the subluxed lateral bands (Figure 96-3).

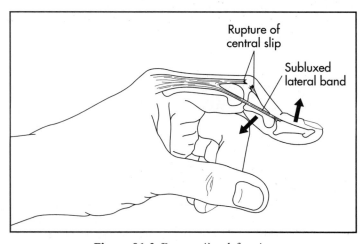

Figure 96-3 Boutonnière deformity.

97 Broken Toe

Presentation

The patient has stubbed, hyperflexed, hyperextended, hyperabducted, or dropped a weight on a toe. He presents with pain, swelling, ecchymosis, and decreased range-of-motion or point tenderness, and there may or may not be any deformity.

What To Do:

✔ Examine the toe, particularly for lacerations that could become infected, prolonged capillary filling time in the injured or other toes that could indicate poor circulation, or decreased sensation in the injured or other toes that could indicate peripheral neuropathy and may interfere with healing.

✔ **X-rays are not essential but are often necessary to provide patient satisfaction.** They have little effect on the initial treatment but may help predict the duration of pain and disability (e.g., fractures entering the joint space).

✔ **Displaced or angulated phalangeal fractures must be reduced with linear traction after a digital block or injection of the fracture hematoma.** Angulation can be further corrected by using a finger as a fulcrum to reverse the direction of the distal fragment. **The broken toe should fall into its normal position when it is released after reduction.**

✔ **Splint the broken toe by taping it to an adjacent nonaffected toe,** padding between toes with gauze or Webril, and using half-inch tape. Give the patient additional padding and tape, so he may revise the splinting, and (if there is a fracture) advise him that he will require such immobilization for approximately 1 week, by which time there should be good callus formation around the fracture and less pain with motion. Inform the patient that he must keep the padding dry between his toes while they are taped together, or the skin will become macerated and will break down. If the toe required reduction, warn him not to separate his toes when replacing the padding.

✔ **Also treat with rest, ice, elevation, and antiinflammatory medication. A cane, crutches, or hard-soled shoes that minimize toe flexion may all provide comfort. Let the patient know that in many cases a soft slipper or an old sneaker with the toe cut out may be more comfortable.**

✔ If the fracture is not of a phalanx but of the metatarsal, buddy taping is not effective. Instead, construct a pad for the sole with space cut out under the fracture site and the distal metatarsal head either taped to the foot or ideally inside a roomy cast shoe used for walking casts.

✔ **Arrange for follow-up if the toe is not much better within 1 week.**

What Not To Do:

✗ Do not tape toes together without padding between them. Friction and wetness will macerate the skin between.

✗ Do not let the patient overdo ice, which should not be applied directly to skin and should not be used for more than 10 to 20 minutes per hour.

✗ Do not overlook the possibility of acute gouty arthritis, which sometimes follows minor trauma after a delay of a few hours.

 DISCUSSION

If there is no toe fracture, the treatment is the same, but the pain, swelling, and ability to walk may improve in 3 days rather than 1 to 2 weeks. Although patients still come to the emergency department asking whether the toe is broken, if there is no deformity, they can usually be managed adequately over the telephone to be seen the next day.

98 Bursitis

Presentation

Following minimal trauma or repetitive motion, a nonarticular synovial sac or bursa protecting a tendon or prominent bone becomes swollen, tender, and inflamed. The elbow, hip, knee, and shoulder are most commonly involved. Because there is no joint involved, there is usually little decreased range of motion, except in the shoulder, where bursitis can produce dramatic limitation. If the tendon sheath is involved, there may be some stiffness and pain with motion. Olecranon bursitis often occurs in people who lean on their elbows, and prepatellar bursitis or "housemaid's knee" occurs in those who kneel for long periods of time. Swelling is less evident when the bursa is deep.

What To Do:

✔ Obtain a detailed history of the injury or precipitating activity, document a thorough physical examination, and rule out a joint effusion (see Chapter 133).

✔ **If there is swelling and fluctuance to suggest an effusion in the bursa, or erythema, warmth, and tenderness to suggest infection, prepare the skin with alcohol and antiseptic solution and anesthetize the skin with 1% lidocaine and a 30-gauge needle or spray with Ethyl Chloride. Puncture the swollen bursa with an 18- or 20-gauge needle, using aseptic technique, and withdraw some fluid to drain the effusion and rule out a bacterial infection.**

✔ Examine a Gram's stain of the effusion and send a sample for leukocyte count and culture. With or without fluid to examine, if there is any sign of a bacterial infection, prescribe appropriate oral antibiotics. **Bacterial infections tend to be gram-positive cocci and respond well to cephalexin (Keflex) or dicloxacillin (Dynapen) 500 mg tid × 10 to 15 days.**

✔ **When there is no indication of a bacterial infection, inflammatory bursitis may respond to injection of local anesthetics like lidocaine (Xylocaine) or bupivacaine (Marcaine) 2 to 5 ml mixed with corticosteroids like methylprednisolone (Depo-Medrol) 40 mg or betamethasone (Celestone Soluspan) 1 ml. Use a 25-gauge, 1¼-inch needle and review the anatomy so the needle can be carefully pushed through the lowest density tissue and the shortest** pathway, causing the least amount of pain while probing for the bursa sac. For olecranon bursitis, perform the injection with the arm in extension and penetrate the sac parallel to the ulna on the lateral side, away from the ulnar nerve. Approach the subacromial and greater trochanteric bursae from the lateral and posterior side. After injection, it may take several minutes or longer for patients to perceive pain relief and regain lost range-of-motion.

✔ **For knee and elbow, apply a bulky compressive dressing for protection and comfort. Construct a splint and instruct the patient in rest, elevation, and ice packing. A sling should suffice for the shoulder. Prescribe NSAIDs and arrange for follow-up.** Fluid may reaccumulate and require additional aspiration.

What Not To Do:

✘ Do not inject corticosteroids into an infected bursa. The infection is likely to worsen and spread.

✘ Do not puncture an olecranon bursitis by needling perpendicular to the ulna. Flexion and trauma may produce a chronic sinus.

 DISCUSSION

Common sites for bursitis include the subacromial bursa of the shoulder, the prepatellar bursa of the knee, the olecranon bursa of the elbow, and the trochanteric bursa of the hip. In shoulder bursitis, x-rays may reveal a calcific bursitis, and there may be bony spurs in olecranon bursitis, but these images are not needed for routine emergency therapy.

Patients with septic bursitis, unlike those with septic arthritis, can often be safely discharged on oral antibiotics because the risk of permanent damage is much less when there is no joint involvement. Severe cases with extensive cellulitis or lymphangitis, however, may require hospitalization and IV antibiotics. Immunocompromised patients may require longer courses of antibiotics. Reaspirate grossly purulent fluid that reaccumulates.

Some long-acting corticosteroid preparations can produce a rebound bursitis several hours after injection, after the local anesthetic wears off, but before the corticosteroid crystals dissolve. Patients should be so informed.

Prevent recurrence by wearing knee or elbow pads at work, avoiding pressure and trauma to vulnerable areas, and caring for skin wounds near bursae.

SUGGESTED READINGS

Pien FD, Ching D, Kim E: Septic bursitis: experience in a community practice, *Orthopedics* 14:981–984, 1991.
Smith DL, McAfee JH, Lucas LM, et al: Treatment of nonseptic olecranon bursitis, *Arch Intern Med* 149:2527–2530, 1989.

99

Carpal Tunnel Syndrome

Presentation

The patient complains of pain, tingling, or a "pins and needles" sensation in the hand or fingers. Onset may have been abrupt or gradual, but the problem is most noticeable on awakening or after extended use of the hand. The sensation may be bilateral, may include pain in the wrist or forearm, and is usually ascribed to the entire hand until specific physical examination localizes it to the median nerve distribution. Strenuous use of the hand almost always aggravates the symptoms. More established cases may include weakness of the thumb and atrophy of the thenar eminence.

Physical examination localizes paresthesia and decreased sensation to the median nerve distribution (which may vary) (Figure 99-1) and motor weakness, if present, to intrinsic muscles with median innervation. Innervation varies widely, but the muscles most reliably innervated by the median nerve are the abductors and opponens of the thumb (Figure 99-2).

What To Do:

✔ Perform and document a complete examination, sketching the area of decreased sensation and grading (on a scale of 1-5) the strength of the hand.

✔ **Have the patient passively drop both wrists to 90 degrees of flexion for 60 seconds, to see if this reproduces symptoms.** This is known as Phalen's test (Figure 99-3), is more sensitive than the reverse (hyperextending the wrist), and more specific than tapping over the volar carpal ligament to elicit paresthesia (Tinel's sign).

✔ Explain the nerve-compression etiology to the patient and arrange for additional evaluation and follow-up. Borderline diagnoses may be established with electromyography (EMG), but cases with pronounced pain or weakness may require early surgical decompression. **Antiinflammatory medication, elevation of the affected hand, ice, immobilization with a volar splint in a neutral position, and rest may all help to reduce symptoms.**

✔ **A 2-week course of oral prednisone (e.g., 20 mg daily for 1 week then 10 mg) may offer short-term relief in mild-to-moderate cases.**

✔ **Alternatively, injections of corticosteroids can often dramatically alleviate symptoms.** Using a 1-inch, 25-gauge needle with 20 mg of methylprednisolone (Depo-Medrol) or 0.5 ml of betamethasone (Celestone Soluspan) along with 5 ml of

267

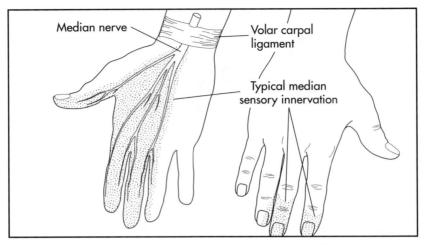

Figure 99-1 Sensory abnormalities are found along the median nerve distribution.

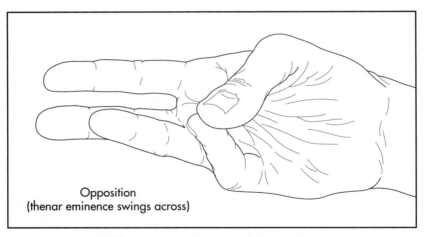

Figure 99-2 Test the strength of thumb abductors and opponens muscles.

bupivacaine (Marcaine), inject on the ulnar side of the palmaris longus tendon, midway between the flexor carpi radialis and the flexor carpi ulnaris tendons, just proximal to the flexor crease of the wrist, distally into the central portion of the flexor tendon mass (Figure 99-4). Avoid injecting either the median or ulnar nerve or radial or ulnar artery. If injection produces paresthesia in the distribution of the median or ulnar nerve, withdraw the needle and redirect it to avoid intraneural injection. After 1 day of wrist splinting, the patient can expect symptomatic relief, but the maximum effect may come a few days later. Warn the patient that his hand will feel somewhat numb for a few hours, and that a rebound phenomenon or flare may develop within 12 hours after the injection. NSAIDs, elevation, and ice packs will help if this rebound pain occurs.

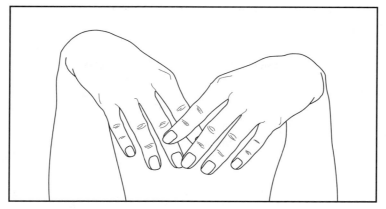

Figure 99-3 Phalen's test.

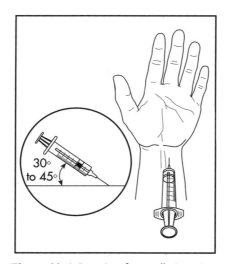

Figure 99-4 Location for needle insertion.

What Not To Do:

✗ Do not rule out thumb weakness just because the thumb can touch the little finger. Thumb flexors may be innervated by the ulnar nerve. Test abduction and opposition: can the thumb rise from the plane of the palm, and can the thumb pad meet the little finger pad?

✗ Do not diagnose carpal tunnel syndrome solely on the basis of a positive Tinel's sign. Paresthesia can be produced in the distribution of any nerve if one taps hard enough.

✗ Do not perform Phalen's test for more than 60 seconds; maintaining a flexed wrist for longer may produce paresthesia in a normal hand.

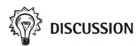

DISCUSSION

There is little space to spare where the median nerve and digit flexors pass beneath the volar carpal ligament, and very little swelling may produce this specific neuropathy. Repetitive use of the arm or hand, trauma, arthritis, pregnancy, diabetes mellitus, and weight gain are among the many factors that can precipitate this syndrome. Carpal tunnel syndrome is one of the most common causes of hand pain, particularly in middle-aged women.

Indications for surgery include severe or long-standing symptoms, persistent dysesthesia, thenar weakness or atrophy, and acute median neurapraxia caused by the closed compartment compression.

Less often, the median nerve can be entrapped more proximally, where it enters the medial antecubital fossa through the pronator teres. Symptoms of this cubital tunnel syndrome may be reproduced with elbow extension and forearm pronation.

SUGGESTED READINGS

Burke DT, Burke MM, Stewart GW, et al: Splinting for carpal tunnel syndrome: in search of the optimal angle, *Arch Phys Med Rehab* 75:1241–1244, 1994.

Kuhlman KA, Hennessey WJ: Sensitivity and specificity of carpal tunnel syndrome signs, *Am J Phys Med Rehab* 76:451–457, 1997.

100

Cervical Strain
(Whiplash)

Presentation

The patient may arrive directly from a car accident, arrive the following day (complaining of increased neck stiffness and pain), or arrive long after (to have injuries documented). The injury occurred when the neck was subjected to sudden extension and flexion when the car was struck from the rear, possibly injuring intervertebral joints, discs, and ligaments; cervical muscles; or even nerve roots. As with other strains and sprains, the stiffness and pain may tend to peak on the day after the injury.

What To Do:

✔ Obtain a detailed history to determine the mechanism and severity of the injury. Was the patient wearing a seat belt? Was the headrest up? Were eyeglasses thrown into the rear seat? Was the seat broken? Was the car damaged? Was the car driveable afterwards? Was the windshield shattered? Was there intrusion into the passenger compartment?

✔ To evaluate the possibility of head trauma, ask about loss of consciousness or amnesia, and check the patient's orientation, cranial nerves, and strength and sensation in the legs as well.

✔ **Examine the patient for involuntary splinting, point tenderness over the spinous processes of the cervical vertebrae, cervical muscle spasm or tenderness, and strength, sensation, and reflexes in the arms (to evaluate the cervical nerve roots).**

✔ If there is any question at all of an unstable neck injury because of focal neurologic deficits, altered mentation, moderate to severe neck pain, or distracting injuries, start the evaluation with a cross-table lateral radiograph of the cervical spine while maintaining cervical immobilization with a rigid collar. If necessary, the AP view and open-mouth view of the odontoid can also be obtained before the patient is moved.

✔ **If any of the above suggest injury to the cervical spine, obtain three x-ray views of the cervical spine: AP, lateral, and open mouth odontoid.** If there is clinical nerve root impairment, or if more detail of the posterior elements of the vertebrae needs to be seen, oblique views may also be useful. Flexion and extension views may be needed to evaluate stability of joints and ligaments but should only be done under careful supervision, so the spinal cord is not injured in the process.

✔ **If x-rays show no fracture or dislocation, and if history and physical examination are consistent with stable joint, ligament, and muscle injury, explain to the patient that the stiffness and pain are often worse after 24 hours but usually begin to resolve over the next 3 to 5 days. Most patients are back to normal in 1 week, although some have persistent pain for 6 weeks.**

✔ **Provide 1 or 2 days of intermittent immobilization by fitting a soft cervical collar to wear when out of bed.** Place the wide side of the cervical collar either anterior or posterior based on the position of maximum comfort. If neither position improves comfort, omit the collar.

✔ **Instruct the patient to apply topical ice for the first day, apply heat for the later spasm, and take OTC antiinflammatory analgesics like aspirin, ibuprofen, or naproxen. Arrange follow-up as necessary.**

What Not To Do:

✘ Do not forget to tell the patient her symptoms may well be worse the day after the injury.

✘ Do not skimp recording the history and physical. This sort of injury may end up in litigation, and a detailed record can obviate your being subpoenaed to testify in person.

✘ Do not x-ray every neck. A thousand negative cervical spine x-rays are cost effective if they prevent one paraplegic from an occult unstable fracture, but several studies have shown that patients who have no neck pain or stiffness, are not intoxicated, do not have an altered mental status, and are not distracted by other injuries are not likely to have an unstable cervical spine fracture or dislocation and do not have to be x-rayed just because they were in an auto accident, fell, or hit their head.

 DISCUSSION

Blunt trauma carries the risk of associated cervical spine injury, which is not increased by the presence of face or neck injury. X-ray results for neck injuries seldom add much to the clinical assessment, but the sequelae of unrecognized cervical spine injuries are so severe that it is still worth while to x-ray relatively mild injuries, in contrast to skull and lumbosacral spine radiographs, which should be ordered far less often. It is often useful to discuss the pros and cons of x-rays with the patient, who may prefer to do without, or conversely may be in the office purely to obtain radiologic documentation of her injuries.

The term *whiplash* is probably best reserved for describing the mechanism of injury and is of little value as a diagnosis. Because of the many undesirable legal connotations that surround this term it may be advisable to substitute "flexion/extension injury."

The use of soft cervical collars should be based on each patient's perception of the collar's effectiveness. Studies have shown that soft cervical collars do not influence the duration or degree of persistent pain.

SUGGESTED READINGS

Borchgrevink GE, Kaasa A, McDonagh D, et al: Acute treatment of whiplash neck sprain injuries: a randomized trial of treatment during the first 14 days after a car accident, *Spine* 23:25-31, 1998.

Gennis P, Miller L, Gallagher J, et al: The effect of soft cervical collars on persistent neck pain in patients with whiplash injury, *Acad Emerg Med* 3:568-573, 1996.

101 Cheiralgia Paresthetica (Handcuff Neuropathy)

Presentation

The patient may complain of pain around the thumb while tight handcuffs were in place. The pain decreased with handcuff removal, but there is residual paresthesia or decreased sensation over the radial side of the thumb metacarpal (or a more extensive distribution). The same injury may also be produced by pulling on a ligature around the wrist or wearing a tight watchband.

What To Do:

✔ **Carefully examine and document the motor and sensory function of the hand. Draw the area of paresthesia or decreased sensation as demonstrated by light touch or two-point discrimination.** Document that there is no weakness or area of complete anesthesia.

✔ **Explain to the patient that the nerve has been bruised and that its function should return as it regenerates, but that the process is slow, requiring about 2 months.**

✔ Arrange for follow-up if needed. Bandages, splints, or physical therapy are usually not necessary.

What Not To Do:

✘ Do not overlook more extensive injuries, such as a complete transection of the nerve (with complete anesthesia) or a more proximal radial nerve palsy (see Chapter 124). Do not forget alternative causes, such as peripheral neuropathy, de Quervain's tenosynovitis (see Chapter 131), carpal tunnel syndrome (see Chapter 99), scaphoid fracture (see Chapter 125), or a gamekeeper's thumb (see Chapter 127).

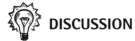 **DISCUSSION**

A superficial, sensory, cutaneous twig of the radial nerve is the branch most easily injured by constriction of the wrist. Its area of innervation can vary widely (Figure 101-1). Axonal regeneration of contused nerves proceeds at about I mm per day (or about an inch per month); thus recovery may require 2 months (measuring from site of injury in wrist to end of area of paresthesia). Patients may want this injury documented as evidence of "police brutality," but it can be a product of their own struggling as much as too-tight handcuffs.

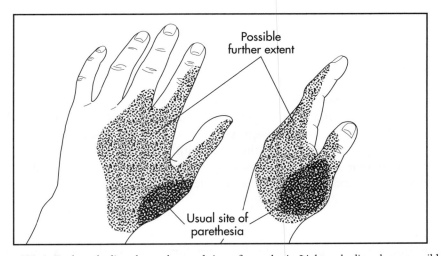

Figure 101-1 Darkest shading shows the usual sites of paresthesia. Lighter shading shows possible further extent.

c h a p t e r

102

Clavicle (Collarbone) Fracture

Presentation

The patient has fallen onto her shoulder or outstretched arm or, more commonly, has received a direct blow to the clavicle and now presents with pain to direct palpation over the clavicle and with movement of the arm or neck. Patients therefore cannot raise their arm due to pain at the fracture site. There may be deformity of the bone with swelling and ecchymosis. An infant or small child might present after a fall not moving the arm, but examination of the arm will be normal and only further examination of the clavicle will reveal the actual site of the injury.

What To Do:

✔ After completing a musculoskeletal examination, evaluate the neurovascular status of the arm.

✔ **Obtain x-rays to rule out other injuries and document the fracture for follow-up.** Fractures or dislocations at the sternal end of the clavicle are often difficult to see on plain radiographs but are well visualized on CT scans.

✔ **Obtain orthopedic consultation if there is any evidence of neurovascular compromise. Fractures of the lateral clavicle at the acromioclavicular joint, if displaced more than one centimeter, also require orthopedic consultation to consider surgical reduction.**

✔ **Fit arm for a sling or clavicle strap that comfortably immobilizes the arm. Patients probably experience fewer complications and less pain with a simple sling, and there is no difference in healing time.**

✔ **Prescribe analgesics,** usually antiinflammatories like ibuprofen or naproxen, but narcotics when significant pain is present or anticipated.

✔ Inform the patient that she may be more comfortable sleeping in a semi-upright position.

✔ Arrange for orthopedic follow-up in 1 week to evaluate healing and begin pendulum exercises of the shoulder.

What Not To Do:

✗ Do not apply a figure-of-eight dressing or clavicle strap if this form of splinting increases patient discomfort.

✗ Do not leave an arm immobilized in a sling for more than 1 week. This can result in loss of range-of-motion or "frozen shoulder."

 DISCUSSION

In children, fracture of the clavicle requires very little force and usually heals rapidly and without complication. In adults, however, this fracture usually results from a greater force and is associated with other injuries and complications. Clavicle fractures are sometimes associated with a hematoma from the subclavian vein, but other nearby structures, including the carotid artery, brachial plexus, and lung, are usually protected by the underlying anterior scalene muscle and the tendency of the sternocleidomastoid muscle to pull up the medial fragment of bone. A great deal of angulation deformity and distraction on x-ray are usually acceptable because the clavicle mends and re-forms itself so well and does not have to support the body in the meantime. As with rib fractures, respiration prevents full immobilization, so the relief that comes with callus formation may be delayed an additional week.

SUGGESTED READINGS

Anderson K, Jensen PO, Lauritzen J: Treatment of clavicular fractures: figure-of-eight bandage versus a simple sling, *Acta Orthop Scand* 58:71-74, 1987.

Eskola A, Vainionpaa S, Myllynen P, et al: Outcome of clavicular fracture in 89 patients, *Arch Orthop Trauma Surg* 105:337-338, 1986.

Stanley D, Norris SH: Recovery following fractures of the clavicle treated conservatively, *Injury* 19:162-164, 1988.

103

Coccyx Fracture (Tailbone Fracture)

Presentation

The patient fell on his buttocks or tailbone and now complains of pain that is worse with sitting, and perhaps with defecation. There should be little or no pain with standing, but walking may be uncomfortable. On physical examination, there is point tenderness and perhaps deformity of the coccyx that is best palpated by examining through the rectum with a finger (Figure 103-1).

What To Do:

✔ Verify the history (was this actually a straddle injury?) and examine thoroughly, including the lumbar spine, pelvis, and legs. **Palpate the coccyx from inside and out, feeling primarily for point tenderness and/or pain on motion.**

✔ **X-rays are optional.** Any noticed variation can be an old fracture or an anatomic variant, and a fractured coccyx can appear within normal limits.

✔ **Instruct the patient in how to sit forward, resting his weight on ischial tuberosities and thighs, instead of on the coccyx.** A foam-rubber doughnut cushion may help. **If necessary, prescribe antiinflammatory pain medications and stool softeners.**

✔ Inform the patient that the pain will gradually improve over 1 week, as bony callus forms and motion decreases, and arrange for follow-up as needed. Chronic pain is rare but treatable by surgically removing the coccyx.

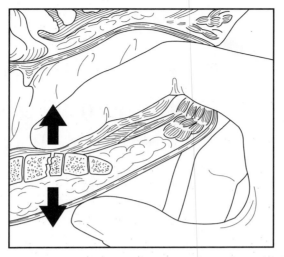

Figure 103-1 Finger palpating the coccyx via rectal examination.

Extensor Tendon Avulsion—Distal Phalanx (Baseball or Mallet Finger)

Presentation

There is a history of a sudden resisted flexion of the distal interphalangeal (DIP) joint, such as when the finger tip is struck by a ball, resulting in pain and tender ecchymotic discoloration over the dorsum of the base of the distal phalanx. When the finger is held in extension, the injured DIP joint remains in slight flexion (Figure 104–1).

What To Do:

✔ **Obtain an x-ray with anteroposterior and lateral views, which may or may not demonstrate an avulsion fracture.**

✔ Test for stability of the collateral ligaments of the DIP joint with varus and valgus stress. **With the proximal interphalangeal joint (PIP) held in extension, test for both active extension and flexion of the DIP joint.** There should be a loss of full active extension while active flexion and passive range-of-motion remain intact.

✔ **Apply a finger splint that will hold the DIP joint in neutral position or slight hyperextension and firmly tape it in place.** Either a dorsal or a volar splint of aluminum and foam may be used. Plastic finger-tip splints are manufactured in various sizes (e.g., Stax extension splints) (Figures 104-2 to 104-4).

✔ **Instruct the patient to keep the splint in place continuously and seek orthopedic follow-up care within 1 week.**

✔ Prescribe an analgesic as needed.

What Not To Do:

✘ Do not assume there is no significant injury just because the x-ray is negative. The clue to this injury is persistent drooping of the distal phalanx and tenderness over the bony

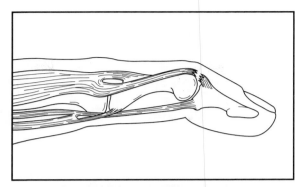

Figure 104–1 Injured DIP joint in slight flexion.

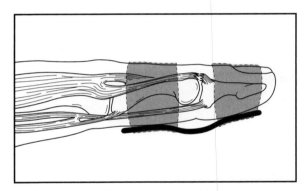

Figure 104–2 Commercial concave aluminum splint.

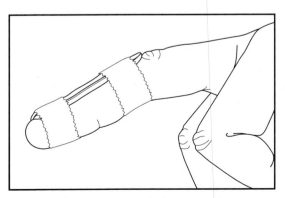

Figure 104–3 Dorsal aluminum splint.

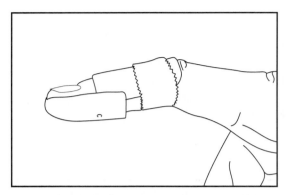

Figure 104-4 Commercial Stax extension splint.

insertion of the extensor tendon. With or without a fracture the tendon avulsion requires splinting.

✗ Do not forcefully hyperextend the joint. This can result in ischemia and skin breakdown over the joint.

✗ Do not unnecessarily impair the movement of the PIP joint.

 DISCUSSION

Adequate splinting usually restores near full range and strength to DIP joint extension, but the patient will require 6 weeks of immobilization, and should be informed that healing might be inadequate, requiring surgical repair. The splint should remain in place at all times. If a patient needs to remove it for any reason, instruct him to have someone hold his finger in extension until he can replace the splint. If the DIP joint is allowed to flex at any time—and it will drop into flexion on its own—healing of the injured tendon will be interrupted and the chance of a poor result increased.

A wide variety of splints are commercially available for splinting this injury (e.g., Stax hyperextension splint, padded aluminum frog splint) but, in a pinch, a tape-covered paper clip will do (Figure 104-5). A dorsal splint allows more use of the finger but requires more padding and may contribute to ischemia of the skin overlying the DIP joint. Figure-of-eight taping also provides some limitation of flexion.

Injuries in which there is a large, widely displaced fracture require open reduction and Kirschner wire fixation, especially if there is associated volar subluxation of the joint. If the diagnosis of an extensor tendon avulsion is initially missed, treatment by splinting is still possible as late as 6 to 10 weeks after injury. The result, however, is usually not as satisfactory as it is with early diagnosis and treatment.

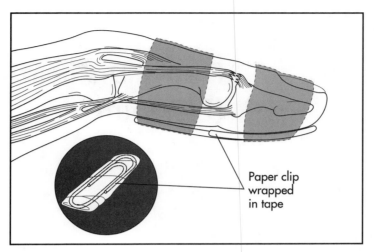

Paper clip
wrapped
in tape

Figure 104–5 Tape-covered paper clip splint.

105

Finger Dislocation
(PIP Joint)

Presentation

The patient will have jammed his finger, causing a hyperextension injury that forces the middle phalanx dorsally and proximally out of articulation with the distal end of the proximal phalanx. An obvious deformity will be seen unless the patient or a bystander has reduced the dislocation on his own. There should be no sensory or vascular compromise.

What To Do:

✔ **Unless there is a bony instability and a shaft fracture is suspected, x-rays may be deferred and joint reduction can be carried out first.**

✔ **If there has been significant delay in seeking help or if the patient is suffering considerable discomfort, a digital block over the proximal phalanx or 1% lidocaine injected directly into the joint will allow for a more comfortable reduction.**

✔ **To reduce the joint, do not pull on the finger tip; instead, with the joint slightly extended, push the base of the middle phalanx distally using a thumb until the middle phalanx slides smoothly into its natural anatomic position** (Figure 105-1).

✔ Now test the finger for collateral ligament instability by applying varus and valgus stress in full extension and 30 degrees of flexion, and then test for avulsion of the central extensor tendon slip (see Chapter 96). The patient should be able to extend his finger at the PIP joint. Testing for avulsion of the volar carpal plate, you will be able to hyperextend the PIP joint more than that of the same finger on the uninjured hand. If any of these associated injuries exist, orthopedic consultation should be sought and prolonged splinting and rehabilitation may be required.

✔ Postreduction x-rays should be taken. "Chip fractures" may represent tendon or ligament avulsions.

✔ **If the joint feels unstable with a tendency to dislocate when extended, then splint the finger 20 degrees short of full extension with a padded dorsal splint for 3 to 4 weeks and provide follow-up for active range-of-motion exercises to restore normal joint mobility** (Figure 105-2).

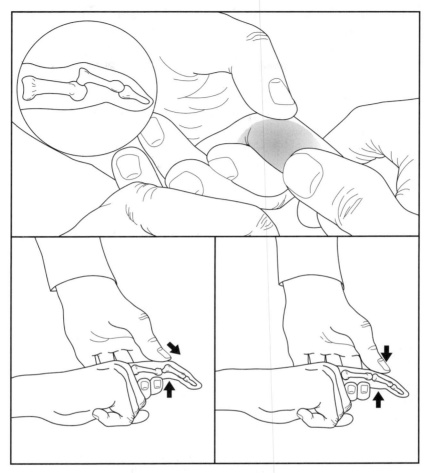

Figure 105–1 PIP joint reduction.

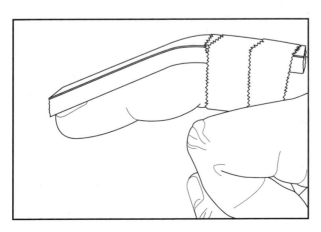

Figure 105–2 Dorsal extension block splint for PIP dislocation.

✔ **If the joint feels stable, "buddy taping" to adjacent digits is an acceptable immobilization technique** (Figure 105-3). The tape should be removed at night or if the skin becomes wet (to prevent skin maceration). Have the patient dry the skin thoroughly prior to retaping. Cotton padding placed between fingers can also be used to prevent skin breakdown.

✔ Inform the patient that joint swelling and stiffness may persist for months after the initial injury. Prophylactic nighttime PIP extension splinting can be used to prevent the mild PIP joint flexion contractures that are common consequences of these injuries.

✔ Remind the patient to keep the injured finger elevated. Recommend ice application for 20 minutes three to four times over the next 24 hours and NSAIDs for pain.

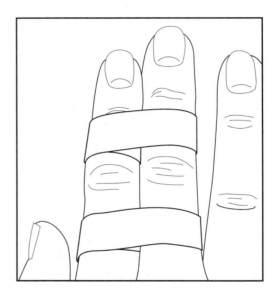

Figure 105-3 Buddy taping.

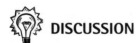

DISCUSSION

If there is any doubt as to the competence of the central extensor slip or the volar carpal plate, the joint may be splinted in full extension for 3 to 4 weeks (see Chapter 96). Irreducible dislocation of the PIP joint is usually caused by a complete tear of one of the collateral ligaments or a slip of the extensor or flexor tendon that prevents closed reduction and requires arthrotomy.

106

Finger Sprain
(PIP Joint)

Presentation

During sports activity or a fall, the patient's finger is jammed or hyperextended, resulting in a painful, swollen, possibly ecchymotic PIP joint. There may have been an initial dislocation, which was reduced by the patient or a bystander.

What To Do:

✔ Get a detailed history of the exact mechanism of injury.

✔ **Palpate to locate precise areas of tenderness. Pay particular attention to the collateral ligaments, the volar plate, and the insertion of the central slip of the extensor tendon at the base of the middle phalanx** (see Chapter 96). Note any associated injuries above and below the PIP joint.

✔ Test both extensor and flexor function at the PIP joint and note normal sensation distal to the injury.

✔ If pain precludes active motion testing, consider using a 1% lidocaine digital block or joint injection.

✔ **Assess stability by stress testing the injured joint in all directions—radial, ulnar, volar, and dorsal—performed with the joint at 30 degrees of flexion.**

✔ **Obtain anteroposterior and lateral x-ray views of the finger.**

✔ **When there is no loss of function and no significant joint instability, immobilize the joint by buddy taping adjacent digits.** Have the patient remove the tape while sleeping or if the hand becomes wet (to prevent maceration of the skin) and have him dry the skin thoroughly prior to retaping. Prophylactic nighttime PIP extension splinting can be used with the more serious sprains to prevent the mild PIP joint flexion contractures that are common consequences of these injuries. Minor sprains may not require any special splinting.

✔ **Instruct the patient to use ice, elevation, and NSAIDs for pain.**

✔ Inform the patient that swelling, stiffness, and discomfort may persist for months and provide follow-up for continued care or physical therapy.

287

What Not To Do:

✖ Do not miss joint instability or tendon avulsion—these injuries require special splinting and orthopedic referral.

 DISCUSSION

The major complications of PIP joint injuries are stiffness, joint enlargement, ligamentous laxity, and boutonnière deformity. Stiffness and joint enlargement are to be expected for most PIP joint dislocations. Boutonnière deformity (see Chapter 96) can be prevented by adequate examination and diagnosis of volar dislocation. Ligamentous laxity is not common, but if there is significant laxity, which usually affects the index or small finger, the ligament can be surgically reattached or reconstructed.

107

Finger-Tip (Tuft) Fractures

Presentation

The patient seeks help after a crushing injury to the finger tip such as catching it in a closing car door. The finger tip will be swollen and painful, with ecchymosis. There may or may not be a subungual hematoma, open nailbed injury, or finger pad laceration.

What To Do:

✔ Assess for associated injuries and DIP joint instability.

✔ **Obtain finger x-rays with anteroposterior and lateral views.**

✔ If there are open wounds, perform a digital block (see Appendix B), thoroughly cleanse and debride any open wounds, and repair any nailbed lacerations (see Chapter 144).

✔ **For open tuft fractures with gross contamination and marginally viable tissue, give prophylactic antibiotics like cefazolin (Ancef) 1000 mg IV followed by cephalexin (Keflex) 500 mg qid PO × 5 days.**

✔ **Apply a sterile, nonadhesive protective dressing to open wounds, and provide an aluminum finger-tip splint to prevent further injury and pain.**

✔ **If necessary, provide oral analgesics** and advise the patient to elevate the injury above the heart to minimize swelling.

✔ Insure follow-up to monitor the patient's recovery, and in the case of open fracture, to intervene in the event of infection.

What Not To Do:

✗ Do not prescribe prophylactic antibiotics for clean and uncomplicated open fractures of the distal tuft. Prophylactic antibiotics have been shown to be of no benefit when aggressive irrigation and debridement have been provided.

SUGGESTED READINGS

Sloan JP, Dove AF, Maheson M, et al: Antibiotics in open fracture of the distal phalanx? *J Hand Surg* 12:123-124, 1987.

Suprock MD, Hood JM, Lubahn JD: Role of antibiotics in open fractures of the finger, *J Hand Surg* 15:761-764, 1990.

Ganglion Cysts

Presentation

The patient is concerned about a rubbery, rounded swelling emerging from the general area of a tendon sheath of the wrist or hand. It may have appeared abruptly, been present for years, or fluctuated, suddenly resolving and gradually returning in pretty much the same place. There is usually little tenderness, inflammation, or interference with function, but ganglion cysts are bothersome when they get in the way and painful when repeatedly traumatized.

What To Do:

✔ Undertake a thorough history and physical examination of the hand to ascertain that everything else is normal. **X-rays are of no value unless there is some question of bony pathology.**

✔ **Although most ganglions can be diagnosed easily on physical examination, ultrasound may be helpful in diagnosing a small or questionable lesion.**

✔ Explain to the patient that this is a fluid-filled cyst, spontaneously arising from bursa, ligament, or tendon sheath, and posing no particular danger. **Treatment options include the following: (1) hitting it with a large book to rupture the cyst, with a fair chance of recurrence; (2) draining the contents of the cyst with an 18-gauge needle to reduce its size and then injecting corticosteroid, also with good chance of recurrence; (3) arranging for a surgical excision,** which will provide definitive pathologic diagnosis, but the dissection is sometimes unexpectedly extensive and still allows some chance of recurrence; and **(4) doing nothing,** in which case the cyst may spontaneously drain and may recur.

✔ Follow the wishes of the patient regarding treatment and arrange for follow-up.

✔ **If the patient requests immediate decompression, prep the skin, anesthetize the skin and cyst wall using a 30-gauge needle with 1% lidocaine, and then with an 18-gauge needle on a 10-ml syringe, aspirate the mucinous contents. Optionally, instill a long-acting corticosteroid like 1 ml betamethasone (Celestone Soluspan).**

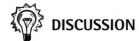

DISCUSSION

Ganglion cysts are outpouchings of bursae, ligament, or tendon sheaths, with no clear etiology and no relation to nerve ganglia. Perhaps ganglion cysts got their name because their contents are like "glue." Reassurance about their insignificance is often the best we can offer patients. Ganglion cysts recur over 50% of the time after simple aspiration. Other techniques of aspiration and injection have reported recurrence rates from 13% to 100%. After surgical excision, 0% to 50% recur. With no treatment, 38% to 58% have been reported to disappear spontaneously.

SUGGESTED READINGS

Zubowicz VN, Ishii CH: Management of ganglion cysts of the hand by simple aspiration, *J Hand Surg* 12:618-620, 1987.

109

Gouty Arthritis, Acute

Presentation

Usually a male patient over 50 years of age with an established diagnosis of gout or hyper-uricemia rapidly develops an intensely painful monarticular arthritis, often in the middle of the night, but sometimes a few hours following a minor trauma. Any joint may be affected, but most common is the metatarsophalangeal joint of the great toe (podagra). The joint is red, hot, swollen, and intensely tender to touch or movement. There is usually no fever, rash, or other sign of systemic illness. The patient may have predisposing factors that increase his risk of develop-ing gout, like obesity, moderate-to-heavy alcohol intake, high blood pressure, diabetes, and ab-normal kidney function, or he may be taking certain drugs including thiazide diuretics, low-dose aspirin, and tuberculosis medications (pyrazinamide and ethambutol).

What To Do:

✔ **If the patient has not been previously diagnosed by arthrocentesis that showed crystals, then tap the involved joint as described in acute monarticular arthri-tis** (see Chapter 114). In addition to ruling out infection, look under the microscope for crystals in the joint fluid. Urate crystals look like needles and may be in white cells. The calcium pyrophosphate dihydrate crystals of pseudogout are rhomboids. Polarizing filters above and below the sample help distinguish the negatively birefringent crystals of sodium urate from the weakly positively birefringent calcium pyrophosphate dihydrate.

✔ **Provide rapid pain relief with loading doses of NSAIDs such as ketorolac (Toradol) 60 mg IM, indomethacin (Indocin) 50 mg PO, ibuprofen (Motrin) 800 mg PO, or naproxen (Anaprox) 825 mg PO, then tapering, once pain is relieved, to maintenance doses for the next 4 to 5 days (e.g., indomethacin 25 mg tid, ibuprofen 600 mg qid, naproxen 500 mg bid).** Excruciating pain may require one dose of narcotics while the antiinflammatory drugs take effect.

✔ **An alternative treatment for acute gouty arthritis is colchicine 0.6 mg PO qh un-til pain is relieved, the patient develops nausea, vomiting, or diarrhea, or a max-imum dose of 6 mg is reached. Colchicine can also be given IV 2 mg q6h to a maximum of 4 mg.** After these maximum doses, no more colchicine should be pre-scribed for 1 week to avoid toxicity. IV administration provides faster relief and lower gastric toxicity but greater hepatic toxicity, and extravasation can cause tissue necrosis. These doses should be halved in renal insufficiency and elderly patients.

✔ **If the patient has a medical problem** (e.g., peptic ulcer or gastritis, liver or kidney disease) **that might contraindicate use of the NSAIDs or colchicine but has no infection, uncontrolled diabetes, or hypertension, use parenteral, oral, or intraarticular corticosteroids, like triamcinolone (Aristocort) 60 mg IM or prednisone (Deltasone) 30 to 50 mg PO qd for 5 days or betamethasone (Celestone Soluspan) 0.5 to 1.0 ml intraarticularly.**

✔ Adrenocorticotropic hormone (ACTH) 80 USP Units IM is also effective in about 3 hours.

✔ **Delay injecting corticosteroids into the joint until the possibility of infection is eliminated.** After draining excess fluid from the joint, instill an aqueous suspension of betamethasone (as above) or methylprednisolone (Depo-Medrol), about 20 to 40 mg mixed in an appropriate volume of bupivacaine (Marcaine).

✔ Instruct the patient to elevate and rest the painful extremity, apply ice packs, and arrange for follow-up.

What Not To Do:

✘ Do not depend on serum uric acid to diagnose acute gouty arthritis—it may or may not be elevated (>8 mg/dl) at the time of an acute attack. Hyperuricemia will be found in 70% of patients with their first attack of gout.

✘ Do not use NSAIDs when a patient has a history of active peptic ulcer disease with bleeding. Relative contraindications include renal insufficiency, volume depletion, gastritis, inflammatory bowel disease, asthma, and congestive heart disease.

✘ Do not start maintenance NSAID doses for an acute inflammation. It will take 1 day or more to reach therapeutic levels and pain relief.

✘ Do not insist on reconfirming an established diagnosis of gout by ordering serum uric acid levels (which are often normal during the acute attack) or tapping an exquisitely painful joint at every attack in a patient with known gout and a typical presentation.

✘ Do not, on the other hand, miss a septic arthritis in a patient with gout.

✘ Do not attempt to reduce the serum uric acid level with probenecid, allopurinol, or sulfinpyrazone during an acute attack of gouty arthritis. This will not help the arthritis and may even be counterproductive. Leave it for follow-up.

 DISCUSSION

Gout is almost exclusively a disease of adult men, and it is rare in premenopausal women and prepubertal children. While hyperuricemia may indicate an increased risk of gout, the relationship between serum uric acid and arthritis is unclear. Many patients with hyperuricemia

293

Continued

DISCUSSION—cont'd

do not develop gout, while some patients with repeated attacks of gout have normal or low uric acid levels.

In addition to the first metatarsophalangeal joint involved in podagra, gout can strike ankles, knees, wrists, fingers, and elbows. These painful attacks usually subside in hours to days with or without treatment. Most patients with gout experience repeated attacks of arthritis over the years. Conditions other than septic arthritis that can mimic gout include psoriatic arthritis, rheumatoid arthritis, and pseudogout (in which crystals of calcium pyrophosphate dihydrate replace uric acid).

Uric acid–lowering medications like allopurinol, probenecid, or sulfinpyrazone are useful for prophylaxis but can actually worsen an attack when used acutely. If patients are already taking maintenance doses, they may be continued and need not be held during an acute attack. Colchicine may also be used for prophylaxis in the smaller dose of 0.6 mg PO qd, especially in the first few months of treatment with allopurinol, probenecid, or sulfinpyrazone, which lower uric acid but can initially precipitate attacks.

110 Knee Sprain

Presentation

After twisting the knee from a slip and fall or some sports injury, the patient complains of knee pain and variable ability to bear weight. There may be a tense effusion or spasm of the quadriceps forcing the patient to hold the knee at 10 to 20 degrees of flexion.

What To Do:

✔ **If there is going to be any delay in examining the knee, provide ice, a compression dressing, and elevation above the level of the heart.**

✔ **For severe pain, provide immediate analgesia with NSAIDs like ibuprofen (Motrin) 800 mg PO along with a narcotic like oxycodone (Percocet, Tylox).**

✔ Ask about the mechanism of injury, which is often the key to the diagnosis. Ask about any previous injuries, the time of the injury, and any treatment so far.

✔ **Suspect a tear to the anterior cruciate ligament (ACL) if the knee gave way with an audible "pop" or "snap" while decelerating, cutting, sidestepping, or landing from a jump.** The patient may describe the anterior dislocation of the tibia on the femur, followed by immediate effusion and loss of function.

✔ **Valgus and varus stresses can tear the medial collateral ligament (MCL) and lateral collateral ligament (LCL), respectively.** These injuries occur in football, other contact sports, and when a skier hooks the inside edge of a ski tip in the snow. There is usually no audible sound, and swelling may peak about 6 hours after the injury.

✔ **Injury to the posterior cruciate ligament (PCL) may result from a blow to the anterior tibia with the knee flexed,** as when it strikes the dashboard in an automobile accident.

✔ **A tear to the meniscal cartilage may result from a direct blow when the foot is firmly planted and the knee is rotated and forcefully extended.**

✔ Inspect the knee for swelling, ecchymosis, or disruption of skin. Look for injuries of the back and pelvis. Check hip flexion, extension, and rotation. Thump the sole of the foot as an axial loading clue to a tibia or fibula fracture. Document any effusion, discoloration, heat, deformity, or loss of function, circulation, sensation, or movement.

✔ Stress the four major knee ligaments, comparing the injured to the uninjured knee to determine if there is any instability.

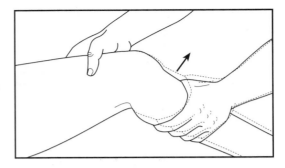

Figure 110-1 Lachman's test.

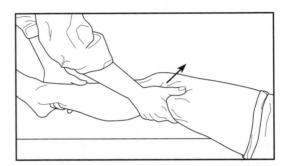

Figure 110-2 Varus stress test.

✔ **Perform a Lachman's test to diagnose injury of the ACL** (Figure 110-1). With the knee flexed 15 to 20 degrees, place one hand on the proximal tibia and the other on the distal femur. Stabilize the femur, grasp the tibia, and pull it anteriorly. Increased anterior displacement of the tibia compared to the uninjured side and a soft or incomplete end point indicate ACL disruption.

✔ **Test MCL stability with the valgus stress test.** With the knee still flexed 15 to 20 degrees, grasp the tibia distally to stabilize the lower leg, then apply direct, firm pressure in a medial direction from the lateral femoral condyle.

✔ **Test LCL stability with the varus stress test** (Figure 110-2), **pressing laterally on the medial femoral condyle.** If there is varus laxity, also check the function of the peroneal nerve by asking the patient to dorsiflex the big toe.

✔ **Test the integrity of the PCL and posterior capsule with the posterior drawer test** (Figure 110-3). Flex the knee to 90 degrees and apply firm direct pressure in a posterior direction to the anteroproximal tibia. Look for increased posterior displacement of the tibia and a soft or mushy end point. This test may be difficult to perform if there is a large effusion.

✔ **Examine for an injury to the medial or lateral meniscal cartilage with McMurray's test** (Figure 110-4). With the patient supine, hold the knee anteriorly at the femoral condyle with one hand, fingers positioned along the joint line, and hold the foot with the other hand. While externally rotating the lower leg, flex the knee and hip,

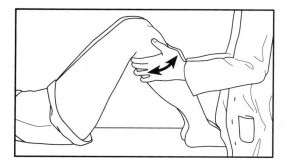

Figure 110–3 Posterior drawer test.

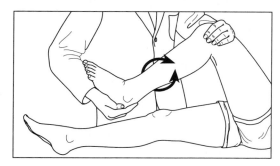

Figure 110–4 McMurray's test.

then slowly extend, then repeat with the lower leg internally rotated. Pain associated with audible sounds or palpable crepitus suggests a tear of the meniscus. **This test may be difficult to complete if there is acute pain and muscle spasm.**

✔ After examining for ligamentous and meniscal injuries, palpate the knee to localize areas of point tenderness and determine the extent of any joint effusion. **Tenderness from meniscal tears is localized along the joint line,** most prominently at or posterior to the collateral ligament. **Palpate the patella and head of the fibula looking for tenderness associated with fracture. Assess for effusion** by placing a finger lightly on the patella with the knee fully extended and, with the other hand, gently pinching the soft tissue on both sides of the patella feeling for a fluid wave. In the presence of an intraarticular effusion, the patella can also be bounced or ballotted against the underlying femoral condyle.

✔ **X-rays to rule out fracture may be deferred or avoided if the patient does not meet one of the following Ottawa criteria:**
- 55 years of age or older
- Tenderness at the head of the fibula
- Isolated tenderness of the patella
- Inability to flex the knee to 90 degrees
- Inability to bear weight (four steps) both immediately after injury and at initial physical assessment

297

✔ These criteria do not apply to patients younger than 18 years of age or patients with an altered level of consciousness, multiple painful injuries, paraplegia, or diminished limb sensation.

✔ **Minor (grade one) sprains that do not exhibit any joint instability or intraarticular effusion can be treated with rest, elevation, ice (20-minute periods three or four times a day for 3 days), and NSAIDs (ibuprofen, naproxen).** The patient can usually return to her previous activities as rapidly as pain allows. Provide follow-up if symptoms do not improve in 5 to 7 days.

✔ **Moderate (grade II) and severe (grade III) sprains with partial or complete ligament tears, meniscal tears, joint effusion, or instability should be treated with rest and ice as above, but also immobilized with a bulky compression splint or knee immobilizer and made nonweight-bearing with crutches.** Patients should keep the leg elevated above the heart as much as possible to minimize swelling. **Narcotic analgesics may be added to NSAIDs, and patients should be referred for orthopedic assessment within 5 to 7 days.** Instruct the patient that additional injuries may become apparent as the spasm and effusion abate.

What Not To Do:

✘ Do not assume that a negative radiograph means a major injury does not exist.

✘ Do not rely on magnetic resonance imaging (MRI) to assess all injured knees. MRI is not cost-effective or superior to clinical assessment in accuracy.

✘ Do not inject or prescribe corticosteroids for acute knee injuries. These drugs may retard soft tissue healing.

 DISCUSSION

The vast majority of patients with a knee injury suffer soft tissue damage, including ligament, tendon, meniscal cartilage, and muscle tears. In most cases, plain radiographs do little to aid diagnosis of soft tissue injury. Physicians must rely on physical examination to identify patients with serious knee injuries that require orthopedic referral. Joint aspiration of hemarthrosis to reduce severe pain should be reserved for patients with very large or tense effusions and should be performed with sterile technique. Fat globules in bloody joint fluid suggest occult fracture.

In general, a patient who has had a knee injury can be given the go-ahead to resume sports activities when examination demonstrates that the cruciate and collateral ligaments are intact, the knee is capable of moving from full extension to flexion of 120 degrees, and there is no effusion. The patient's pain should be markedly diminished, and there should be no locking or limp.

SUGGESTED READINGS

Bauer SJ, Hollander JE, Fuchs SH, et al: A clinical decision rule in the evaluation of acute knee injuries, *J Emerg Med* 13:611-615, 1995.

Gelb HJ, Glasgow SG, Sapega AA, et al: Magnetic resonance imaging of knee disorders: clinical value and cost-effectiveness in a sports medicine practice, *Am J Sports Med* 24:99-103, 1996.

Johnson LL, Johnson AL, Colquitt JA, et al: Is it possible to make an accurate diagnosis based only on a medical history? A pilot study on women's knee joints, *Arthroscopy* 12:709-714, 1996.

Muellner T, Weinstabl R, Schabus R, et al: The diagnosis of meniscal tears in athletes: a comparison of clinical and magnetic resonance imaging investigations, *Am J Sports Med* 25:7-12, 1997.

O'Shea KJ, Murphy KP, Heekin RD, et al: The diagnostic accuracy of history, physical examination and radiographs in the evaluation of traumatic knee disorders, *Am J Sports Med* 24:164, 1996.

Stiell IG, Greeberg GH, Wells GA, et al: Derivation of a decision rule for the use of radiography in acute knee injuries, *Ann Emerg Med* 26:405-414, 1995.

Stiell IG, Greeberg GH, Wells GA, et al: Prospective validation of a decision rule for the use of radiography in acute knee injuries, *JAMA* 275:611-615, 1996.

Stiell IG, Wells GA, Hoag RH, et al: Implementation of the Ottawa knee rule for the use of radiography in acute knee injuries, *JAMA* 278:2071-2079, 1997.

Weber JE, Jackson RE, Peacock WF, et al: Clinical decision rules discriminate between fractures and nonfractures in acute isolated knee trauma, *Ann Emerg Med* 26:429-433, 1995.

111

Ligament Sprains (Including Joint Capsule Injuries)

Presentation

A joint is distorted beyond its normal anatomic limits (as when an ankle is inverted or a shoulder is dislocated and reduced). The patient may complain of a snapping or popping noise at the time of injury, immediate swelling, and loss of function (suggestive of second- or third-degree sprain or a fracture), or he may come in hours to days after the injury, complaining of gradually increasing swelling and resulting pain and stiffness (suggestive of a first- or second-degree sprain and development of a traumatic effusion).

What To Do:

✔ Obtain a detailed history of the mechanism of injury, and examine the joint for structural integrity, function, and point tenderness. Inability to fully extend an elbow is a strong indicator of significant injury. Use the uninjured limb as a control.

✔ Obtain x-rays (these can be deferred if findings are minimal with full range–of–motion without bony tenderness or if specific criteria are not met, as for knee and ankle sprains).

✔ **With first- and second-degree sprains, gently immobilize the joint using an elastic bandage alone or in combination with a cotton roll or plaster splint, as discomfort demands. Dynamic bracing (such as ankle stirrup splints and hinge knee braces) should be used with stable injuries when available.** Most upper extremity injuries can be immobilized by a sling alone or in combination with a soft or rigid splint.

✔ **Consider prescribing antiinflammatory pain medication when the patient complains of pain at rest and provide crutches when discomfort will not allow weight-bearing.**

✔ **If there is a fracture or ligament tear with instability, the limb is usually best immobilized in a splint or cast. Splint ankles at 90 degrees, wrists in extension, fingers at slight flexion.**

✔ **Instruct the patient in rest, elevation above the level of the heart, and application of ice 10 to 20 minutes each hour for the first few hours then three or four times a day for 3 days. Minor injuries may need only 1 day of treatment.**

✔ Explain to the patient that swelling in acute musculoskeletal injuries usually increases for the first 24 hours, and then decreases over the next 2 to 4 days (longer if the treatment above is not employed), and that some swelling and discomfort may persist for several weeks and at times for several months.

✔ **Advocate early mobilization and early return to normal functions for first- and second-degree sprains.**

✔ Explain the possibility of occult injuries, the necessity for follow-up, and the slow healing of injured ligaments (usually 6 months until full strength is regained).

What Not To Do:

✘ Do not obtain x-rays before the history or physical examination. Films of the wrong spot can be very misleading. For example, physicians have been steered away from the diagnosis of an avulsion fracture of the base of the fifth metatarsal by the presence of normal ankle films.

✘ Do not base the diagnosis on x-rays. They should be used as confirmatory evidence.

✘ Do not obtain routine comparison views on pediatric patients. They usually do not improve diagnostic accuracy.

 DISCUSSION

Ligamentous injuries are classified as first-degree (minimal stretching); second-degree (a partial tear with functional loss and bleeding but still holding); and third-degree (complete tear with ligamentous instability, often requiring a cast). A tense joint effusion will limit the physical examination (and is one reason to require reevaluation after the swelling has decreased) but also suggests less than a third-degree ligamentous injury, which is normally accompanied by a tear of the joint capsule, and release of any tense effusion.

112

Locked Knee

Presentation

A patient, usually with a history of a previous knee injury, and often with previous knee locking, suddenly develops a mechanical inability to extend her knee fully. The knee may flex but not extend and may be causing mild-to-moderate pain.

What To Do:

✔ Perform a complete knee examination, checking for point tenderness, effusion, meniscal tear, and joint stability. **If comfort allows, gently and repeatedly perform the maneuvers of McMurray's test** (see Chapter 110). **This alone may release the locked knee. If not, continue as described below.**

✔ **Obtain knee x-rays** looking for a osteocartilaginous loose body or other pathology.

✔ Prep the knee with povidone-iodine solution and, at a point just superior and lateral to the patella, using a 25-gauge 1-inch needle, inject 10 ml of 0.5% bupivacaine (Marcaine) into the joint space.

✔ **With the knee thus anesthetized, place a roll of towels under the heel and ankle to serve as a fulcrum. Leave the patient supine so gravity will aid in extension and have the patient gently rock and rotate the knee for 20 minutes.**

✔ **When the mechanical block is dislodged and the knee extended, place the patient in a knee immobilizer, keep her nonweight-bearing with crutches, and refer her to an orthopedic surgeon for early arthroscopic examination and definitive treatment.**

What Not To Do:

✘ Do not forcefully manipulate the knee. This may produce further intraarticular injury.

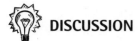 **DISCUSSION**

Knee locking is usually caused by previous injuries that include meniscal tears, partial or complete anterior cruciate ligament tears, osteocartilaginous loose bodies, pathologic medial plicae, and foreign bodies. Less commonly, locking can occur without a history of trauma. In such cases, the cause may be torsion of the infrapatellar fat pad or an intraarticular tumor such as a ganglion. In a locked knee, one of those structures has become entrapped between the tibial plateau and the femoral condyles, mechanically blocking extension of the joint.

113

Lumbar Strain ("Mechanical" Low Back Pain, Sacroiliac Dysfunction), Acute

Presentation

Suddenly or gradually after lifting, sneezing, bending, or other movement, the patient develops a steady pain in one or both sides of the lower back. At times, this pain can be severe and incapacitating. It is usually better on lying down, worse with movement, and will perhaps radiate around the abdomen or down the thigh but no farther. There is insufficient trauma to suspect bony injury (e.g., a fall or direct blow), and no evidence of systemic disease that would make bony pathology likely (e.g., osteoporosis, metastatic carcinoma, multiple myeloma). On physical examination, there may be spasm in the paraspinous muscles (i.e., contraction that does not relax, even when the patient is supine or when the opposing muscle groups contract, as with walking in place), but there is no point tenderness over the spinous processes of lumbar vertebrae and no nerve root signs such as pain or paresthesia in dermatomes below the knee (especially with straight leg raising), no foot weakness, and no loss of the ankle jerk. There may be point tenderness to firm palpation or percussion over the sacroiliac joint, especially if the pain is on that side.

What To Do:

✔ Perform a complete history and physical examination of the abdomen, back, and legs, looking for alternative causes for the back pain.

✔ Consider plain x-rays of the lumbosacral spine of patients who have suffered injury sufficient to cause bony injury (even mild trauma over 50 years of age), patients under 20 years of age or over 50 years of age who have had pain more than a month, patients who are on long-term corticosteroid medication, patients with a history of osteoporosis or cancer, and patients over 70 years of age. A negative x-ray does not rule out disease.

✔ Order an erythrocyte sedimentation rate (ESR) on patients with a history of cancer or IV drug abuse or signs or symptoms of underlying systemic disease (e.g., unexplained weight loss, fatigue, night sweats, fever, lymphadenopathy, and back pain at night or unrelieved by bed rest). Bone scans, CT scans, or MRI may be better than plain radiographs in these patients.

✔ **For point tenderness over a sacroiliac joint with no neurologic findings to suggest nerve root compression or any indication of underlying systemic disease, try an intraarticular injection of a local anesthetic mixed with a corticosteroid.** Improvement of pain is both diagnostic and therapeutic. Draw up 10 ml of 0.5% bupivacaine (Marcaine) mixed with 1 ml (40 mg) of methylprednisolone (Depo-Medrol) or 1 to 2 ml (6 to 12 mg) of betamethasone (Celestone Soluspan). Using a 1¼-inch, 25-gauge needle and sterile technique, inject deeply into the sacroiliac joint at the point of maximal tenderness or into the dimple immediately lateral to the sacrum (Figure 113-1). When the needle is in the joint there should be a free flow of medication from the syringe without causing soft tissue swelling. During the injection, the patient may feel a brief increase of pain, followed by dramatic relief in 5 to 20 minutes that is usually permanent. Warn the patient that there may be a flare in pain when the anesthetic wears off that could last for 24 to 48 hours.

✔ **For point tenderness of the lumbosacral muscles, inject 10 to 20 ml of 0.25% to 0.5% bupivacaine (Marcaine) deeply into the points of maximal tenderness of the erector spinae and quadratus lumborum muscles,** using a 1¼-inch, 25-gauge needle. Quickly puncture the skin, drive the needle into the muscle belly, and inject the anesthetic, slowly advancing or withdrawing, fanning out the medication. Often one fan block can reduce symptoms by 95% after injection and yield a 75% permanent reduction of painful spasms. Following injection, teach stretching exercises.

✔ **For severe pain that cannot be relieved by injections of local anesthetic, it may be necessary to provide the patient with 1 to 2 days of bed rest, although the majority of patients with acute low back pain recover more rapidly by continuing ordinary activities** within the limits permitted by their pain than with bed rest or back-mobilizing exercises.

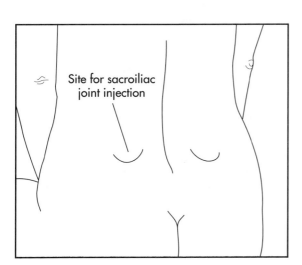

Site for sacroiliac
joint injection

Figure 113-1 The dimple on either side of the sacrum can serve as a landmark for injecting a painful sacroiliac joint.

✔ **Consider disk herniation when leg pain overshadows the back pain.** Back pain may subside as leg pain worsens. This pain tends to worsen with coughing, Valsalva maneuver, trunk flexion, and prolonged sitting or standing. Look for weakness of ankle or great toe dorsiflexion (drooping of the big toe and inability to heel walk) and sensory changes over the medial dorsal foot when there is compression of the fifth lumbar nerve root. Look for weak plantarflexion (inability to toe walk), diminished ankle reflex, and paresthesias of the lateral foot when there is first sacral root compression. Raise each leg 30 degrees from the horizontal and consider the test positive for nerve root compression if it produces pain down the leg along a nerve root distribution, rather than pain in the back, increased by dorsiflexion of the foot and relieved by plantarflexion. Ipsilateral straight-leg raising is a moderately sensitive but not a specific test. A herniated intervertebral disk is more strongly indicated when contralateral radicular pain is reproduced in one leg by raising the opposite leg. If nerve root compression is suspected, prescribe short-term bed rest and NSAIDs and arrange for general medical, orthopedic, or neurosurgical referral. Some consultants recommend short-term corticosteroid treatment such as prednisone 50 mg qd × 5 days. The patient should try 4 to 6 weeks of conservative treatment before submitting to an operation on the herniated disk. Eighty per cent of patients with sciatica recover with or without surgery. The rare cauda equina syndrome is the only complication of lumbar disk herniation that calls for emergent surgical referral. It occurs when a massive extrusion of disk nucleus compresses the caudal sac containing lumbar and sacral nerve roots, producing bilateral radicular leg pain or weakness, bladder or bowel dysfunction, perineal or perianal anesthesia, decreased rectal sphincter tone in 60% to 80% of cases, and urinary retention in 90% of cases. An emergent MRI is the study of choice for confirming this diagnosis.

✔ **Prescribe a short course of antiinflammatory analgesics (aspirin, ibuprofen, naproxen) for patients who are not already taking NSAIDs.** Because gastric bleeding and renal insufficiency are common with long-term use of NSAIDs, consider substituting acetaminophen (Tylenol) 1000 mg q4-6h (maximum four doses daily) or salsalate (Disalcid) two 750 mg tabs bid or two 500 mg tabs tid.

✔ **Prescribe ice to the acutely injured area, 20 minutes per hour for the first day.** (This therapy is unconventional but works as well as it does for any other musculoskeletal injury.)

✔ **Refer patients with uncomplicated back pain to their primary care provider for follow-up care in 3 to 7 days. Reassure patients that back pain is seldom disabling and that it usually resolves rapidly with their return to normal activity.** Tell patients that the pain may be recurrent and that cigarette smoking, sedentary activity, and obesity are risk factors for back pain. Teach them to avoid twisting and bending when lifting, and show them how to lift with the back vertical, using thigh muscles and holding heavy objects close to their chest to avoid reinjury. Encourage them to return to work or resume normal activities as soon as possible and to participate in an aerobic exercise program when the pain has subsided.

What Not To Do:

✘ Do not be eager to use narcotic pain medicines. The sensation of pain from an acute musculoskeletal injury reminds the patient not to use the damaged part and exacerbate the injury but instead to keep it at rest and speed healing. Narcotics are also apt to make the patient constipated, and straining at stool can be especially uncomfortable with a back injury.

✘ Do not be too eager to use antispasm medicines. Many have sedative or anticholinergic side effects.

✘ Do not apply lumbar traction. It has not been proven to be any better than placebo for relieving back pain. Do not provide orthotics, back braces, or lumbar cushions. They have no proven benefit. Lumbar supports have not been proven to reduce the incidence of low back pain in industrial workers and should not be routinely recommended for the prevention of low back pain.

✘ Do not recommend bed rest for more than 4 days. It is not helpful and may further debilitate the patient.

DISCUSSION

Low back pain is a common and sometimes chronic problem that accounts for an enormous amount of disability and time lost from work. The approach discussed here is geared only to the management of acute injuries and flareups, from which most people recover on their own, which leaves only about 10% developing chronic problems. With acute pain, reassurance plus limited medication may be the most useful intervention.

History and physical examination are essential to rule out serious pathologic conditions that can present as low back pain but require quite different treatment—aortic aneurysm, pyelonephritis, pancreatitis, pelvic inflammatory disease, ectopic pregnancy, retroperitoneal or epidural abscess.

The standard five-view x-ray study of the lumbosacral spine may entail 500 mrem of radiation and yet only 1 in 2500 lumbar spine plain films of adults below 50 years of age show an unexpected abnormality. In fact, many radiographic anomalies such as spina bifida occulta, single-disk narrowing, spondylosis, facet joint abnormalities, and several congenital anomalies are equally common in symptomatic and asymptomatic individuals. It is estimated that the gonadal dose of radiation absorbed from a five-view lumbosacral series is equivalent to that from 6 years of daily AP and lateral chest films. The World Health Organization now recommends that oblique views be reserved for problems remaining after review of AP and lateral films. For simple cases of low back pain, even with radicular findings, both CT scans and MRI are overly sensitive and often reveal anatomic abnormalities that have no clinical significance.

While adults are more apt to have disk abnormalities, muscle strain, and degenerative changes associated with low back pain, athletically active adolescents are more likely to have

307

Continued

DISCUSSION—cont'd

posterior element derangements like stress fractures of the pars interarticularis. Early recognition of this spondylolysis and treatment by bracing and limitation of activity may prevent nonunion, persistent pain, and disability.

Malingering and drug-seeking are major psychological components to consider in patients who have frequent visits for back pain and whose responses seem overly dramatic or otherwise inappropriate. These patients may move around with little difficulty when they do not know they are being observed. They may complain of generalized superficial tenderness when you lightly pinch the skin over the affected lumbar area. If suspicious that the patient's pain is psychosomatic or nonorganic, use the axial loading test, in which the head of the standing person is gently pressed down on. This should not cause significant musculoskeletal back pain. The rotation test can also be performed, in which the patient stands with his arms at his sides. Hold his wrists next to his hips and turn his body from side to side, passively rotating his shoulders, trunk, and pelvis as a unit. This maneuver creates the illusion that the spinal rotation is being tested, but in fact the spinal axis has not been altered and any complaint of back pain should be suspect.

SUGGESTED READINGS

Carey TS, Garrett J, Jackman A, et al: The outcomes and costs of care for acute low back pain among patients seen by primary care practitioners, chiropractors and orthopedic surgeons. *N Engl J Med* 333:913-917, 1995.

Deyo RA, Diehl AK, Rosenthal M: How many days of bed rest for acute low back pain? *N Engl J Med* 315:1064-1070, 1986.

Deyo RA, Rainville J, Kent DL: What can the history and physical examination tell us about low back pain? *JAMA* 268:760-765, 1992.

Elam KC, Cherkin DC, Deyo RA: How emergency physicians approach low back pain: choosing costly options, *J Emerg Med* 13:143-150, 1995.

Malmivaara A, Hakkinen U, Aro T, et al: The treatment of acute low back pain: bed rest, exercise, or ordinary activity? *N Engl J Med* 332:351-355, 1995.

Suarez-Almazor ME, Belseck E, Russell AS, et al: Use of lumbar radiographs for the early diagnosis of low back pain: proposed guidelines would increase utilization, *JAMA* 277:1782-1786, 1997.

van Poppel MNM, Koes BW, van der Ploeg T, et al: Lumbar supports and education for the prevention of low back pain in industry: a randomized controlled trial, *JAMA* 279:1789-1794, 1998. (editorial 1826-1827)

van Tulder MW, Assendelft WJ, Koes BW, et al: Spinal radiographic findings and nonspecific low back pain. A systematic review of observational studies, *Spine* 22:427-434, 1997.

van Tulder MW, Koes BW, Bouter LM: Conservative treatment of acute and chronic nonspecific low back pain. A systematic review of randomized controlled trials of the most common interventions, *Spine* 22:2128-2156, 1997.

van Tulder MW, Koes BW, Bouter LM, et al: Management of chronic nonspecific low back pain in primary care: a descriptive study, *Spine* 22:76-82, 1997.

114

Monarticular Arthritis, Acute

Presentation

The patient complains of one joint that has become acutely red, swollen, hot, painful, and stiff, with pain on minimal range of motion. Rapid onset with fever and local warmth suggests the possibility of septic arthritis. A migratory tendonitis or arthritis often precedes gonococcal monoarthritis. A history of similar attacks, especially of the first metatarsophalangeal joint, suggests the possibility of gouty arthritis. A history of recurrent knee swelling with minimal erythema and gradual onset after overuse or minor trauma is more likely associated with osteoarthritis and pseudogout.

What To Do:

✔ Ask about previous, similar episodes in this or other joints, as well as trauma, systemic illness, tick bites (Lyme arthritis), sexual risk factors, IV drug use, infections, or rashes, and ask for any history of gout (see Chapter 109). Perform a thorough physical examination, looking for evidence of the above. Obtain cervical or urethral swabs for culture and Gram stain when you suspect gonococcal arthritis because cultures of synovial fluid are positive in only about a quarter of patients.

✔ Examine the affected joint and document the extent of effusion, involvement of adjacent structures, and degree of erythema, tenderness, heat, and limitation of range of motion. Fluid can often be detected by pressing on one side of the affected joint and at the same time palpating a wavelike fluctuance on the opposite side of the joint.

✔ Send a blood sample for complete blood count and ESR. When sepsis is suspected, obtain blood cultures. Serum uric acid measurement is not always helpful and may be misleading. Lyme antibodies may be appropriate when there is a reasonable clinical suspicion.

✔ **Obtain x-rays of the affected joint to detect possible unsuspected fractures or evidence of chronic disease, such as rheumatoid, crystal-induced chondrocalcinosis of pseudogout arthritis or osteoarthritis.**

✔ **Perform arthrocentesis to remove joint fluid for analysis, to relieve pain and, in the case of septic or crystal-induced arthritis, to reduce the bacterial and crystal load within the joint.** Using sterile technique throughout, cleanse the skin over the

309

most superficial area of the joint effusion with alcohol and povidone-iodine (Betadine), anesthetize the skin with 1% plain buffered lidocaine, and aspirate as much joint fluid as possible through an 18- to 20-gauge needle. The joint space of the **knee** (Figure 114-1, *A*) may be entered medially or laterally with the leg fully extended and the patient lying supine. Hold the needle parallel to the bed surface and direct it just posterior to the patella, into the subpatellar space. The **elbow** joint (Figure 114-1, *B*) is best entered at about 30 degrees of flexion, with the needle introduced proximal to the olecranon process of the ulna and just below the lateral epicondyle. Advance the needle medially into the joint space. The best site for needle entry of the **wrist** is on the dorsal radial aspect, at the proximal end of the anatomic snuff box and the distal articulation of the radius. Place the wrist in about 20 degrees of flexion and introduce the needle perpendicular to the skin, advancing it toward the ulna, into the joint space (Figure 114-1, *C*). The **ankle** joint (Figure 114-1, *D*) may be entered with the patient supine, the knee ex-

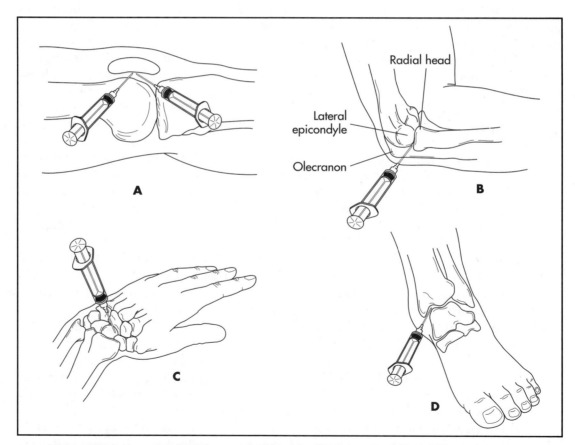

Figure 114-1 Entry sites for arthrocentesis. (*A and **D**, Illustrations provided by Dr. D.H. Neustadt. **B** and **C**, Adapted from Akins CM: Aspiration and injection of joints, bursae and tendons. In Vander Salm et al, editors:* Atlas of bedside procedures, *ed 2, Boston, 1988, Little Brown & Co.)*

tended, and the foot plantarflexed. Find the small depression that is just medial to the extensor hallucis longus and tibialis anterior tendons, inferior to the distal tibia, then direct your needle into the tibiotalar articulation. For small joints, enter the midline on the dorsolateral aspect and advance a small needle into the joint space. Joints of the digits may have to be distracted by pulling on the end to enlarge the joint space. Fluoroscopy may be valuable in guiding needle placement for hip or shoulder joint aspiration.

✔ Grossly examine the joint aspirate. Clear, light-yellow fluid is characteristic of osteoarthritis or mild inflammatory or traumatic effusions. Grossly cloudy fluid is characteristic of more severe inflammation or bacterial infection. Blood in the joint is characteristic of trauma (a fracture or tear inside the synovial capsule) or bleeding from hemophilia or anticoagulants.

✔ One drop of joint fluid may be used for a crude string or mucin clot test. Wet the tips of two gloved fingers with joint fluid, and repeatedly touch them together and slowly draw them apart. As this maneuver is repeated 10 or 20 times, and the joint fluid dries, normal synovial fluid will form longer and longer strings, usually to 5 to 10 cm in length. Inflammation inhibits this string formation. This is a nonspecific test but may aid decision-making at the bedside.

✔ **The most important laboratory tests on joint fluid consist of a Gram's stain and culture for possible septic arthritis.** Gram-positive bacteria can be seen in 80% of culture-positive synovial fluid, but gram-negative bacteria are seen less often; gram-negative diplococci are seen rarely.

✔ **A joint fluid total and differential leukocyte count is the next most useful test to order. A count greater than 50,000 WBC/mm³ is characteristic of bacterial infection** (especially when >90% are polymorphonuclear neutrophils). In **osteoarthritis,** there are usually fewer than 2000 WBC/mm³, and **inflammatory arthritis** (such as gout and rheumatoid arthritis) falls in the middle range of 2000 to 50,000 WBC/mm³.

✔ **Send a wet prep looking for crystals.** Identification of crystals can establish a diagnosis of gout or pseudogout and avoid unnecessary hospitalization for suspected infectious arthritis.

✔ If there is more fluid, send it to the lab for a glucose level, which will be less than half the serum level if there is a joint infection.

✔ **If there is any suspicion of a bacterial infection (based on fever, elevated ESR, cellulitis, lymphangitis, or the joint fluid results) start the patient on appropriate antibiotics based on the results of the Gram's stain.** Adequate treatment should include aspiration of synovial fluid on a daily basis and hospitalization for IV antibiotics. In older patients, use nafcillin (Unipen) or cefuroxime (Zinacef), plus gentamicin (Garamycin). For penicillin-allergic patients and patients with *Staphylococcus aureus* on Gram's stain and rheumatoid arthritis, use vancomycin (Vancocin) or clindamycin (Cleocin). For patients with suspected gonococcus, use ceftriaxone (Rocephin). For children less than 3 years of age, prescribe nafcillin (Unipen) or oxacillin (Prostaphlin) plus cefotaxime (Claforan).

✔ **Inflammatory arthritis may be treated with NSAIDs, beginning with a loading dose such as indomethacin (Indocin) 50 mg or ibuprofen (Motrin) 800 mg,**

311

tapered to usual maintenance doses. If infection can be confidently excluded from the diagnosis, then intraarticular injections of depot preparations of corticosteroids can be a useful adjunctive or alternative therapy. Using aseptic technique, prep the skin with povidone-iodine and alcohol. Using the techniques described above, with a 3- to 5-ml syringe and a 1¼-inch needle, inject 1 to 2 ml of 40 mg/ml methylprednisolone (Depo-Medrol) with 2 to 4 ml of bupivacaine (Marcaine) into the affected joint. For finger or toe joints, use a smaller volume (0.2 to 0.5 ml) of the more concentrated (80 mg/ml) methylprednisolone along with a lesser volume of bupivacaine. Warn patients of the 10% to 15% risk of postinjection flare or recurrent pain for 24 to 48 hours after the local anesthetic wears off.

✔ **When joint fluid cannot be obtained to rule out infection, it may be a good tactic to treat simultaneously for infectious and inflammatory arthritis.**

✔ **Splint and elevate the affected joint and arrange for admission or follow-up.**

What Not To Do:

✘ Do not tap a joint through an area of obvious contamination such as subcutaneous cellulitis. Synovial fluid may consequently be inoculated with bacteria.

✘ Do not be misled by bursitis, tenosynovitis, or myositis without joint involvement. An infected or inflamed joint will have a reactive effusion, which may be evident as fullness, fluctuance, reduced range of motion, or joint fluid that can be drawn off with a needle. It is usually difficult to tap a joint in the absence of a joint effusion.

✘ Do not treat hyperuricemia with drugs that lower uric acid levels, such as allopurinol or probenecid, during an acute attack of gout (see Chapter 109).

✘ Do not use NSAIDs when a patient has a history of active peptic ulcer disease with bleeding. Relative contraindications include renal insufficiency, volume depletion, gastritis, inflammatory bowel disease, asthma, and congestive heart disease.

✘ Do not start maintenance NSAID doses for an acute inflammation. It will take 1 day or more to reach therapeutic levels and pain relief.

 DISCUSSION

The urgent reason for tapping a joint effusion is to rule out a bacterial infection, which could destroy the joint cartilage in as little as 1 or 2 days. Beyond identifying an infection (with Gram's stain, culture, and WBC) further diagnosis of the cause of arthritis is not particularly accurate nor is it necessary to decide on specific acute treatment. Reducing the volume of the effusion may alleviate pain and stiffness, but this effect is usually short-lived, as the effusion reaccummulates within hours. Identification of crystals is essential for the diagnosis of gout or pseudogout, but one acute attack may be treated the same as another inflammatory arthritis, and exact diagnosis may be deferred to follow-up.

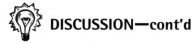

DISCUSSION—cont'd

Infants and young children may present with fever and reluctance to walk from septic arthritis of the hip or knee, and arthrocentesis may require sedation or general anesthesia.

Acute arthritis in prosthetic joints is always of concern. Infections in prostheses are disastrous and require urgent consultation.

SUGGESTED READINGS

Baker DG, Schumacher HR: Acute monoarthritis, *N Engl J Med* 329:1013-1020, 1993.

115 Muscle Cramps

Presentation

The patient complains of painful, visible, palpable muscle contractions, often affecting the gastrocnemius muscle or small muscles of the foot or hand. Ordinary cramps occur chiefly at rest or after trivial movement but also can occur after forceful muscle contraction. Other muscle cramps are associated with exercise in the heat, occupations that cause overuse, and drug or alcohol use. Most cramps are transient in nature, but they are likely to recur after a severe episode. Following this, the muscles may be tender and painful for some time.

What To Do:

✔ **Look for a specific underlying cause. Unaccustomed exercise and salt depletion from sweating are common precipitating causes. Drug-induced cramps can include those from alcohol, lithium, cimetidine, nifedipine, antipsychotic medications** (see Chapter 2), **clofibrate, and others. Hyponatremia, hypokalemia, hyperkalemia, hypocalcemia, hypomagnesemia, and respiratory alkalosis** (see Chapter 3) **can all cause muscle cramping.**

✔ **Address any specific cause. IV fluids with electrolyte replacement will help with heat cramps and alcohol-induced cramps.**

✔ Ordinary muscle cramps can be treated with passive stretching.

✔ **For severe, persistent cramping, try muscle relaxants like cyclobenzaprine (Flexeril) 10 mg tid, methocarbamol (Robaxin) 750 mg qid, or orphenadrine (Norflex) 100 mg bid.**

✔ Provide appropriate follow-up to patients who have more than benign self-limited cramps.

What Not To Do:

✗ Do not ignore muscle weakness, fasciculations, and wasting, which are signs of lower motor neuron disorders including amyotrophic lateral sclerosis, polyneuropathy, peripheral nerve injury, and nerve root compression.

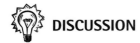 **DISCUSSION**

Most muscle cramps are thought to be caused by hyperactivity of the peripheral or central nervous system rather than the muscle itself. The pain results from a combination of ischemia, accumulation of metabolites, and possible damage to the muscle fibers. Electromyographic studies indicate that during ordinary muscle cramps, motor units fire at about 300/second, far more rapidly than any voluntary contraction. This rapid firing rate causes the muscle tightness and pain.

There are reports that nitroglycerin paste applied to the overlying skin may relieve a muscle cramp rapidly, but the dose must be small to avoid hypotension, headache, and flushing.

116

Muscle Strains and Tears

Presentation

Strains are acute injuries to muscle-tendon units that result from overstretching or overexerting. Strains may occur in the trapezius or paravertebral muscles during an automobile accident with a whiplash-type injury to the neck, or in the hamstring group or gastrocnemius muscle while accelerating, running, or playing in a sport like tennis. There may be an insidious development of pain and tightness, which is worse with use and better with rest, or with more severe injury the pain may be immediate and disabling. Tears of the muscle belly tend to be partial, with sudden onset of pain and partial loss of function. Often a tear occurs with considerable bleeding, which can lead to remarkable hematomas, causing swelling at the site and dissecting along tissue planes to create ecchymoses at distant, uninvolved sites. Complete tears are more likely in the tendinous part of the muscle and produce immediate loss of function and retraction of the torn end, creating a deformity and bulge.

What To Do:

✔ Obtain a history of the mechanism of injury and test individual muscle functions. **A complete tear of a muscle merits orthopedic consultation.**

✔ Even for a partial tear of a muscle belly, try to refine the diagnosis to a specific muscle or muscle group to help exclude other possibilities.

✔ **For mild-to-moderate muscle strains, provide soft splinting, NSAIDs, and instruct the patient to apply warm, moist compresses for comfort.** Soak towels in hot water or put damp towels in a microwave oven and apply for 20 to 30 minutes at a time, reheating every 5 minutes.

✔ **Ice massage may be preferable to heat in the first 1 to 3 days.** Freeze water in a small paper or styrofoam cup, tear off the upper rim to expose the ice, then massage the injured muscle with the ice using slow circular strokes for 5 to 20 minutes, using the cup as an insulator.

✔ **For muscle tears, construct a loose splint to immobilize the injured part and instruct the patient in rest, NSAIDs, elevation, and ice compresses.**

✔ When pain requires maximum immobilization, add a soft cervical collar, sling, or crutches but encourage the patient to resume movement as soon as comfortable.

✔ Warn the patient that partial tears can become complete and that blood will change color and percolate to the skin at distant sites, where it does not imply additional injury. Arrange for follow-up.

What Not To Do:

✗ Do not order x-rays when the injury is clearly isolated to a muscle or tendon and there is no bony involvement.

 ## DISCUSSION

Some restrict the terms *strain* for muscle injuries and *sprain* for ligament injuries. Grading the severity of strains is similar to judging the severity of sprains. In mild strains, muscles or tendons develop a few torn fibers. The patient can contract the muscle forcefully, but the movement brings pain. More tearing occurs in moderate strains, and pain and weakness are present when the patient contracts the muscle. Complete rupture of the muscle or tendon is a severe strain.

Heat and cold treatments facilitate early range of motion, relieve pain, and encourage an earlier return to normal function. It may be helpful to alternate heat and cold treatments and allow the patient to choose which is better for relieving pain or improving range of motion.

A complete tear of the plantaris tendon in the leg is difficult to differentiate from a partial tear of the medial head of the gastrocnemius muscle, but the treatment for both is the same (see Chapter 120).

117

Myofascial Syndrome (Fibromyalgia, Trigger Points)

Presentation

In myofascial syndrome, the patient, generally 25 to 50 years of age, will be troubled by the gradual onset of fibromuscular pain that at times can be immobilizing. There may be a previous history of acute strain, muscle spasm, or nerve root irritation (e.g., whiplash injury of the neck or low back strain). The areas most commonly affected include the posterior muscles of the neck and scapula, the soft tissues lateral to the thoracic and lumbar spine, and the sacroiliac joints.

The patient with fibromyalgia is often depressed or under emotional or physical stress, has associated fatigue with disturbed sleep, and has sensations of numbness or swelling in the hands and feet. Cold weather may be one of the precipitating causes of pain.

In both syndromes, there should be no swelling, erythema, or heat over the painful areas, but applying firm pressure over the site with an examining finger will cause the patient to wince with pain. This tender "trigger point" is usually no larger than a finger tip and when pressed will cause local pain, referred pain, or both. There may be a subtle palpable swelling at the point of maximum tenderness.

What To Do:

✔ **When a trigger point is found, map out its exact location (point of maximum tenderness) and place an X over the site with a marker or ball-point pen.** If the trigger point is diffuse, there is no need to outline its location (Figure 117-1).

✔ Obtain a careful history and perform a general physical examination to help exclude the possibility of a serious underlying disorder, such as rheumatoid arthritis or cancer.

✔ With any suspicion that an underlying problem exists, obtain an x-ray or an erythrocyte sedimentation rate. These studies should be normal in both fibromyalgia and myofascial syndrome.

✔ **Where trigger points are diffuse, prescribe an NSAID** such as naproxen (Anaprox) 275 mg two tablets stat then one qid, or ibuprofen (Motrin) 800 mg stat then 600 mg qid × 5 days. A muscle relaxant like cyclobenzaprine (Flexeril) 10 mg tid may also be helpful.

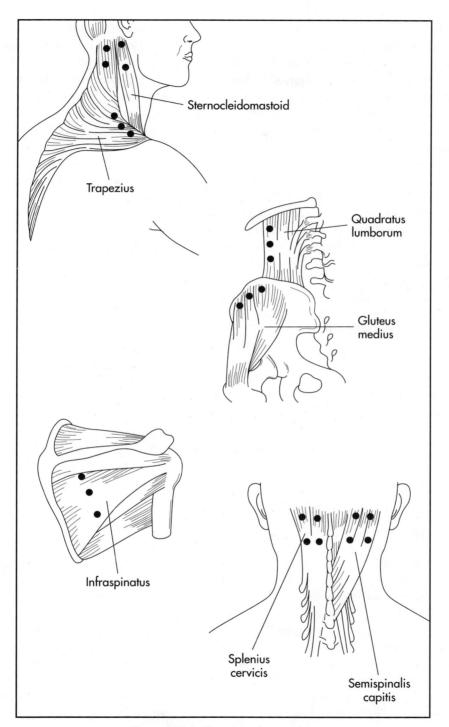

Figure 117-1 Common trigger points.

✔ **When a focal trigger point is present, suggest that the patient may get immediate relief with an injection. Inject 2 to 5 ml of l% lidocaine (Xylocaine) or longer-acting 0.5% bupivacaine (Marcaine) along with 20 to 40 mg of methylprednisolone (Depo Medrol) or 2 to 5 mg of triamcinolone (Aristospan) through the mark you placed on the skin, directly into the painful site.** Be sure you are not in a blood vessel or pleural cavity and then "fan" the needle in all directions while injecting the trigger point. In addition, massage the area after the injection is complete to ensure total coverage. The patient will often get complete or near-complete pain relief, which helps to confirm the diagnosis of fibromyalgia or myofascial syndrome. The beneficial effect of this injection may last for weeks or months. A supplementary 5-day course of NSAIDs is optional.

✔ Moist, hot compresses and massage may also be comforting to the patient after discharge.

✔ **Inform the patient that after trigger point injection there may be a transient painful rebound. Antiinflammatory analgesics will help to reduce this potential discomfort.**

✔ Provide follow-up care for patients in the event that their symptoms do not clear and they require further diagnostic evaluation and therapy. For example, hypothyroidism and polymyalgia rheumatica coexist with or predispose to fibromyalgia, or the patient may develop dermatomyositis.

What Not To Do:

✘ Do not attempt to inject a very diffuse trigger point (more than two square centimeters) or multiple scattered sites as found in true fibromyalgia syndrome. Results are generally unsatisfactory.

✘ Do not prescribe narcotic analgesics or systemic steroids. They are no more effective and add side effects and the risk of dependence.

 DISCUSSION

Although the pathophysiology of fibromyalgia is unknown, it is a very real syndrome. Treatment may provide only partial symptomatic relief. True fibromyalgia syndrome usually occurs in women and is manifested by multiple tender sites over the limbs, pain on both sides of the body above and below the waist, weakness, insomnia, gastrointestinal problems, headaches, depression, and menstrual irregularity. It is a chronic condition requiring long-term management that may include physical therapy, exercise, patient education, and reassurance, along with sleep-enhancing medications like low-dose tricyclic antidepressants. NSAIDs and corticosteroids may be of little benefit.

Emergency physicians more often see trigger points associated with simple self-limiting regional myofascial pain syndromes, which appear to arise from muscles, muscle-tendon junc-

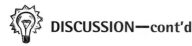

DISCUSSION—cont'd

tions, or tendon-bone junctions. Myofascial disease can result in severe pain, but it is typically in a limited distribution, without the systemic feature of fatigue, and without the multiple somatic complaints of fibromyalgia. When symptoms recur or persist after the basic therapy above or are accompanied by generalized complaints, emergency physicians should refer the patient to a rheumatologist or primary care physician for follow-up.

When the quadratus lumborum muscle is involved, there is often confusion as to whether or not the patient has a renal, abdominal, or pulmonary ailment. The reason for this is the muscle's proximity to the flank and abdomen, as well as its attachment to the twelfth rib, which when tender, can create pleuritic symptoms. A careful physical examination reproducing symptoms through palpation, active contraction, and passive stretching of this muscle can save this patient from a multitude of laboratory and x-ray studies.

118

Patellar Dislocation

Presentation

After a direct blow to the medial aspect of the patella or a sudden cutting motion to the oppo-site side of the planted foot (with contraction of the quadriceps and external rotation of the tibia on the femur), the patient's kneecap dislocates laterally. She is brought in with the knee slightly flexed, in severe pain, with the patella situated lateral to the lateral femoral condyle, creating an obvious lateral deformity (Figure 118-1). There may have been a spontaneous reduction, and the patient reports that the knee or kneecap slipped back into place.

What To Do:

✔ **For a persistent dislocation, provide immediate reduction. Gain the patient's confidence and cooperation while gently grasping the patella and stabilizing it by applying mild lateral traction and maintaining its position to prevent sudden motion. Have the patient gradually extend the knee. When it is fully extended, slowly release traction on the patella and gently let it slip into its normal anatomic position. This technique rarely requires any analgesia or sedation.**

✔ **Order knee x-rays, including patellar views,** to rule out an avulsion fracture of the superomedial pole of the patella, an osteochondral fracture of the lateral femoral condyle, or a fracture of the posterior patellar articular surface. There are associated fractures in 28% to 50% of patellar dislocations, which can lead to degenerative arthritis.

✔ **Fit the patient for crutches and a knee immobilizer that will keep the knee straight, provide analgesia, and instruct on the use of ice and elevation.** Teach nonweight-bearing walking with crutches.

✔ **Provide orthopedic follow-up in 1 to 3 days.**

What Not To Do:

✗ Do not try to force the patella to move medially. This may succeed in reduction but is unnecessarily painful and can cause harm.

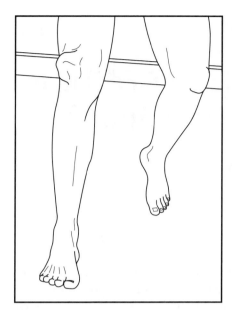

Figure 118-1 Patellar dislocation.

 DISCUSSION

Unlike medial collateral ligament injury, patellar dislocation disrupts the knee joint capsule. The resulting hemarthrosis, when it occurs, extravasates into the surrounding tissue and may cause swelling over the entire knee. Recurrent dislocations or associated fractures may require operative intervention.

119

Plantar Fasciitis ("Heel Spur")

Presentation

Patients seek help because of gradually increasing heel pain that has progressed to the point of inhibiting their normal daily activities. This fasciitis can develop in anyone who is ambulatory but appears to be more common in athletes (especially runners), those over 30 years of age, and the overweight. There is no defining episode of trauma. The most distinctive clue is exquisite pain in the plantar aspect of the heel when taking the first step in the morning. There is gradual improvement with walking, but as the day progresses, the pain may increase. First-step pain is also present after the patient has been sitting. The heel is tender to palpation over the medial calcaneal tubercle, exacerbated by dorsiflexion of the ankle and toes, particularly the great toe, which creates tension on the plantar fascia. Often the mid-fascia is tender to palpation too. There is generally no swelling or discoloration.

What To Do:

✔ **Obtain x-rays** to look for stress fractures of the metatarsals, calcifications, or osteophytes (spurs).

✔ **Prescribe NSAIDs for 2 to 3 weeks.**

✔ **Have the patient wear soft (viscoelastic) heel cushions like Bauerfeind Viscoheel** and a sports shoe with a firm impact-resistant heel counter and longitudinal arch support.

✔ **Ice massage can be helpful.** The patient can roll his heel over a can of frozen juice concentrate, followed by stretching.

✔ **Athletes should practice stretching the Achilles tendon before running by placing the sole flat, leaning forward against a counter or table, and slowly squatting while keeping the heel on the ground.** Others may stand, wearing tennis shoes, on the edge of a step, facing up stairs, slowly lowering their heels until they feel a pulling sensation in their upper calf. Hold for ½ to 1 minute or until there is pain. Repeat three times daily, increasing the stretch time to a maximum of 3 minutes per session. Although there may be a transient increase in pain after beginning this program, the heel pain usually begins to resolve within several weeks.

✔ **Have the patient reduce his ambulatory activities.** Have runners decrease their mileage by 25% to 75% and avoid sprinting, running on hard surfaces, and running up-hill. A program of cross training incorporating swimming and bicycling maintains cardiovascular fitness while decreasing stress on the feet.

✔ **When there is an exquisitely tender area on the medial calcaneus, local corticosteroid injection can speed recovery.** Palpate the heel pad to locate the point of maximum tenderness, cleanse the skin with povidone-iodine, and using a 25-gauge 1-inch needle, inject the area with 4 ml of bupivacaine (Marcaine) along with 1 ml of triamcinolone (Aristocort), betamethasone (Celestone Soluspan), or methylprednisolone (Depo-Medrol). **Enter medially and advance the needle parallel to the plantar fascia until you can feel its thick and gritty substance.** Inject half of the mixture at this exterior location and then punch through the fascia and inject the remainder deeper. Finish by massaging the heel pad to spread the medication (Figure 119-1).

What Not To Do:

✘ Do not inject into the heel pad itself, which may cause fat atrophy. Two or three injections at intervals of several weeks may be necessary.

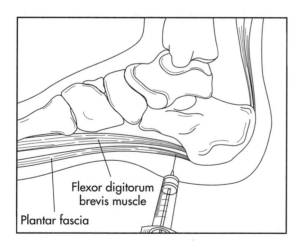

Plantar fascia

Flexor digitorum brevis muscle

Figure 119-1 Proper location for injection.

 DISCUSSION

Tightness of the Achilles tendon contributes to increased tension on the plantar fascia during walking or running and is therefore an important contributor to plantar fasciitis.

X-ray examination will reveal a calcaneal spur in 50% to 60% of patients with plantar fasciitis, but the heel spur is not the cause of the patient's pain. The pain is the result of chronic inflammation. The spur is formed by the traction of the plantar fascia where it attaches to the calcaneus and is seen in about 15% of asymptomatic feet.

Continued

DISCUSSION—cont'd

If a patient has persistent bilateral involvement, systemic disease may be the cause. Ankylosing spondylitis, Reiter's disease, rheumatoid arthritis, systemic lupus erythematosus, and gouty arthritis all may cause medial calcaneal pain.

In most patients with plantar fasciitis, conservative therapy works best. For the 10% or fewer with heel pain that persists for at least 1 year despite treatment, surgery should be considered. Chronic recurrences may indicate biomechanical imbalances in the foot, which may resolve with custom orthotics from a podiatrist.

120

"Plantaris Tendon" Rupture

Presentation

The patient will come in limping, having suffered a whiplike sting in her calf while stepping off hard on her foot or charging the net during a game of tennis or similar activity. She may have actually heard or felt a "snap" at the time of injury or may think someone kicked her or shot her in the calf. The deep calf pain persists and may be accompanied by mild-to-moderate swelling and ecchymosis. Neurovascular function will be intact.

What To Do:

✔ **Rule out an Achilles tendon rupture.** Test for strength in plantar flexion (can the patient walk on her toes?). **Palpate the Achilles tendon for a tender deformity that represents a torn segment. Squeeze the gastrocnemius muscle just distal to its widest girth, with the patient kneeling on a chair or lying prone on a stretcher with the legs overhanging the end, and look for the normal plantar flexion of the foot. This movement will be totally absent with a complete Achilles tendon tear** (Figure 120-1). With any Achilles tendon tear, orthopedic consultation is necessary.

✔ **When an Achilles tendon rupture has been ruled out, provide the patient with elastic support (e.g., Ace bandage, TEDs stocking, Tubigrip) from the foot to the tibial tuberosity and reassure her about the benign nature of this injury and an expected full recovery.**

✔ **Provide the patient with crutches for several days.** Permit weight-bearing only as comfort allows.

✔ Have the patient keep the leg elevated and at rest for the next 24 to 48 hours, initially applying cold packs, and after 48 hours alternating with heat every few hours.

✔ **An analgesic such as hydrocodone (e.g., Lorcet, Lortab) may be helpful initially, as well as NSAIDs.**

✔ The temporary use of a heel lift may also provide immediate comfort. Encourage patients to return to a heel-toe walking sequence as quickly as possible. When this is achieved, they can discontinue using the heel lift.

327

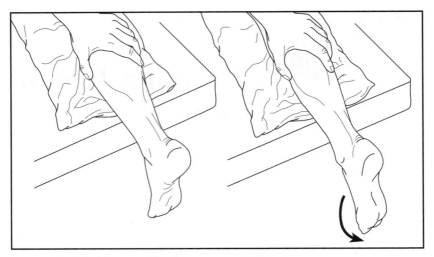

Figure 120-1 Thompson or "calf squeeze" test.

What Not To Do:

✗ Do not bother getting x-rays of the area unless there is a suspected associated bony injury. This is a soft tissue injury that is not generally associated with fractures.

✗ Do not attempt to evaluate Achilles tendon function merely by asking the patient to plantarflex the foot. Achilles tendon function is only isolated with the calf squeeze test.

 DISCUSSION

The plantaris muscle is a pencil-sized structure tapering down to a fine tendon that runs beneath the gastrocnemius and soleus muscles to attach to the Achilles tendon or to the medial side of the tubercle of the calcaneus. The function of the muscle is of little importance and, with rupture of either the muscle or the tendon, the transient disability is due only to the pain of the torn fibers or swelling from the hemorrhage. Clinical differentiation from complete rupture of the Achilles tendon is sometimes difficult to make. Most instances of "tennis leg" are now felt to be due to partial tears of the medial belly of the gastrocnemius muscle or to ruptures of blood vessels within that muscle. The greater the initial pain and swelling, the longer one can expect the disability to last.

The diagnosis of Achilles tendon rupture is missed in up to 25% of patients by the initial examiner. One misleading finding is that the patient is able to plantarflex the foot with no resistance because several other muscles (toe flexors, peroneus) also perform this action. The expected defect in the tendon may also be obscured by edema or hemorrhage. The squeeze test (Thompson test) is the only infallible sign of complete rupture.

121

Polymyalgia Rheumatica

Presentation

An elderly patient (more commonly female) complains of a month or more of morning stiffness, which may interfere with her ability to rise from bed, but improves during the day. She has had pain across her neck, shoulder girdle, and pelvic girdle. She may ascribe her problem to muscle weakness or joint pains, but physical examination discloses that symmetric pain and tenderness of neck, shoulder, and hip muscles are the actual source of any "weakness." There may be some mild arthritis of several peripheral joints, but the rest of the physical examination is negative other than appearing fatigued.

What To Do:

✔ Perform a complete history and physical examination, particularly of the cervical and lumbar spines and nerve roots (strength, sensation, and deep tendon reflexes in the distal limbs should be intact with polymyalgia rheumatica [PMR]). Confirm the diagnosis of PMR by palpating tender shoulder muscles (perhaps also hips, and less commonly, neck).

✔ **Confirm the diagnosis by obtaining an ESR, which should be in the 30 to 100 mm/hour range.** (An especially high ESR, over 100/hour, suggests more severe autoimmune disease or malignancy.)

✔ **Mild and borderline cases may respond to NSAIDs (ibuprofen, naproxen). More severe cases will respond to prednisone 10 to 60 mg qd within 1 to 2 weeks, after which the dose should be tapered.** Failure to respond to corticosteroid therapy suggests some other diagnosis.

✔ To allay a patient's fears of long-term steroids, inform her that once her sedimentation rate becomes normal, her dose can be gradually reduced.

✔ Explain the syndrome to the patient and arrange for follow-up.

What Not To Do:

✘ Do not miss temporal arteritis, a common component of the PMR syndrome and a clue to the existence of ophthalmic and cerebral arteritis, which can have dire neurologic consequences. Palpate the temporal arteries for tenderness, swelling, or induration, and ask about transient neurologic signs.

✗ Do not postpone diagnosis or treatment of temporal arteritis pending results of a temporal artery biopsy showing giant cell arteritis. The lesion typically skips areas, making biopsy an insensitive diagnostic procedure.

 DISCUSSION

Stiffness, pain, and weakness are common complaints in older patients, but polymyalgia rheumatica may respond dramatically to treatment. Rheumatoid arthritis produces morning stiffness but is usually present in more peripheral joints, and without muscle tenderness. Polymyositis is usually characterized by increased serum muscle enzymes with a normal ESR, and may include a skin rash (dermatomyositis). Often, a therapeutic trial of prednisone helps make the diagnosis. Giant cell arteritis can be a serious and occasionally fatal illness, with sudden irreversible visual loss, permanent hearing loss, or aortic dissection. Larger doses of corticosteroids are required than for polymyalgia rheumatica.

SUGGESTED READINGS

Evans JM, Vukov LF, Hunder GG: Polymyalgia rheumatica and giant cell arteritis in emergency department patients, *Ann Emerg Med* 22:1633-1635, 1993.

Radial Head Fracture

Presentation

A patient has fallen on an outstretched hand and has a normal, nonpainful shoulder, wrist, and hand but pain in the elbow joint. The joint may be intact, with full range of flexion, but there is pain or decreased range of motion on extension, supination, and pronation. Tenderness is greatest over the radial head and lateral condyle. X-rays may show a fracture or dislocation of the head of the radius. In all views, a line down the center of the radius should point to the capitellum of the lateral condyle. Often, however, no fracture is visible, and the only x-ray signs are of an elbow effusion or hemarthrosis pushing the posterior fat pad out of the olecranon fossa and the anterior fat pad out of its normal position on the lateral view (Figure 122-1).

What To Do:

✔ Obtain a detailed history of the mechanism of injury and a physical examination, looking for the features described, and x-rays of the elbow, looking for visible fat pads, as well as fracture lines.

✔ **If there is any question of a radial head fracture, immobilize the elbow (preventing pronation and supination of the hand) with a gutter splint extending from proximal humerus to hand, and then place in a sling for the next week** (Figure 122-2).

✔ Explain to the patient the probability of a fracture, despite x-rays that only demonstrate an effusion, and arrange for follow-up, with reevaluation in 2 to 3 days.

What Not To Do:

✗ Do not jump to the diagnosis of "tennis elbow or "sprained elbow" simply on the basis of an x-ray that does not show a fracture.

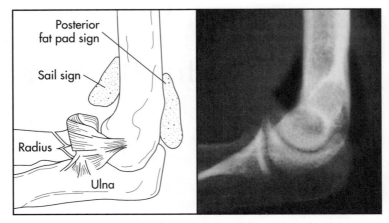

Figure 122–1 Radiologic evidence of elbow hemarthrosis.

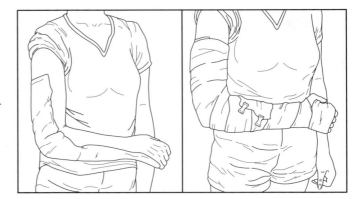

Figure 122–2 Long arm gutter splint.

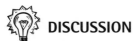

DISCUSSION

Small, nondisplaced fractures of the radial head may show up on x-rays weeks later or never at all. Because pronation and supination of the hand are achieved by rotating the radial head on the capitellum of the humerus, very small imperfections in the healing of the radial head may produce enormous impairment of hand function, which may be only partly improved by surgical excision of the radial head. Immobilization at the first question of a radial head fracture may help preserve essential pronation and supination. Early orthopedic referral is essential because treatment is controversial. Management of radial head fractures depends on the severity of the fracture and associated injuries, and includes early motion, open reduction and internal fixation with screws and wires, immediate and delayed excision, and a prosthesis. Tennis elbow (see Chapter 130) is a tenosynovitis of the common insertion of the wrist extensors on the lateral condyle and results in pain on wrist extension rather than on pronation and supination.

123

Radial Head Subluxation (RHS or Nursemaid's Elbow)

Presentation

A toddler has received a sudden jerk on his arm, causing enough pain that he holds it motionless. Circumstances surrounding the injury may be obvious (such as a parent pulling the child up out of a puddle) or obscure (the baby-sitter who reports that the child "just fell down"). The patient and family may not be accurate about localizing the injury and think that the child has injured his shoulder or wrist. The patient is comfortable at rest, splinting his arm limply at the side with mild flexion at the elbow and pronation of the forearm. There should be no deformity, crepitation, swelling, or discoloration of the arm. There is also no palpable tenderness except possibly over the radiohumeral joint; the child will start to cry with any movement of the elbow, especially attempted supination.

What To Do:

✔ Rule out any history of significant trauma, such as a fall from a height.

✔ Thoroughly examine the entire extremity, including the shoulder girdle, hand, and wrist.

✔ **If there is any suspicion of a fracture, get an x-ray.**

✔ **When subluxation is suspected, place the patient in the parent's lap and inform the mother or father that it appears their child's elbow is slightly out of place and that you are going to put it back in place. Warn them that this is going to hurt for a few moments.**

✔ **Put your thumb over the head of the radius and press down while you smoothly and fully supinate the forearm and extend the elbow. Complete the procedure by fully flexing the elbow while your thumb remains pressing against the radial head and the forearm remains supinated** (Figure 123-1). At some point you should feel a click beneath your thumb. The patient will usually scream for a while at this point. Leave for about 10 minutes, then return and reexamine the elbow to see that the child has fully recovered. This recovery may take as much as 30 minutes. **Postreduction immobilization is unnecessary.**

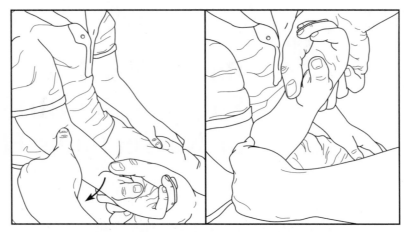

Figure 123-1 Technique for RHS reduction.

✔ Reassure the parents, explain the mechanism involved in the injury, and teach them how to prevent and treat recurrences.

✔ **If there is not full recovery, place the patient in a sling and have him return in 24 hours.** Repeat the above maneuver. If there is not full recovery in 30 minutes, examine again for possible injury to the clavicle or humerus (particularly the lateral condyle) and obtain appropriate x-rays. Consider an underlying osteomyelitis, septic arthritis, or tumor and arrange for consultation or referral.

What Not To Do:

✘ Do not attempt to reduce an elbow where the possibility exists of fracture or dislocation.

✘ Do not get unnecessary x-rays when all the findings are consistent with nursemaid's elbow. The x-rays may appear normal even when the radial head is indeed subluxed. Associated fractures occur but are not common.

✘ Do not confuse nursemaid's elbow with the more serious brachial plexus injury, which occurs after much greater stress and results in a flaccid paralysis of the arm.

 DISCUSSION

RHS is a common emergent problem and represents one fifth of upper-extremity injuries in children. The injury is an anterior subluxation of the radial head away from the capitellum through the annular ligament and occurs almost exclusively among children between 18 months and 3 years of age. RHS is more common in girls and in the left arm. About one third have had a prior episode.

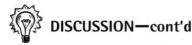

DISCUSSION—cont'd

The assessment of the young child is especially challenging because the child cannot relate a coherent history, has difficulty localizing pain, and often is frightened and uncooperative, hindering physical examination. The diagnosis is nonetheless made by history and physical examination and confirmed by prompt reuse of the affected arm following reduction. X-rays cannot be relied on. The subluxation is subtle and requires measurement or comparison to appreciate. (Draw a line down the axis of the radius. It should bisect the capitellum of the lateral humerus.)

RHS should be considered in any toddler presenting with arm injury without obvious evidence of trauma. The key to diagnosis is the observation that the child is not in pain; has no swelling, ecchymosis, or deformity; holds the elbow in a slightly flexed position with wrist pronated; refuses to use the arm; and resists supination. When history and physical examination suggest RHS, it is appropriate to attempt reduction without obtaining x-rays. Successful reduction is more likely when a click is felt. On occasion, if the subluxation has been present for several hours, edema, pain, and natural splinting will continue even after reduction or may prevent reduction.

SUGGESTED READINGS

Frumkin K: Nursemaid's elbow: a radiographic demonstration, *Ann Emerg Med* 14:690-693, 1985.

Quan L, Marcuse EK: The epidemiology and treatment of radial head subluxation, *Am J Dis Child* 139:1194–1197, 1985.

Schunk JE: Radial head subluxation: epidemiology and treatment of 87 episodes, *Ann Emerg Med* 19:1019-1023, 1990.

Schutzman SA, Teach S: Upper-extremity impairment in young children, *Ann Emerg Med* 26:474-479, 1995.

124

Radial Neuropathy
(Saturday Night Palsy)

Presentation

The patient has injured his upper arm, usually by sleeping with his arm over the back of a chair, and now presents holding the affected hand and wrist with his good hand, complaining of decreased or absent sensation on the radial and dorsal side of his hand and wrist, and of inability to extend his wrist, thumb, and finger joints. With the hand supinated (palm up) and the extensors aided by gravity, hand function may appear normal, but when the hand is pronated (palm down), the wrist and hand will drop (Figure 124-1).

What To Do:

✔ Look for associated injuries. This sort of nerve injury may be associated with cervical spine fracture, injury to the brachial plexus in the axilla, or fracture of the humerus.

✔ Document in detail all motor and sensory impairment. Draw a diagram of the area of decreased sensation, and grade muscle strength of various groups (flexors, extensors, and so on) on a scale of 1-5.

✔ **If there is complete paralysis or complete anesthesia, arrange for additional neurologic evaluation and treatment right away. Incomplete lesions may be satisfactorily referred for follow-up evaluation and physical therapy.**

✔ **Construct a splint, extending from proximal forearm to just beyond the metacarpophalangeal joint (leaving the thumb free), which holds the wrist in 90-degree extension.** This and a sling will help protect the hand, also preventing edema and distortion of tendons, ligaments, and joint capsules, which can result in loss of hand function after strength returns (Figure 124-2).

✔ Explain to the patient the nature of his nerve injury, the slow rate of regeneration, and the importance of splinting and physical therapy for preservation of eventual function. Arrange for follow-up.

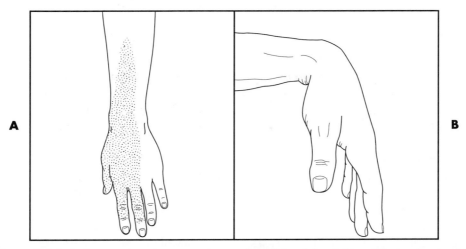

Figure 124-1 A, Decreased or absent sensation on the radial and dorsal sides of the hand and wrist. **B,** Hand will drop when positioned palm down.

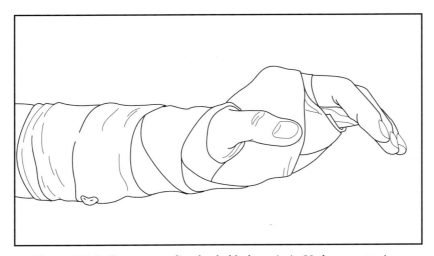

Figure 124-2 Construct a splint that holds the wrist in 90-degree extension.

What Not To Do:

✗ Do not be misled by the patient's ability to extend the interphalangeal joints of the fingers, which may be accomplished by the ulnar-innervated interosseus muscles.

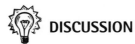 **DISCUSSION**

This neuropathy is produced by compression of the radial nerve as it spirals around the humerus. Most commonly it occurs when a person falls asleep intoxicated, and is held up by his arm thrown over the back of a chair. Because drunkenness apparently predisposes a person to prolonged sleep in one position (without the movement typical of normal sleep) the weight of the body may exert pressure on the arm for enough time to produce wallerian degeneration of nerve fibers. Less severe forms may befall the swain who keeps his arm on his date's chair back for an entire double feature, ignoring the growing pain and paresis. If the injury to the radial nerve is at the elbow or just below, there may be sparing of the wrist radial extensors, as well as the radial nerve autonomous sensation. The deficient groups will be the wrist ulnar extensors as well as the metacarpophalangeal extensors. A high radial palsy in the axilla (e.g., from leaning on crutches) will involve all of the radial nerve innervations, including the triceps. In the majority of cases, the Saturday night palsy resolves spontaneously and completely over the course of a few months. A wrist splint and passive range-of-motion exercises are usually sufficient treatment.

125

Scaphoid (Carpal Navicular) Fracture

Presentation

The patient (usually 14 to 40 years of age) fell on an outstretched hand with the wrist held rigid and extended and now complains of pain, swelling, and decreased range of motion in the wrist, particularly on the radial side. Physical examination discloses no deformity but shows pain with motion and palpation and often swelling, especially in the anatomic snuff box, the hollow seen on the radial aspect of the wrist when the thumb is in full extension (between the tendon of the extensor pollicis longus and the tendons of the abductor pollicis longus and extensor pollicis brevis) (Figure 125-1). A good maneuver is axial loading along the proximal phalanx of the thumb, eliciting pain at the base of the first metacarpal.

What To Do:

✔ Apply ice and a temporary splint or sling, check for distal sensation and movement and other injuries, and **order x-rays of the wrist, with special attention to the scaphoid bone and its fat pad.**

✔ **Regardless of whether a scaphoid fracture shows on x-ray, when there is pain and swelling as described above, splint or cast the wrist in extension, with the thumb out in opposition, and immobilized distally to its interphalangeal joint (e.g., a short arm thumb spica splint)** (Figure 125-2).

✔ Explain to the patient the common difficulty of visualizing scaphoid fractures on x-rays, the common difficulty in healing of scaphoid fractures due to variable blood supply, and the resultant necessity of keeping this splint or cast in place until reevaluated by an orthopedic specialist.

✔ **Provide a sling to keep the elbow flexed at 90 degrees and prescribe NSAIDs, adding narcotics when necessary.**

✔ As with any acute injury, have the patient apply ice for 15 to 20 minutes three or four times per day and maintain elevation above the level of the heart as much as possible.

✔ **Arrange for reevaluation and further treatment within the next few days. Bone scans after 3 days or repeat x-rays after 2 weeks may reveal a fracture that was initially occult.**

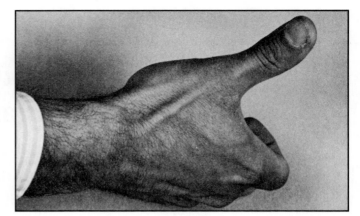

Figure 125-1 Examine for swelling or tenderness within the anatomic snuff box.

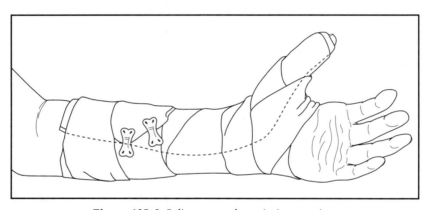

Figure 125-2 Splint or cast the wrist in extension.

What Not To Do:

✗ Do not assume a wrist injury is "just a sprain" when x-rays are negative. Any wrist injury with significant tenderness, pain on range of motion, and swelling should be splinted and referred for further evaluation.

 DISCUSSION

Because fractures of the scaphoid bone are common, because as many as 15% are invisible on x-rays until weeks later, because the blood supply to the fractured area may be tenuous and nonunion or avascular necrosis likely, and because the resultant pain and arthritis may severely limit hand function, it is prudent practice to splint or cast all potential scaphoid frac-

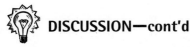

DISCUSSION—cont'd

tures with a thumb spica until orthopedic reevaluation. The blood supply to the scaphoid bone originates at the end of the bone and then flows to the proximal pole. The more proximal the fracture, the greater the chance of delayed union or avascular necrosis. Fracture fragments that are widely separated or rotated may require surgical pinning. Call for immediate orthopedic consultation.

SUGGESTED READINGS

Murphy DG, Eisenhauer MA, Powe J, et al: Can a 4 day bone scan accurately determine the presence or absence of scaphoid fracture? *Ann Emerg Med* 26:434-438, 1995.

Waeckerle JF: A prospective study identifying the sensitivity of radiographic findings and the efficacy of clinical findings in carpal navicular fractures, *Ann Emerg Med* 16:733-737, 1987.

126

Shoulder Dislocation

Presentation

The patient was holding her shoulder abducted horizontally to the side when a blow knocked the humeral head anteriorly. She arrives holding the shoulder abducted ten degrees from her side, unable to move it without increasing the pain. Recurrent dislocations may be the result of relatively minor forces such as those produced when reaching into the back seat of a car from the driver's seat or rolling over while asleep. The delto-pectoral groove becomes a bulge (caused by the dislocated head of the humerus) and the acromion is prominent laterally, with a depression below (where the head of the humerus normally sits on the undislocated shoulder) (Figure 126-1).

What To Do:

✔ **Provide analgesia.** Ketorolac (Toradol) 60 mg IM or 30 mg IV is good, but IV narcotics may be needed. To abolish muscle spasm and provide conscious sedation for a difficult reduction, but have the patient awake enough to go home in an hour, one recommended regimen is titrating IV midazolam (Versed) 5 mg and fentanyl (Sublimaze) 0.1 mg, given 10 minutes before attempting reduction, with continuous pulse oximetry, EKG monitoring, IV fluids running, and the physician by the bedside with bag-valve-mask and endotracheal intubation kit ready. **Many shoulders, however, can be reduced without conscious sedation.**

✔ **When analgesia is required, another alternative is the use of intraarticular lidocaine.** After preparing the skin with povidone-iodine, using a 1½-inch 20-gauge needle, inject 20 ml of 1% lidocaine 2 cm inferiorly and directly lateral to the acromion, in the lateral sulcus left by the absent humeral head.

✔ **If available, obtain a prereduction x-ray to rule out fractures or unreduceable injuries. This image may be deferred if the injury was recurrent and relatively atraumatic.**

✔ **Test and record the sensation over the deltoid to establish if there is an injury of the axillary nerve (rare)** and confirm the circulation, sensation, and movement in the elbow, wrist, and hand. **Reexamine after the shoulder is reduced.**

✔ **To reduce a dislocation, gain the patient's confidence by holding her arm securely, asking her to relax, telling her that she will not be moved suddenly, and**

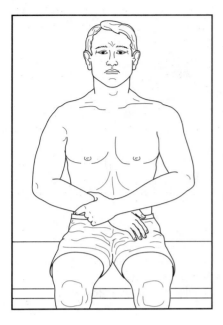

Figure 126-1 Shoulder dislocation with loss of the normal deltoid bulge. *(From Ruiz E, Cicero JJ:* Emergency management of skeletal injuries, *St Louis, 1995, Mosby.)*

that if any pain occurs you will stop. Then in a very calm and gentle manner ask her to let his muscles go loose so his shoulder can stretch out.

✔ **With the elbow flexed at 90 degrees, apply steady traction at the distal humerus. Pull inferiorly and at the same time externally rotate the forearm very, very slowly. If the patient complains of pain, stop rotating, allow him to relax, and let the shoulder muscles stretch while traction is maintained along the humerus. Resume external rotation when he is comfortable again. Using this method, full external rotation alone will reduce most anterior shoulder dislocations** (Figure 126-2, *A*).

✔ If the shoulder joint is not felt or seen to reduce, then while maintaining traction and external rotation, slowly and gently adduct the humerus until it is against the anterior chest wall and then very slowly internally rotate the forearm against the anterior chest. The vast majority of shoulder dislocations can be reduced comfortably this way, often without the use of any analgesics (Figure 126-2, *B*).

✔ An alternative technique when the lateral border of the scapula can be palpated is reduction by scapular manipulation. With the patient sitting up, place the uninjured shoulder firmly against an immovable support such as a wall or the raised head of the stretcher. Have an assistant face the patient and gently lift the outstretched wrist of the affected arm until it is horizontal. The assistant then places the palm of her free hand against the midclavicular area of the injured shoulder as counterbalance, and then gently but firmly pulls the patient's arm towards her. At the same time, manipulate the scapula by adducting the inferior tip using thumb pressure, while stabilizing the superior aspect with the upper hand (Figure 126-3).

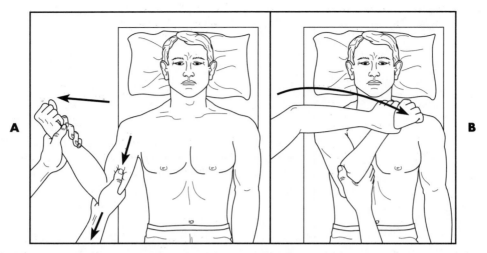

Figure 126-2 A, Slow and gentle external rotation technique. **B,** Slow and gentle adduction followed by gradual internal rotation will reduce the majority of dislocations that do not respond to external rotation alone. *(From Ruiz E, Cicero JJ:* Emergency management of skeletal injuries, *St Louis, 1995, Mosby.)*

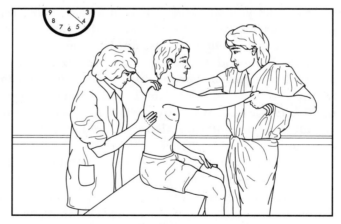

Figure 126-3 Scapular technique.

✔ **When the patient is comfortable and range of motion has been restored, secure the reduction in a sling and a swath around the arm and chest. Obtain postreduction x-rays, and discharge the patient once he is alert, with a prescription for analgesics as needed and an appointment for orthopedic follow-up in 1 week (sooner if any problem).**

What Not To Do:

✘ Do not use the forearm as a lever to force reduction and possibly fracture the neck of the humerus.

✘ Do not redislocate the shoulder by repeating the motions of the mechanism of injury.

 DISCUSSION

The strategy is to relocate the shoulder with minimal damage to the joint capsule and anterior labrum of the glenoid fossa, hoping the patient does not become a chronic dislocator with an unstable shoulder. Chronic dislocators are easier to reduce, and come less often to the emergency department, because they learn how to relocate their own shoulders. Of patients whose first shoulder dislocation occurs before 20 years of age, 90% will have a recurrent dislocation. Only 14% of first dislocations after 40 years of age recur.

Posterior dislocations are caused by internal rotation of the shoulder, as during a seizure, and are more subtle to diagnose. Subglenoid dislocation or luxatio erecta is rare and unmistakable, with the arm raised and abducted with no external rotation possible.

SUGGESTED READINGS

Garnavos C: Technical note: modifications and improvements of the Milch technique for the reduction of anterior dislocation of the shoulder without premedication, *J Trauma* 32:801-803, 1992.

Hendey GW, Kinlaw K: Clinically significant abnormalities in postreduction radiographs after anterior shoulder dislocation, *Ann Emerg Med* 28:39-402, 1996.

Matthews DE: Intra-articular lidocaine versus intravenous analgesic for reduction of acute anterior shoulder dislocation: a prospective randomized study, *Am J Sports Med* 23:54-58, 1995.

McNamara RM: Reduction of anterior shoulder dislocation by scapular manipulation, *Ann Emerg Med* 22:1140-1144, 1993.

Riebel GD, McCabe JB: Anterior shoulder dislocation: a review of reduction techniques, *Am J Emerg Med* 9:180-188, 1991.

Westin CD, Gill EA, Noyes ME, et al: Anterior shoulder dislocation: a simple and rapid method for reduction, *Am J Sports Med* 23:369-371, 1995.

127

Third-Degree Tear of Ulnar Collateral Ligament (Ski Pole or Gamekeeper's Thumb)

Presentation

The patient fell while holding onto a ski pole, banister, or other fixed object, forcing his thumb radially into abduction. (This same lesion may be produced by the repeated breaking of the necks of game birds—hence the name.) The metacarpophalangeal joint of the thumb is swollen, tender, and stiff, but when tested for stability can be deformed towards the radial (or palmar) aspect more than the metacarpophalangeal joint of the other thumb. The patient's power pinch between the thumb and index finger, if possible at all, is less strong than with the other hand.

What To Do:

✔ **Examine thoroughly and obtain x-rays,** which should be negative or show a small avulsion fracture at the insertion of the ulnar collateral ligament.

✔ **Treat with ice, elevation, rest, antiinflammatory medications, and immobilization in a radial gutter splint, including the thumb.**

✔ Explain to the patient that this particular injury may not heal with closed immobilization but sometimes requires operative repair. Arrange for reexamination and orthopedic referral after a few days, when the swelling is decreased.

 DISCUSSION

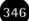

The ulnar collateral ligament of the metacarpophalangeal joint of the thumb, once completely torn, may retract its torn ends under other structures, where they are no longer apposed and cannot be depended on to heal. An operation may be required to reappose the two ends of the ligament or reattach an avulsed insertion, but this is not usually done immediately.

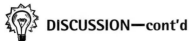

DISCUSSION—cont'd

Left unrepaired, a gamekeeper's thumb remains unstable and weak in pinching and holding. For minor sprains or partial ligament tears, an elastic wrap that incorporates the thumb may be all that is required to reduce mobility and provide comfort.

128

Splay Finger (Avulsion of Flexor Digitorum Profundus Tendon)

Presentation

The patient has injured his fingertip by falling backward and striking it on the floor, causing sudden and forceful hyperextension at the distal interphalangeal (DIP) joint. Alternatively, this injury can befall a football player trying to tackle the ball carrier but only catching the jersey or belt with the last joint of one finger (Figure 128-1). Both mechanisms can avulse the insertion of the flexor tendon on the distal phalanx. The patient may feel a pop, followed by immediate pain and swelling. The finger becomes swollen, often with ecchymosis on the volar side. The patient is often unaware that he cannot flex the DIP joint.

What To Do:

✔ **Have the patient try to close the fingers against the palm in a loose fist.** All the fingers will readily flex into the palm, but the DIP joint of the injured digit is unable to bend, and the patient cannot bring the fingertip into the palm.

✔ **Obtain x-rays of the finger** with anteroposterior and lateral views. The x-ray is usually normal, although occasionally a small avulsion fracture may be visible on the proximal volar aspect of the distal phalanx.

✔ **Request consultation from a hand surgeon for early surgical repair. If this injury is not treated within 3 weeks, the tendon will shorten and retract into the palm.**

What Not To Do:

✘ Do not assume a simple sprain exists because of negative x-rays. When there is marked swelling of the distal finger pad following a grabbing injury, be mindful of the possibility of a flexor digitorum profundus avulsion.

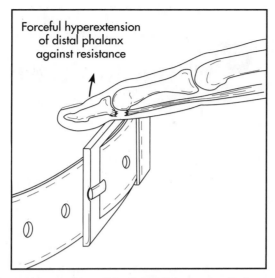

Forceful hyperextension
of distal phalanx
against resistance

Figure 128-1 Avulsion of the flexor digitorum profundus tendon.

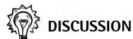 **DISCUSSION**

Avulsion of the insertion of the flexor digitorum profundus tendon results from the sudden forced extension of a finger when the tendon is contracting. Unless the physician specifically examines for flexion of the DIP joint, the opportunity to repair the tendinous insertion may be lost.

129 Tendonitis

Presentation

There is pain along the involved tendon, often poorly localized, but worse with motion, resisted contraction, or passive stretching. A vibratory crepitus may be felt on palpation during tendon movement. Common sites include the thumb side of the wrist (de Quervain's disease, see Chapter 131) and the lateral elbow (tennis elbow, see Chapter 130). There may be a history of repetitive overuse of the tendon or of a single sudden pull. Older patients participating in occasional sports are particularly prone to tendon injuries.

What To Do:

✔ If there is swelling, erythema, fever, puncture of the skin, gonorrhea, or marked pain, rule out infection. Send blood for CBC and ESR and request consultation.

✔ **X-rays are usually of little diagnostic value.** They may reveal calcifications, osteochondritis, or osteophytes that suggest chronic inflammation, but do not necessarily correlate with symptoms.

✔ **Instruct the patient to avoid the precipitating activity and prescribe an NSAID** unless it is contraindicated by allergy, bleeding, gastritis, or renal insufficiency.

✔ **Splint the involved joint for a few days to prevent or minimize the painful motion. Have the patient try heat for comfort.**

What Not To Do:

✘ Do not inject corticosteroids directly into the tendon or provide repeat steroid injections, which may potentiate infection, weaken the tendon, or cause it to rupture. Repeated subfascial or subcutaneous injections can result in atrophy of the skin and subcutaneous tissue and loss of pigmentation. Reserve steroid injection of the tendon sheath or peritendinous tissue for patients who fail conservative treatment and practitioners experienced in the procedure.

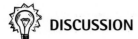 **DISCUSSION**

Tendonitis can be difficult to distinguish from bursitis (see Chapter 98), and often the two co-exist. If the tendon must be injected, withdraw the needle from the tendon and into the peritendinous tissue. Do not inject if there is resistance to flow.

130

Tennis Elbow (Lateral Epicondylitis)

Presentation

The patient complains of pain in the lateral elbow. Flexion, extension, pronation, and supination are slightly painful, but the real discomfort is with extension of the wrist and fingers. Holding lightweight objects such as a cup may be difficult. The common origin of the extensor muscles anterior and distal to the lateral epicondyle of the humerus is tender to palpation, especially the tendinous origin of the extensor carpi radialis brevis muscle.

What To Do:

✔ Examine thoroughly to rule out infection, fracture, or loss of function. Ask about vigorous or repetitive activities that could have precipitated the epicondylitis.

✔ **Prescribe an NSAID unless it is contraindicated** by allergy, bleeding, gastritis, or renal insufficiency.

✔ **Application of moist heat or ice may be comforting.**

✔ **For a severe case, splint the elbow with a sling for a few days to prevent or minimize the painful motion. To provide immediate and prolonged pain relief, consider injecting the point of maximum tenderness with a combination of bupivacaine 0.5% (Marcaine) 3 ml and methylprednisolone (Depo Medrol) 20 to 40 mg using a 1¼-inch 25-gauge needle.** Forewarn patients of a possible flare up of pain when the local anesthetic wears off, which may last for 24 to 48 hours.

✔ **For long-term treatment, prescribe a circumferential forearm band just below the elbow.** This compresses the extensor muscles and reduces the strain. Commercial tennis elbow straps are easily obtained at any sports shop.

What Not To Do:

✗ Do not order x-rays for a classic presentation. Reserve them for questions of bony pathology.

✗ Do not inject corticosteroids repeatedly into the tendon. They cause it to weaken or rupture.

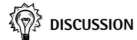 **DISCUSSION**

Tennis elbow usually affects patients from 30 to 60 years of age, with a peak incidence in the 40s. The name comes from one sports medicine etiology: poor form for the backhand stroke, extending the wrist when striking the ball instead of holding the wrist and elbow immobile and swinging from the shoulder. One solution is a two-handed backstroke. Other mechanisms that require rotation of the forearm and extension of the wrist include turning a screwdriver or painting a wall, both of which can result in overuse of the forearm muscles. A direct blow can also trigger tennis elbow.

131

Thumb Tenosynovitis (de Quervain's)

Presentation

The patient, usually a middle-aged woman, has difficulty with tasks like opening jars because of pain at the base of the thumb, which may also be present on awakening. On examination, there is little or no swelling and no deformity, just tenderness on palpating or stretching the extensor pollicis brevis and abductor pollicis longus tendons bordering the palmar side, or less commonly, the extensor pollicis longus tendon bordering the dorsal side of the anatomic snuff box.

What To Do:

✔ Document normal circulation, sensation, and movement. Compress the thumb metacarpal onto the scaphoid (see Chapter 125) to see if it is fractured. Look for carpal tunnel syndrome (see Chapter 99) with Phalen's test.

✔ **Have the patient fold the thumb into the palm, close the fingers over it into a fist, then ulnar deviate the wrist. This is known as the Finklestein test, and reproduces the pain of de Quervain's tenosynovitis of the extensor pollicis brevis and abductor pollicis longus tendons.**

✔ **Prescribe antiinflammatory analgesics and apply a radial gutter splint to immobilize the thumb distally to the interphalangeal joint. Arrange for rehabilitation.**

✔ **Tendon sheath injection is a technique that can be used by the more experienced clinician to help ensure a more rapid recovery.** Using a 25-gauge, 1-inch needle, slowly penetrate the skin and soft tissue, aiming for the middle of the tendon. When the tendon is hit, it may produce a muscle reflex, increased resistance to advancement of the needle, and pain, which are signals to withdraw the needle slightly. Move the muscle-tendon unit so it slides back and forth and readvance the needle until the tendon is felt slightly scraping the point. Back off one millimeter, steady the syringe and needle, and inject 1 ml of betamethasone (Celestone) or 20 mg of triamcinolone (Aristocort) along with 2 ml of bupivacaine (Marcaine) 0.5%. While injecting, palpate the tendon, feeling for a "sausaging" effect as the mixture inflates the sheath. Splint the thumb at night and expect resolution of symptoms in 1 to 2 days. Warn the patient that there may be a transient flare in pain when the anesthetic wears off, which may last 24 to 48 hours.

What Not To Do:

✗ Do not inject directly into the tendon. This may weaken the tendon and lead to future rupture.

 DISCUSSION

Symptoms of de Quervain's syndrome are related to overuse. They are often seen in super-market cashiers and piecework factory workers, and after intensive computer keyboarding. It is important to have the patient avoid the activity that brought on the condition. Tendon sheath injections are well tolerated and can be repeated safely at least three times, spaced several months apart. Half the time, one injection is effective.

SUGGESTED READINGS

Weiss APC, Akelman E, Tabatabai M, et al: Treatment of de Quervain's disease, *J Hand Surg* 19:595, 1994.

132

Torticollis (Wry Neck)

Presentation

The patient complains of neck pain and is unable to turn his head, usually holding it twisted to one side, with some spasm of the neck muscles and the chin pointing to the other side. These symptoms may have developed gradually, after minor turning of the head, after vigorous movement or injury, or during sleep. The pain may be in the neck muscles or down the spine, from the occiput to between the scapulae. Spasm in the occipitalis, sternocleidomastoid, trapezius, splenius cervicis, or levator scapulae muscles can be the primary cause of the torticollis, or it can be secondary to a slipped facet, herniated disk, or viral or bacterial infection (Figure 132-1).

What To Do:

✔ Ask the patient about precipitating factors, and perform a thorough physical examination, looking for muscle spasm, point tenderness, signs of injury, nerve root compression, masses, or infection. Include a careful nasopharyngeal examination, as well as a basic neurologic examination.

✔ **When forceful trauma is involved, and fracture, dislocation, or subluxation is possible, obtain lateral, anteroposterior, and odontoid x-ray views of the cervical spine.** If there are neurologic deficits, CT scan or MRI may be better to visualize nerve involvement (as well as herniated disk, hematoma, or epidural abscess).

✔ **When there is no suspicion of a serious illness or injury, apply heat (e.g., a Hydrocolator pack wrapped in several thicknesses of towel) and give antiinflammatory analgesics (e.g., aspirin, ibuprofen, naproxen) and perhaps oral cyclobenzaprine (Flexeril) or diazepam (Valium). Alternating heat with ice massages may also be helpful, as well as gentle range-of-motion exercises.**

✔ If there is point tenderness posterior to the sternocleidomastoid muscle (over the vertebral facets) and the head cannot turn toward the side of the point tenderness, suspect a facet syndrome, obtain x-rays, and gently test neck motion again after a few minutes of manual traction along a longitudinal axis (sometimes this provides some relief).

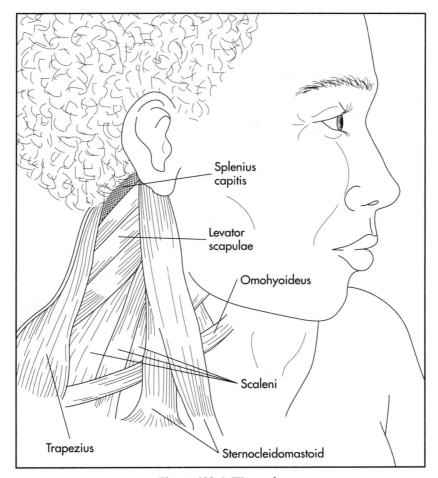

Figure 132-1 Wry neck.

✔ **If a localized trigger point is discovered, treat this as any other source of myo-fascial pain** (see Chapter 117). **Trigger point injection can often partially or completely relieve the symptoms of torticollis.**

✔ If there is any arm weakness or paresthesia corresponding to a cervical dermatome, suspect nerve root compression as the underlying cause, and arrange for x-rays, MRI, and neurosurgical or orthopedic consultation.

✔ With signs and symptoms of infection (e.g., fever, toxic appearance, lymphadenopathy, tonsillar swelling, trismus, pharyngitis, or dysphagia) take soft tissue lateral neck films and consider obtaining a complete blood count and ESR to help rule out early abscess formation. Arrange for specialty consultation.

✔ **For minor causes, discharge the patient with a soft cervical collar if this provides relief and arrange for x-rays and follow-up if the torticollis has not fully resolved in 1 or 2 days.**

What Not To Do:

✗ Do not overlook infectious etiologies presenting as torticollis, especially the pharyngo-tonsillitis of young children, which can soften the atlantoaxial ligaments and allow sub-luxation.

✗ Do not undertake violent spinal manipulations in the emergency department, which can make an acute torticollis worse.

✗ Do not confuse torticollis with a dystonic drug reaction (see Chapter 2) from pheno-thiazines or butyrophenones.

 DISCUSSION

Although torticollis may signal some underlying pathology, usually it is a local musculoskeletal problem—only more frightening and noticeable for being in the neck—and need not always be worked up comprehensively when it first presents to the clinician.

Traumatic Effusion

Presentation

Either immediately or 1 to 2 days after an injury such as a contusion of a bursa or the deformation of a joint, the patient complains of swelling, pain, and (in the case of a joint injury) decreased range of motion. Physical examination shows minimal or absent redness and heat, but there is a palpable or visible effusion, which may interfere with evaluation of bony or ligamentous tenderness or stability. The loss of full extension of the elbow is a reliable indicator of significant injuries (e.g., joint effusion or fractures).

What To Do:

✔ Obtain a complete history, including the mechanism of injury and subsequent treatments, and as complete a physical examination as possible.

✔ **Obtain x-rays (these may be deferred—see decision rules for ankle and knee sprains)** (see Chapters 95 and 110).

✔ If it is necessary to rule out infection, relieve severe pain, or demonstrate a complete (third-degree) ligamentous tear that will be repaired operatively in the next few days, then prep the skin, tap the effusion, examine the fluid, and instill 1% plain lidocaine (Xylocaine) or 0.5% bupivacaine (Marcaine) and reexamine the joint for stability.

✔ **Instruct the patient on rest, ice application for 10 to 20 minutes per hour for the first 24 to 72 hours, and the use of crutches if appropriate. Immobilize the joint with a bulky dressing, sling, or splint and elevate the injured part above the heart until the swelling is decreased. Prescribe NSAIDs for the pain, swelling, inflammation, and stiffness. Arrange follow-up in 3 to 4 days.**

What Not To Do:

✗ Do not forget to warn patients with acute musculoskeletal injuries that stiffness, effusions, and edema typically peak at 24 to 48 hours. The patient who is not prepared for this may return unnecessarily, convinced he is getting worse.

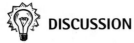 **DISCUSSION**

An effusion in 1 hour suggests a disruption and hemorrhage, while an effusion that developed gradually over 24 hours is probably caused by inflammation. Although a tense joint effusion interferes with testing of associated ligaments, its existence at least proves the joint capsule is intact, and implies that the contiguous ligaments are not likely to be completely ruptured (this assurance does not apply to the knee).

Tapping traumatic effusions and hemarthroses does transiently decrease pain, but the fluid usually reaccumulates within a few hours. Fat globules in the effusion indicate an occult fracture. Immediate operative repair of third-degree ligamentous tears is usually reserved for young athletes, who demand maximum function as soon as possible. The majority of joint effusions are not significantly helped by routine arthrocentesis.

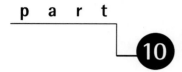

part

10

Soft Tissue Emergencies

c h a p t e r

134

Bicycle Spoke Injury

Presentation

A small child, riding on the back of a friend's bike, gets her foot caught between the spinning spokes and the frame or fender supports. The skin over the lateral or medial aspect of the foot or ankle is crushed and abraded with underlying soft tissue swelling (Figure 134-1). s

What To Do:

✔ Cleanse the area with a gentle scrub (SurClens, Betadine).

✔ Provide any tetanus prophylaxis required and apply a temporary normal saline dressing (see Chapter 151).

✔ **Get radiographic studies to rule out any fracture.**

✔ **Dress the wound with antibiotic ointment and a nonadherent cover, such as Adaptic gauze. Incorporate a bulky compressive dressing consisting of gauze fluffs, Kerlex, and a mildly compressive Ace wrap.**

✔ **Have the patient keep the foot strictly elevated over the next 24 hours and schedule her for a wound check within 48 hours.**

✔ Inform the parents that the crushed skin is not a simple abrasion and may not survive. They should understand that a slow-healing sore might result or skin grafting might be required, and therefore careful surgical follow-up is necessary.

What Not To Do:

✘ Do not assume that the injury is merely a simple abrasion because the x-rays are negative.

 DISCUSSION

Bicycle spoke injuries are similar to but not as serious as wringer injuries. Fractures are not commonly associated with these injuries, but often there is severe soft tissue injury. Consequences of a crush injury can be minimized by the use of compression dressings, elevation, and early follow-up.

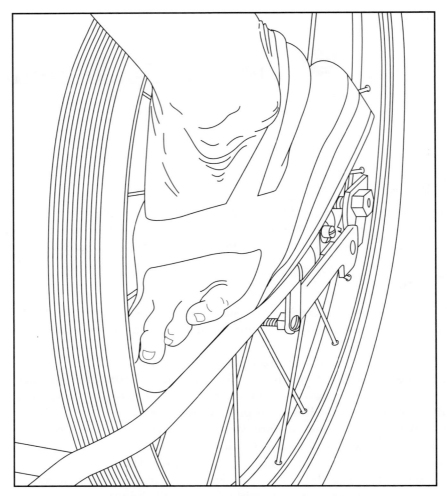

Figure 134–1 Foot caught in bicycle spokes.

135

Bites

Presentation

Histories of animal bites are usually volunteered, but the history of a human bite, such as one obtained over the knuckle during a fight, is more likely to be denied or explained only after questioning. A single bite may contain various types of injury, including underlying fractures and tendon and nerve injuries, not all of which are immediately apparent.

What To Do:

✔ Obtain a complete history, including the type of animal that bit, whether or not the attack was provoked (a rabid animal is more likely to make an unprovoked attack), what time the injury occurred, the current health status and vaccination record of the animal, and whether or not the animal has been captured and is being held for observation. Report the bite to the police or appropriate local authorities.

✔ Assess the wound for any damage to deep structures, any need for surgical consultation, and any risk of infection. Look for bone and joint involvement and, if present, obtain appropriate imaging studies (dog bites have caused open, depressed skull fractures in small children). Examine for nerve and tendon injury and be aware that crush and puncture wounds, as well as bites on the hands, wrists, and feet, are at higher risk for development of infection and significant complications such as tenosynovitis, septic joints, osteomyelitis, and sepsis, which will require operative debridement and inpatient IV antibiotics. Bites from cats, humans, or other primates are also associated with higher rates of infection. If tissue damage is extensive, then obtain vascular, orthopedic, otorhinolaryngologic, reconstructive, or other consultation.

✔ For crush wounds and contusions, elevate above the heart and apply cold packs.

✔ If the wound requires debridement, or will be painful to cleanse and irrigate, anesthetize with buffered lidocaine (epinephrine will slightly increase infection rates).

✔ If there are already signs of infection, obtain aerobic and anaerobic cultures of any pus.

✔ **Cleanse the wound with antiseptic (10% povidone-iodine solution, diluted 1:10 in normal saline) and sharply debride any debris and nonviable tissue.**

✔ **Irrigate the wound with jet lavage, using a 10-ml syringe, a 19-gauge plastic catheter, or an irrigation shield (ZEROWET SPLASHIELD) and at least 200 ml of sterile saline or the diluted to 1% povine–iodine solution.** This technique demonstrably reduces microscopic debris and bacteria. Use an IV setup to irrigate a large area.

✔ **Prepare every wound as if it would be sutured.**

✔ **For animal bite wounds that are clean, uninfected, and open lacerations, located anywhere other than the hand or foot, staple, tape, or suture them closed. Prophylactic antibiotics are not necessary.** Infection rates in sutured dog bite wounds have compared favorably with those for unsutured wounds and with nonbite lacerations.

✔ **If the wound is infected when first seen, plan either a delayed repair after 3 to 5 days of saline dressings or secondary wound healing without closure. Prescribe antibiotics for 7 to 10 days.** Severe infections require hospitalization for evaluation, immobilization, IV antibiotics, and surgical consultation.

✔ **With human bites; animal bites that are punctures or located on the hand, wrist, or foot; or bites more than 12 hours old, in most cases leave the wounds open, apply a light dressing or saline dressing, and consider delayed primary closure after 2 to 3 days.** Wounds should also be left open on debilitated patients with diabetes, alcoholism, chronic steroid use, organ transplants, vascular insufficiency, splenectomy, HIV, or other immunocompromised condition. **Start prophylactic antibiotics on those wounds and also in patients with artificial or damaged heart valves and implanted prosthetic devices.** The most effective dose is the one that can be given now. **Amoxicillin plus clavulanate (Augmentin) 875/125 mg bid is the current CDC recommendation for all bites.** Alternatives for prophylaxis include: for *dog* bites in adults, clindamycin (Cleocin) 150 to 300 mg qid plus ofloxacin (Floxin) 400 mg bid, for children, clindamycin (Cleocin) plus trimethoprim plus sulfamethoxazole (Bactrim); for *cat* bites in adults, cefuroxime (Ceftin) 500 mg bid or doxycycline 100 mg bid or ceftriaxone (Rocephin) 500 to 2000 mg IM or IV; and for *human* bites, cefoxitin (Mefoxin) 2000 mg q8h IV.

✔ If the patient has had no tetanus toxoid in the past 5 to 10 years, provide prophylaxis (see Chapter 151).

✔ **If the patient was bitten by an oddly behaving domestic animal, or a bat, coyote, fox, opossum, raccoon, or skunk, start rapid rabies vaccination with 20 IU/kg of rabies immune globulin and the first of five 1-ml doses of human diploid strain rabies vaccine.** Reassure the patient that bites of rodents and lagomorphs, including rats, squirrels, hamsters, and rabbits, in America do not usually transmit rabies (see Appendix E).

✔ With human bites, provide hepatitis prophylaxis for patients who have been bitten by known carriers of hepatitis B. Administer hepatitis B immune globulin 0.06 ml/kg IM at the time of injury and schedule a second dose in 30 days.

✔ **Minimize edema (and infection) of hand wounds by splinting and elevation.**

✔ **Have the patient return for a wound check in 2 days, or sooner if there is any sign of infection.** Explain the potential for a serious complication such as septic arthritis, osteomyelitis, and tenosynovitis, which will require specialty consultation.

What Not To Do:

✘ Do not overlook a puncture wound.

✘ Do not infiltrate irrigant solution into tissue planes in puncture wounds.

✘ Do not suture debris, nonviable tissue, or a bacterial inoculum into a wound.

✘ Do not use buried absorbable sutures, which act as a foreign body and cause a reactive inflammation for about a month.

✘ Do not waste time and money obtaining cultures and Gram's stains of fresh wounds. The results of these tests do not correlate well with the organisms that subsequently cause infection.

DISCUSSION

Animal bites are often brought promptly to the attention of medical personnel, if only because of a legal requirement to report the bite, or because of fear of rabies. Bite wounds account for 1% of all emergency department visits in the United States, most caused by dogs and cats. Most dog bites are from household pets rather than strays. A disproportionate number of dog bites are from German shepherds.

Bites occur most commonly among young, poorly supervised children who disturb the animals while they are sleeping or feeding, separate them during a fight, try to hug or kiss an unfamiliar animal, or accidentally frighten it. Malpractice claims and other civil lawsuits often follow bite injuries.

Dog and cat bites both show high rates of infection with staphylococci and streptococci species, as well as *Pasteurella multocida* and many different gram-negative and anaerobic bacteria. In addition to these organisms, 10% to 30% of all human bites are infected with *Eikenella corrodens,* which sometimes shows resistance to the semisynthetic penicillins but sensitivity to penicillin. Adequate debridement and irrigation are clearly more effective than prophylactic antibiotics, and are often all that is required to prevent animal bite infections.

Less than 0.1% of all animal bites result in rabies. For questions on local rabies risk, local public health services may be available and provide valuable support.

SUGGESTED READINGS

Dire DJ, Hogan DE, Riggs MW: A prospective evaluation of risk factors for infections from dog bite wounds, *Acad Emerg Med* 1:258-266, 1994.

Elenbaas RM, McNabney WK, Robinson WA: Evaluation of prophylactic oxacillin in cat bite wounds, *Ann Emerg Med* 13:155-157, 1984.

Rosen RA: The use of antibiotics in the initial management of recent dog bite wounds, *Am J Emerg Med* 3:19-23, 1985.

136

Fingernail or Toenail Avulsion

Presentation

The patient may have had a blow to the nail; the nail may have been torn away by a fan blade or other piece of machinery; or a long hard toenail may have caught on a loop of a shag carpet or other fixed object and been pulled off the nailbed. The nail may be completely avulsed, partially held in place by the nail folds, or adhering only to the distal nailbed. On occasion, an exposed nailbed will have a pearly appearance with minimal bleeding, making it seem as if the nail is still in place when actually it has been completely avulsed.

What To Do:

✔ Obtain x-rays if there was any crushing or high velocity shearing force involved.

✔ **Perform a digital block** (see Appendix B) to anesthetize the entire nailbed.

✔ **Cleanse the nailbed with normal saline and remove any loose cuticular debris. Although it is acceptable simply to cover the nailbed with a nonadherent dressing, the patient is usually more comfortable with a clean nail or surrogate in place while a new nail grows in.** No dressing is truly nonadherent over an exposed nailbed. If the nail or artificial stent is not used, then bring the patient back for an early dressing change in 1 day to prevent painful adherence.

✔ If the partially avulsed nail is still tenuously attached, remove it by separating it from the nailfold using a straight hemostat. **Cleanse the nail thoroughly with normal saline, cut away the distal free edge of the nail, and remove only loose cuticular debris.**

✔ **Inspect the nailbed for lacerations and if present carefully reapproximate with fine (6-0 or 7-0) absorbable sutures.**

✔ Reduce any displaced or angulated fractures of the distal phalanx. If a stable reduction cannot be obtained, consult an orthopedic, hand, or podiatric surgeon for possible pinning.

✔ **Reinsert the nail under the eponychium and apply a finger-tip dressing** (see Appendix C) (Figure 136-1).

✔ **If the nail does not fit tightly under the eponychium, it can be sutured in place at its base** (see Chapter 143). **A loose-fitting nail can also be glued in place using cyanoacrylate topical skin adhesive (Dermabond).**

✔ **If the nail is missing, badly damaged, or contaminated, replace it with a substitute. An artificial nail can be cut out of the sterile aluminum foil found in**

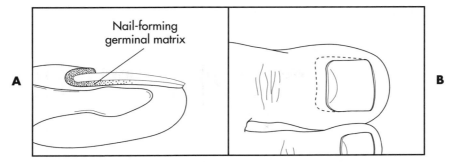

Figure 136-1 A, Nail or stent in place. **B,** Nail under the eponychium.

a suture pack or can be cut from a sheet of vaseline gauze. Insert this stent under the eponychium in place of the nail and apply a finger-tip dressing after it is in place.

✔ Leave these stents in place until the nailbed hardens and the stent separates spontaneously.

✔ Dressings should be changed every 3 to 5 days.

✔ If the wound was contaminated, the tissue crushed, or the patient immunocompromised, prescribe 3 or 4 days of a first-generation cephalosporin as prophylaxis. However, fractures of the distal phalanx do not always require antibiotics.

✔ Provide appropriate tetanus prophylaxis (see Chapter 151).

What Not To Do:

✗ Do not dress an exposed nailbed with an ordinary gauze dressing. It will adhere to the nailbed, require lengthy soaks, and at times cause an extremely painful removal.

✗ Do not ignore nailbed lacerations or fractures of the distal phalanx. The new nail can become deformed or ingrown wherever the bed is not smooth and straight.

✗ Do not debride any portion of the nailbed, sterile matrix, or germinal matrix.

 DISCUSSION

Although the eponychium is unlikely to scar to the nailbed unless there is infection, inflammation, or considerable tissue damage, separating the eponychium from the nail matrix by reinserting the nail or inserting an artificial stent helps to prevent synechiae and future nail deformities from developing. The patient's own nail is also her most comfortable dressing. Minimally traumatized avulsed nails can actually grow normally if carefully replaced in their proper anatomic positions. A gauze stent left in the nail sulcus will be pushed out as the new nail grows. Complete regrowth of an avulsed nail usually requires 4 to 5 months at 1 mm per week.

137

Finger-Tip Avulsion, Superficial

Presentation

The mechanisms of injury can be a knife, a meat slicer, a closing door, a falling manhole cover, spinning fan blades, or turning gears. Depending on the angle of the amputation, varying degrees of tissue loss will occur from the volar pad, or finger tip.

What To Do:

✔ **X-ray any crush injury or an injury caused by a high speed mechanical instrument, such as an electric hedge trimmer.**

✔ **Consider tetanus prophylaxis** (see Chapter 151).

✔ **Perform a digital block to obtain complete anesthesia** (see Appendix B).

✔ Thoroughly debride and irrigate the wound.

✔ **When active bleeding is present, provide a bloodless field** by wrapping the finger from the tip proximally with a Penrose drain. Secure the proximal portion of this wrap with a hemostat and unwrap the tip of the finger. Alternatively, cut the end off of a small sized latex glove finger, place it over the hand, then roll the cut end down over the finger, forming a constricting band. A commercial digital tourniquet (Turnicot) may also be used.

✔ **On a wound with less than one square centimeter of full-thickness tissue loss, apply a simple nonadherent dressing** (see Appendix C) with some gentle compression.

✔ Where there is greater than one square centimeter of full-thickness skin loss there are three options that may be followed after surgical consultation:

- Simply apply the same nonadherent dressing used for a smaller wound.
- If the avulsed piece of tissue is available and it is not severely crushed or contaminated, convert it into a modified full-thickness graft and suture it in place. Any adherent fat and as much cornified epithelium as possible must be cut and scraped away using a scalpel blade. This will produce a thinner, more pliable graft that will have much less tendency to lift off its underlying granulation bed as the cornified epithelium dries and contracts. Leaving long ends on the sutures will allow a compressive pad of moistened cotton to be tied on and help prevent fluid accumulation under the graft. A simple finger-tip compression dressing can serve the same purpose (Figure 137-1).

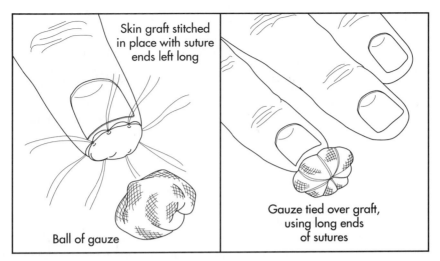

Figure 137-1 Simple finger-tip compression dressing.

- With a large area of tissue loss that has been thoroughly cleaned and debrided and where the avulsed portion has been lost or destroyed, consider a thin split-thickness skin graft on the site. Using buffered 1% Xylocaine, raise an intradermal wheal on the volar aspect of the patient's wrist or hypothenar eminence until it is the size of a quarter. Then, with a #10 scalpel blade, slice off a very thin graft from this site. Apply the graft in the same manner as the full-thickness one (above) with a compression dressing.

✔ **In infants and young children, finger-tip amputations can be sutured back on in their entirety as a composite graft** (i.e., containing more than one type of tissue). In older children and adults, composite grafts will usually fail, and therefore it is important to "defat" the severed portion, as noted above, so that it is more likely to survive as a full-thickness skin graft.

✔ **When the loss of soft tissue has been sufficient to expose bone, simple grafting will be unsuccessful, and surgical consultation is required.**

✔ Schedule a wound check in 2 to 4 days. During that time, the patient should be instructed to keep his finger elevated to the level of his heart and maintained at rest.

✔ Apply a protective four-prong splint for comfort.

✔ Unless the bandage gets wet, a dressing change need not be done for 7 to 10 days. Even then, the innermost layers of gauze may be left in place if the wound appears to be clean and not infected. Always have the patient return immediately with increasing pain or other signs of infection.

✔ If the wound is contaminated, a 3- to 5-day course of an antibiotic like cephalexin (Keflex) 500 mg tid may be effective prophylaxis, but antibiotics are not routinely required even for an uncomplicated open phalanx tip fracture.

✔ Prescribe an analgesic such as acetaminophen plus hydrocodone (Lorcet) 7.5 mg or 10 mg q4h prn pain.

371

What Not To Do:

✘ Do not apply a graft directly over bone or over a potentially devitalized or contaminated bed.

✘ Do not attempt to stop wound bleeding by cautery or ligature, which are likely to increase tissue damage and are probably unnecessary.

✘ Do not forget to remove any constricting tourniquet used to obtain a bloodless field.

 DISCUSSION

The finger tip, being the most distal portion of the hand, is the most susceptible to injury, and thus the most often injured part. Treating small- and medium-sized finger-tip amputations without grafting is becoming increasingly popular. Allowing repair by wound contracture may leave the patient with as good a result and likely better sensation, without the discomfort or minor disfigurement of taking a split-thickness graft.

On the other hand, covering the site with a graft may give the patient a more useful and less sensitive finger tip within a shorter period of time. Unlike the full-thickness graft, a thin split-thickness graft will allow wound contracture and thereby allow for skin with normal sensitivity to be drawn over the end of the finger.

The full-thickness graft, on the other hand, will give an early, tough cover that is insensitive but has a more normal appearance. The technique followed should be determined by the nature of the wound, as well as the special occupational and emotional needs of the patient. Explain the options to the patient, who can help decide the course of action.

138 Fishhook Removal

Presentation

The patient has been snagged with a fishhook and arrives with it embedded in her skin.

What To Do:

✔ Cleanse the hook and puncture wound with povidone-iodine or another antiseptic solution. Provide tetanus prophylaxis as needed (see Chapter 151). **Most patients will benefit from local infiltration of 1% buffered lidocaine using a 27-gauge needle inserted through the same puncture created by the fishhook.**

✔ **For hooks lodged superficially, first try the simple "retrograde" technique.** Push the hook back along the entrance pathway while applying gentle downward pressure on the shank (like the "string" technique, without the string) (Figure 138-2). If the hook does not come out, an 18-gauge needle may be inserted into the puncture hole and used as a miniature scalpel blade. Manipulate the hook into a position so you can cut the bands of connective tissue caught over the barb and release it.

✔ **For more deeply embedded hooks, "needling" the hook is an alternative technique** that requires somewhat greater skill but allows work on an unstable skin surface such as a finger or ear (Figure 138-1). Slide a large gauge (#20 or #18) hypodermic needle through the puncture wound alongside the hook. Now blindly slide the needle opening over the barb of the hook and, holding the hook firmly, lock the two together. Now with the barb covered, remove the hook and needle as one unit. Since the needle does not cut through the dermis, there is often no need for local anesthesia.

✔ **When a single hook is embedded in a stable skin surface such as the back, scalp, or arm, the best way to remove it is by using a simple "string" technique** (Figure 138-2). Align the shaft of the hook so that it is parallel to the skin surface. Press down on the hook with the index finger to disengage the barb. Place a loop of string (fishing line or 1-0 silk) over the wrist and around the hook, and with a quick jerk opposite from the direction the shaft of the hook is running, pop the hook out. When done properly, this procedure is painless and does not require anesthesia. The hook may shoot out in the direction that the string is being pulled, so be careful that no one is standing in the path of the fishhook.

✔ **When the hook is deeply embedded, the barbed end of the hook is protruding through the skin, or the previous techniques cannot be utilized, proceed**

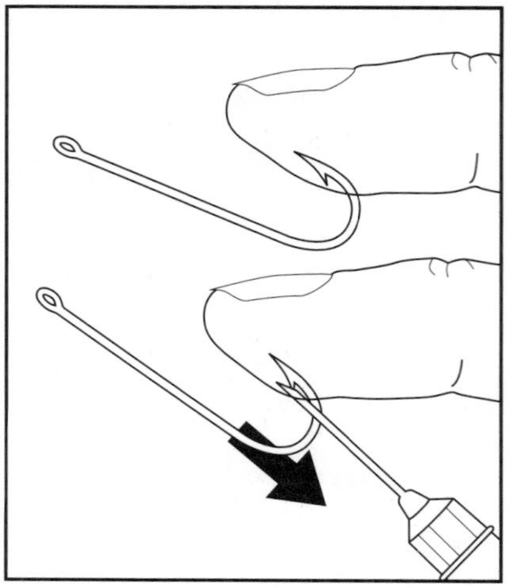

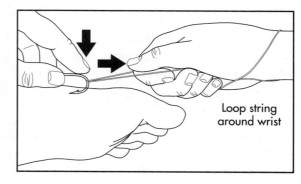

Figure 138-1 Needling hook.

Figure 138-2 "String" technique.

Loop string
around wrist

with the tried and true "push through" maneuver. Locally infiltrate the area with 1% buffered lidocaine and then push the point of the hook along with its barb up through the skin. Now with a pin cutter or metal snip, cut off the tip of the hook and remove the shaft or cut off the shaft of the hook and pull the tip through (Figure 138-3).

✔ **If a multifaceted (treble) hook is embedded, cover the free hooks with corks or use a pin cutter or metal snips to remove the free hooks and protect the patient as well as others from additional harm.** When significant manipulation is anticipated, infiltrate first with 1% buffered lidocaine.

What Not To Do:

✘ Do not try to remove a multiple hook or a fishing lure with more than one hook without first removing the free hooks.

✘ Do not attempt to use the "string" technique if the hook is near the patient's eye.

✘ Do not routinely prescribe prophylactic antibiotics. Even hooks that have been contaminated by fish rarely cause secondary infection.

374

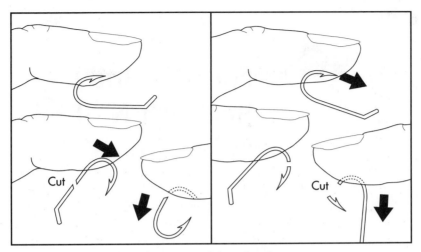

Figure 138-3 Push through techniques.

 DISCUSSION

With the string, retrograde, and needling techniques, there is no lengthening of the puncture track or creation of an additional puncture wound. The quickest and easiest method for removing a fishhook is the string technique. Use it in the field with no special equipment or anesthesia, but it is not recommended when the hook is positioned on a skin surface that is likely to move when the string is pulled, because skin movement will cause the vector of force to change, and the barb may not release.

139

Foreign Body
Beneath Nail

Presentation

The patient complains of a paint chip or wooden sliver under the nail. Often he has unsuccessfully attempted to remove the foreign body, which will be visible beneath the nail.

What To Do (Paint Chip):

✔ **Without anesthesia, remove overlying the nail by shaving it with a #15 scalpel blade** (Figure 139-1).

✔ Cleanse remaining debris with normal saline and trim the nail edges smooth with scissors.

✔ Provide tetanus prophylaxis if necessary (see Chapter 151) and then dress the area with antibiotic ointment and a bandage strip.

What To Do (Sliver):

✔ If the patient is cooperative and can tolerate some discomfort, carve through the nail down to the perimeter of the sliver with a #11 scalpel blade until the overlying nail falls away. The foreign body can now be cleansed away, antibiotic ointment can be applied to the exposed nailbed, and a Band-Aid dressing can be applied (Figure 139-2, *A*).

✔ **For a more extensive excision of a nail wedge, you will need to perform a digital block** (see Appendix B).

✔ **Slide a small straight iris scissors between the nail and nailbed on both sides of the sliver and cut out the overlying wedge of nail** (Figure 139-2, *B*).

✔ Cleanse any remaining debris with normal saline and trim the fingernail until the corners are smooth.

✔ Provide tetanus prophylaxis (see Chapter 151) if needed.

✔ Dress with antibiotic ointment and a bandage. Have the patient redress the area 2 to 3 times daily until healed and keep the fingernail trimmed close.

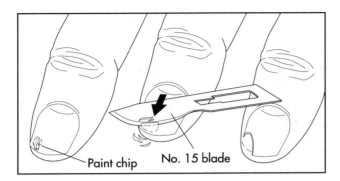

Figure 139-1 Paint chip removal.

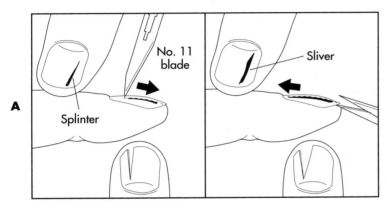

B **Figure 139-2** Sliver removal.

What Not To Do:

✗ Do not run the tip of the scissors into the nailbed while sliding it under the fingernail (instead angle the tip up into the undersurface of the nail).

DISCUSSION

It is usually not possible to remove a long sliver from beneath the fingernail using the "shaving" technique with a scalpel blade without injuring the nailbed and causing the patient considerable discomfort. After providing a digital block, it is sometimes possible to remove the sliver by surrounding it with a hemostat that has been slipped between the nail and nailbed and then pulling out the entire sliver, but if any debris remains visible, then the overlying nail wedge should be removed. It is usually unwise simply to attempt to pull the foreign body from beneath the nail because some debris usually remains and will most likely lead to a nailbed infection.

140

Impalement
Injuries, Minor

Presentation

A sharp metal object such as a needle, heavy wire, nail, or fork is driven into or through a patient's extremity. In some instances, the patient may arrive with a large object attached; for instance, a child who has stepped on a nail going through a board. As minor as most of these injuries are, they tend to create a spectacle and draw a crowd (Figure 140-1).

What To Do:

✔ **If the patient arrives with an impaled object attached to something that is acting like a lever and causing pain with any movement, either quickly cut off this lever or immediately pull the patient's extremity off the sharp object.** (An exposed nail or metal spike can usually be cut with an orthopedic pin cutter [Figure 140-2].)

✔ Obtain x-rays when pain and further damage from a leveraged object are not problems, and when there is a suspicion of an underlying fracture, fragmentation, or hooking of the impaled object, as might occur with a heavy wire that has been thrown from under a lawnmower. **It is not necessary to x-ray a penetrating nail, fork, or other nonmalleable, nonfragile object that will remain intact and is easily removed regardless of its radiographic appearance.**

✔ Examine the extremity for possible neurovascular or tendon injury.

✔ **If surgical debridement is anticipated after removal of the object, then infiltration of an anesthetic should be provided prior to removal.** Otherwise, consider whether or not the patient wants the transient discomfort of local anesthetic before the object is quickly pulled out. Local anesthesia will usually not give complete pain relief when a deeply embedded object is removed; inform the patient of this.

✔ **Objects with small barbs, such as crochet needles and fish spines, can be removed by first anesthetizing the area and then applying firm traction until the barb is revealed through the puncture wound.** The fibrils of connective tissue caught over the barb can then be cut with a scalpel blade or fine scissors.

✔ After removal of the impaled object, the wound should be appropriately debrided and irrigated as described for puncture wounds (see Chapter 147). Tetanus prophylaxis should

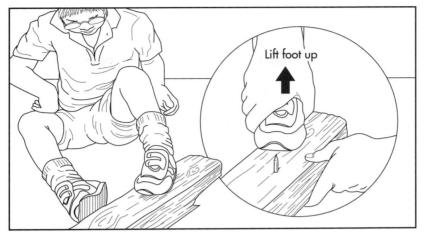

Figure 140–1 Foot stuck to nail with rapid removal.

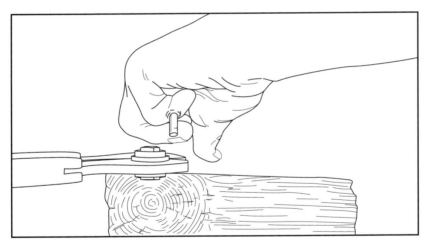

Figure 140–2 Cut an exposed nail with an orthopedic pin cutter.

be provided (see Chapter 151) and, except for contaminated wounds like a fish spine, prophylactic antibiotics should not routinely be prescribed.

What Not To Do:

✘ Do not send a patient to x-ray with a leveraged object impaled, creating further pain and possible injury with every movement.

✘ Do not try to hand-saw off a board attached to an impaled object. The resultant movement will obviously cause unnecessary pain and possibly harm.

DISCUSSION

Simple impalement injuries of the extremities should not be confused with major impalement injuries of the neck and trunk in which the foreign object should not be precipitously removed. With major impalement injuries, careful localization with x-rays is required, and full exposure and vascular control in the operating room are also necessary to prevent rapid exsanguination when the impaled object is removed from the heart or a great vessel. Large impalement injuries of the extremities also require immediate surgical consultation and thorough consideration of potential neurovascular and musculoskeletal injuries.

141

Laceration, Simple

Presentation

There may be a history of being slashed by a knife, glass shard, or other sharp object that results in a clean, straight wound. Impact with a hard object at an angle to the skin may tear up a flap of skin. Crush injury from a direct blow may produce an irregular or stellate laceration with a variable degree of devitalized tissue, abrasion, and visible contamination. Wounds may involve vascular areas of the face and scalp where the risk of infection is low, or extremities where infection becomes a greater risk, along with the possibility of tendon and nerve damage. The elderly and patients on chronic steroid therapy may present with "wet tissue paper" skin tears following relatively minor trauma.

What To Do:

✔ Establish the approximate time of injury. After 4 hours, wounds should be scrubbed to remove the protein coagulum. There is no significant time-related difference in infection rates for wounds closed within 18 hours.

✔ Determine the exact mechanism of injury, which should alert you to the possibility of an underlying fracture, retained foreign body, wound contamination, or tendon or nerve injury.

✔ Investigate for any underlying factors that may increase the risk of wound infection, such as diabetes, malnutrition, morbid obesity, or patients taking chronic immunosuppressive doses of corticosteroids, as well as chemotherapy, AIDS, alcoholism, and renal failure.

✔ Ask about tetanus immunization status and provide prophylaxis where indicated (see Chapter 151).

✔ **Test distal, sensory, and motor function. Test tendon function against resistance. If function is intact but there is pain, suspect a partial tendon laceration.** Tendon and nerve lacerations deserve specialty consultation.

✔ **Consider imaging studies if there might be a radio-opaque retained foreign body.** Most glass fragments will be revealed on ordinary x-rays.

✔ **Consider anxiolytic conscious sedation for children,** such as oral, nasal, or rectal midazolam (Versed) or IM ketamine (Ketalar). Follow your hospital protocol.

✔ **Children may also benefit from a topical anesthetic agent,** especially for scalp and facial lacerations. Lidocaine 4% plus epinephrine 1:1000 plus tetracaine 0.5% (LET) is safe, effective, and inexpensive. Put 3 ml on a cotton ball and press firmly into the wound for 15 minutes either with tape or with the parent's gloved hand. After removing the cotton, test the effectiveness of the anesthesia by touching with a sterile needle. If any sensitivity remains, infiltrate the area with buffered lidocaine as described below.

✔ **Buffer plain lidocaine (Xylocaine) solution by adding 1 ml of sodium bicarbonate solution to every 9 to 10 ml of lidocaine and allow it to approximate body temperature in a pocket.** The maximum safe dose of lidocaine is 5 mg/kg (up to 300 mg). Bupivacaine (Marcaine) is slightly slower in onset but has a much longer duration of action and may be useful for crush injuries and fractures where pain is expected to be prolonged beyond closure of the laceration. Bupivacaine cannot be buffered because it precipitates in alkaline solution. Epinephrine is sometimes added to lidocaine used on the face for its short-lived help with hemostasis and duration of anesthesia, but its use should generally be avoided because of its increased pain on injection and its slower healing and increased infection rate. Bicarbonate inactivates epinephrine.

✔ **To reduce pain, inject subdermally very slowly, begin inside the cut margin of the wound, avoid piercing intact skin,** work from the area already anesthetized, and use a 27- or 30-gauge needle on a 5- or 10-ml syringe.

✔ **Use regional blocks to avoid distorting tissue or where there is no loose areolar tissue to infiltrate, such as the finger tip.**

✔ **Clean the wound after anesthesia is complete. Superficial lacerations with little or no visible contamination, facial lacerations, and scalp lacerations may be cleaned by gentle scrubbing with a gauze sponge soaked in normal saline or a 1% solution of povidone-iodine** (dilute the stock 10% Betadine tenfold with 0.9% NaCl). **Deeper contaminated lacerations may require pressure irrigation with a syringe and splash shield such as ZEROWET SPLASHIELD using the same 1% povidone-iodine solution or plain saline if the patient is allergic to iodine.** All visible debris and devitalized tissue must be removed, either by scraping with the edge of a scalpel blade or by excision with scalpel or scissors. Cosmetic considerations will influence the degree to which facial lacerations are debrided, but excision of contaminated, nonviable wound edges will produce a neater scar.

✔ **Hair generally does not need to be removed. When necessary, shorten hair with scissors rather than shaving with a razor.**

✔ **Simple lacerations seldom require special techniques for hemostasis.** Direct pressure for 10 minutes, correct wound closure, and a compression dressing should almost always stop the bleeding.

✔ Examine the wound free of blood with good lighting. Examine any deep structures such as tendons by direct visualization through their full range-of-motion, looking for partial lacerations. If the wound has been heavily contaminated with debris; crushed, macerated, or neglected for a day; or exposed to pus, feces, saliva, or vaginal discharge, consider excising the entire wound and closing the fresh surgical incision, if practical. Otherwise, provide for open management by packing with sterile, fine-mesh gauze covered with multiple layers of coarse, absorptive gauze, after soaking them in the 1% solution of povidone-iodine. Unless the patient develops a fever, leave the dressing undisturbed for

4 days or have the patient begin cleaning the wound with mild soap and water in 24 to 48 hours. If there are no signs of infection, the granulating wound edges may then be approximated as a delayed primary closure.

✔ **Close the wound primarily only if it is clean and uninfected.** Minimize the amount of suture material buried inside the wound. The less used, the less chance of infection. **Wound closure tapes offer the least risk of infection, and are most successfully used on simple superficial lacerations with minimal tension.** They are the closure material of choice for "wet tissue paper" skin tears. Before application, degrease the skin with alcohol, being careful not to get any into the wound. An adhesive agent such as tincture of benzoin may then be thinly applied to the skin surrounding the laceration (again, avoiding the open wound). Push the wound edges together and apply the tape to maintain approximation. Cyanoacrylate topical skin adhesive (Dermabond) can be used with small wounds as above in a location that does not allow for the application of a length of wound closure tape.

✔ **Most scalp lacerations and many trunk and proximal extremity lacerations that are straight, without edges that curl under (invert), can be most easily repaired using skin staples.** Push edges together and staple so edges evert slightly. Hair does not interfere with this technique and does not cause a problem if caught under a staple.

✔ **For deep or irregular lacerations, or lacerations on hands, feet, and skin over joints, use a monofilament nonabsorbable suture such as nylon or polypropylene, either 4-0, 5-0, or 6-0, using the smallest diameter with sufficient strength.** A good strategy to realign skin and minimize sutures is to begin by approximating the midpoint of the wound and then bisect the remaining gaps. Simple interrupted stitches in most body sites should be about 0.5 cm apart, 0.5 cm deep, and 0.5 cm back from the wound edge. Make each dimension 0.25 cm for cosmetic closure on the face. Angle the needle going in and coming out so it grasps more subcutaneous tissue than skin, and the wound edges should evert so the dermis is aligned level on both sides, thereby minimizing visible scar. Tie each stitch with only enough tension to approximate the edges. A continuous running suture is a more rapid technique of closing a straight laceration. When there is wound-edge inversion, the length of the wound edge can be completely excised, or vertical mattress sutures can be placed between simple interrupted stitches. Unless deep fascial planes are disrupted, avoid buried sutures because they increase the risk of infection.

✔ **After closing the wound with sutures, apply antibiotic ointment and a sterile dressing, which will protect the wound and provide absorption, compression, and immobilization.** Splint lacerations over joints. Scalp lacerations may need a compression dressing only if there is excessive bleeding or swelling. Facial wounds generally do not require special dressings but should be cleaned twice a day with half-strength hydrogen peroxide on a cotton-tipped applicator to prevent crusting between wound edges. This cleaning should be followed by reapplication of antibiotic ointment.

✔ Schedule a wound check in 2 days if the patient is likely to develop any problems with infection, require dressing changes, or need continued wound care. Instruct patients to re-

383

turn at any time for bleeding, loss of function, or signs of infection: increasing pain, pus, fever, swelling, redness, or heat. After 48 hours, most sutured wounds can be redressed with a simple bandage that can be easily removed and replaced by the patient, allowing a shower each day.

✔ Wound closure strips can be left in place until they fall off on their own. Additional tape can be applied if the original closure strips fall off prematurely. A transparent film dressing such as OpSite can be applied over the closure strips when they are first applied to provide a waterproof cover.

✔ **Remove facial sutures in 4 to 5 days to reduce visible stitch marks.** The epidermis should have resealed by this time, but the dermis has not developed much tensile strength, so reinforce the wound edges with woundclosure strips for a few more days.

✔ **Most scalp, chin, trunk, and limb stitches should be removed in 7 days. Sutures may be left in 10 to 14 days where there is tension across wound edges as on the shin and over the extensor surfaces of large joints.** Sutures are easily and painlessly cut with the tip of a #11 or #12 scalpel blade and removed with simple smooth forceps. Cut alternate loops of running sutures.

What Not To Do:

✘ Do not prescribe prophylactic antibiotics for simple lacerations. Antibiotics do not reduce infection rates, and only select for resistant organisms. Most infections can be easily treated when they occur. Limit prophylactic antibiotics to high-risk wounds.

✘ Do not close a laceration if there is visible contamination, debris, nonviable tissue, or signs of infection. Dress it open.

✘ Do not substitute antibiotics for wound cleansing and debridement. Reserve antimicrobials for infections and deep inoculated puncture wounds that cannot be cleaned.

✘ Do not substitute x-rays for meticulous, direct wound examination when a foreign body is suspected by history.

✘ Do not pour topical anesthetic solution on standard wound-dressing sponges for application to the wound. They are designed to absorb liquid rather than deliver it to the wound surface.

✘ Do not use undiluted skin cleansing solution such as 10% povidone-iodine or any skin scrub containing detergents or soap within an open wound. They kill tissue and can even increase the infection rate.

✘ Do not shave an eyebrow. The hair is a useful marker for reapproximating the skin edges and can take months to years to grow back.

✘ Do not remove too much skin or underlying tissue when debriding the face and scalp.

✘ Do not use buried absorbable sutures in a wound with a high risk of infection.

✘ Do not insert drains in simple lacerations. They are more likely to introduce infection than prevent it.

✘ Do not use Neosporin ointment. Many patients are allergic to the neomycin and develop allergic contact dermatitis.

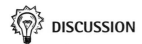 **DISCUSSION**

The most important goal of early wound care is preventing infection. Development of wound infections, failure to detect foreign bodies, and missed injuries of tendons and nerves are common sources of litigation after lacerations. Careful history and wound examination, thorough cleansing, and debridement all reduce these risks. One must strike a balance at times between excising enough tissue to prevent infection but not so much as to create a deformity and limit future options for elective scar revision.

Cyanoacrylate (Dermabond), the less toxic versions of SuperGlue and Crazy Glue, work well for minor pediatric lacerations. The technique is to hold the wound edges together (the same as for tape or staples), squeeze a line of glue over the laceration line, and hold for 30 seconds. For added strength, this may be repeated once or twice. No dressing is required.

Ointments probably facilitate healing and reduce infection by their occlusive, rather than antibiotic, properties. White petrolatum is apparently as good as antibiotic ointment and avoids the risk of allergic reaction. Options for dressings over the ointment have become numerous. It is unclear whether any one dressing is superior to the others, and therefore personal preference and patient convenience should help determine which dressing material to use.

SUGGESTED READINGS

Bruns TB, Simon HK, McLario DJ, et al: Laceration repair using a tissue adhesive in a children's emergency department, *Pediatrics* 98:673-675, 1996.

Cummings P, Del Beccaro MA: Antibiotics to prevent infection of simple wounds: a meta-analysis of randomized studies, *Am J Emerg Med* 13:396-400, 1995.

Ernst AA, Marvez-Valls E, Nick TG, et al: Topical lidocaine adrenaline tetracaine (LAT gel) versus injectable buffered lidocaine for local anesthesia in laceration repair, *West J Med* 167:79-81, 1997.

Mehta PH, Dun KA, Bradfield JF, et al: Contaminated wounds: infection rates with subcutaneous sutures, *Ann Emerg Med* 27:43-48, 1996.

Quinn J, Wells G, Sutcliffe T, et al: A randomized trial comparing octylcyanoacrylate tissue adhesive and sutures in the management of lacerations, *JAMA* 277:1527-1530, 1997.

Scarfone RJ, Jasani M, Gracely EJ: Pain of local anesthetics: rate of administration and buffering, *Ann Emerg Med* 31:36-40, 1998.

Schilling CG, Bank DE, Borchert BA, et al: Tetracaine, epinephrine (adrenaline) and cocaine (TAC) versus lidocaine, epinephrine and tetracaine (LET) for anesthesia of lacerations in children, *Ann Emerg Med* 25:203-208, 1995.

Smack DP, Harrington AC, Dun C, et al: Infection and allergy incidence in ambulatory surgery patients using white petrolatum vs bacitracin ointment: a randomized controlled trial, *JAMA* 276:972-977, 1996.

Marine Envenomations

Presentation

After swimming in the ocean and coming into contact with marine life, the patient may seek medical attention because of local pain, swelling, or skin discoloration. Marine animal envenomations can be divided into two major categories: puncture wounds and focal rashes. Severe envenomations can be accompanied by systemic symptoms such as vomiting, paralysis, seizures, respiratory distress, and hypotension, but this review is limited to the more common injuries with minor local reactions.

Puncture Wounds:

A laceration of the leg with blue edges suggests a **stingray** attack. There is immediate, local, intense pain; edema of soft tissue; and a variable amount of bleeding. The pain peaks after 30 to 60 minutes, may radiate centrally, and may last 48 hours.

A single ischemic puncture wound with a red halo and rapid swelling suggests a **scorpionfish** envenomation. The pain is immediate, intense, and radiating. Untreated, the pain peaks 60 to 90 minutes after the sting, persists for at least 6 to 12 hours, and sometimes lasts for days.

Multiple small punctures in an erratic pattern with or without purple discoloration or retained fragments are typical of a **sea urchin** sting. The venomous spines can inflict immediate and intense burning pain with severe muscle aching. The area surrounding the puncture wounds may be red and swollen.

Focal Rashes:

Contact with a **bristleworm** is followed by an intense, red, itchy rash.

Contact with **feather hydroids** and **sea anemones** induces a mild reaction, consisting of instantaneous burning, itching, and urticaria. The reaction may be delayed and can include the appearance of papules, hemorrhagic vesicles, or zoster-like reactions 4 to 12 hours after contact.

The sting of the **fire coral** induces intense, burning pain, with central radiation and reactive regional lymphadenopathy.

Most of the **jellyfish** with suspended tentacles create "tentacle prints" or a whip-like pattern of darkened reddish brown, purple, or frosted and cross-hatched stripes in the precise areas of skin contact. Vesiculation and skin necrosis may follow.

What To Do:

Puncture wounds:

✔ **To relieve pain and perhaps attenuate some of the thermolabile protein components of the venom, soak the wound in hot (not scalding) water (approximately 45° C or 113° F) for 30 to 90 minutes or longer for pain control.**

✔ During hot water treatment, **infiltrate in or around the wound with 0.5% bupivacaine or 1% or 2% lidocaine without epinephrine to provide further pain control.** When necessary, add narcotic analgesics.

✔ Irrigate larger wounds as soon as possible with normal saline or dilute 1% povidone-iodine solution (add 10% Betadine to 0.9% NaCl in a 1:10 ratio) and remove visible pieces of spine or debris.

✔ **Obtain x-rays if there might be any radio-opaque fragments like retained stingray or sea urchin spines.**

✔ **When anesthesia is complete and pain has been controlled, thoroughly explore, debride, and irrigate open wounds. Remove fragile sea urchin spines using the same technique as for a superficial sliver** (see Chapter 173).

✔ Suture lacerations loosely or, better, pack open for delayed primary closure (see Chapter 151).

✔ Ensure current tetanus prophylaxis (see Chapter 151).

✔ **Prescribe prophylactic antibiotics except for minor abrasions, superficial punctures, and superficial lacerations. Ciprofloxacin (Cipro) 500 to 750 mg bid or doxycycline (Vibramycin) 100 mg bid for adults, and trimethoprim plus sulfamethoxazole (Bactrim) for children, all prescribed for 3 to 5 days, are the most appropriate regimens for coverage of pathogenic marine microbes.** The genus *Vibrio* is particularly common in the ocean and poses a serious risk for immunosuppressed patients. Injuries with potential for serious infection include large lacerations, deep puncture wounds (particularly near joints), and retained foreign material. Recomended initial parenteral antibiotics include cefoperazone, cefotaxime, ceftazidime, chloramphenicol, gentamicin, and tobramycin.

✔ For infected wounds, obtain both aerobic and anaerobic cultures and alert the clinical microbiology laboratory that standard antimicrobial susceptibility testing media may need to be supplemented with NaCl to permit growth of marine bacteria. Institute the above antibiotics except for minor wound infections with the classic appearance of erysipelas, which can be treated with erythromycin or cephalexin. Prescribe antibiotics for 7 to 14 days. Hospitalization may be required for severe infections.

✔ **Provide pain control with NSAIDs and narcotic analgesics as required.**

✔ Follow-up all wounds in 1 to 2 days with periodic revisits until healing is complete.

Focal rashes:

✔ **For fire coral, jellyfish, hydroid, or sea anemone stings, decontaminate the area with a liberal soaking of 5% acetic acid (vinegar).** The leading alternative is 40% to 70% isopropyl (rubbing) alcohol. Apply continuously for 30 minutes or until the pain disappears. Cold compresses may be helpful for relieving edema, erythema, and pruritus.

✔ **After decontamination, remove any visible large tentacles with forceps or double-gloved hands. Remove small particles by applying shaving foam or some equivalent and gently shaving the area with a safety razor, dull knife, or plastic card,** then clean with an antibacterial soap and flush with water or saline solution.

✔ Treat any generalized allergic reactions with antihistamines, corticosteroids, epinephrine, and IV fluids as indicated.

✔ **When irritation from sponges, bristle worms, or other marine creatures causes erythematous or urticarial eruptions, it usually means that tiny spicules and spinules are embedded in the skin.** Apply vinegar compresses to help neutralize toxins and relieve pain. **Dry the skin, apply the sticky side of a piece of adhesive tape to the affected area, and peel the tape back to remove these particles.** Cosmetic deep cleansing strips for skin pores (Bioré Pore Perfect) can also be effective when available.

✔ **Residual inflammation can be treated with topical corticosteroids such as Aristocort A 0.1% or 0.5% cream or Topicort emollient cream or ointment 0.25%** (dispense 15 g and apply tid-qid). **A topical steroid in combination with a topical anesthetic can be additionally soothing** (e.g., Pramosone cream, lotion, or ointment 2.5% tid-qid). Systemic antihistamines will also be helpful, and on occasion, systemic corticosteroids will be required.

✔ Provide pain control with NSAIDs and narcotic analgesics as required.

✔ **Advise the patient on sun avoidance and the use of sun blocks to prevent postinflammatory hyperpigmentation.** Hydroquinone (Eldoquin-Forte) 4% skin bleaching cream can be prescribed to be rubbed in bid when hyperpigmentation occurs.

✔ Check wounds for infection in 2 and 7 days.

What Not To Do:

✘ Do not use fresh water to decontaminate jellyfish stings. It may cause their microscopic cysts to swell, rupture, and trigger additional stinging.

✘ Do not use ammonia as a substitute for vinegar compresses. It is a powerful skin irritant.

✘ Do not use topical or systemic corticosteroids for puncture wounds unless there is an allergic reaction.

✘ Do not constrict limbs tightly.

DISCUSSION

Any wound acquired in the marine environment can become infected, and this is particularly likely if the wound is large, a puncture, or contaminated with bottom sediment or organic matter.

Stingray victims are generally innocent beach walkers who step on the back of the ray, which reflexively strikes upward with its tail, inflicting a penetrating wound along the upper

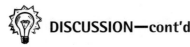

DISCUSSION—cont'd

foot, ankle, or lower leg. The anatomic structure of the stingray's back causes a deep, jagged, painful wound that may contain fragments of the barb that is located proximal to the tail.

Scorpionfish, lionfish, and stonefish stings occur in divers and fisherman, and sometimes keepers of marine aquariums or those involved in illegal tropical fish trade. Catfish stings are common when the fish are handled or kicked. Certain catfish species produce a venom in glands at the base of the dorsal spine, but most do not, and catfish venom causes only mild local pain, redness, and swelling. Of more concern is the wound caused by the spine and the likelihood of infection.

Sea urchin victims are stung when they step on, handle, or brush up against these sessile creatures. The sea urchin secretes a toxin on the surface of its spines that is transferred into the wound when they penetrate the skin. The brittle spines also tend to break off and remain in the wound.

SUGGESTED READINGS

Auerbach PS: Marine envenomations, *N Engl J Med* 325:486–493, 1991.
Schwartz S, Meinking T: Venomous marine animals of Florida: morphology, behavior, health hazards, *J Florida Med Assoc* 84:433–440, 1997.

143

Nail Root Dislocation

Presentation

The patient has caught his finger in a car door or dropped a heavy object like a can of vegetables on a bare toe, with the edge of the can striking the base of the toenail and causing a painful deformity. The base of the nail will be found resting above the eponychium instead of in its normal anatomic position beneath. The cuticular line that had joined the eponychium at the nail fold will remain attached to the nail at its original position (Figure 143-1).

What To Do:

✔ **Take an x-ray to rule out an underlying fracture** (which may require reduction as well as protective splinting).

✔ **Anesthetize the area using a digital block** (see Appendix B).

✔ **Lift the base of the nail off the eponychium and thoroughly cleanse and inspect the nailbed.** Minimally debride loose cuticular tissue and test for a possible avulsion of the extensor tendon (see Chapter 104).

✔ **Repair any nailbed lacerations with a fine absorbable suture like 7-0 or 6-0 Vicryl.**

✔ **Reinsert the root of the nail under the eponychium.**

✔ **Reduce any underlying angulated fracture.**

✔ **If the nail tends to drift out from under the eponychium, it can be sutured in place with two 4-0 nylon or polypropylene stitches in the proximal corners.**

✔ Any nonabsorbable sutures should be removed after 1 week.

✔ Cover the area with a finger-tip dressing (see Appendix C) and splint any underlying fracture.

✔ Provide tetanus prophylaxis (see Chapter 151).

✔ Follow-up should be provided in 3 to 5 days. Instruct patients to return immediately if there is increasing pain or any other sign of infection.

✔ **Prescribe an analgesic like acetaminophen plus hydrocodone (Lorcet).**

✔ Prophylactic antibiotics are not routinely required, even with associated fractures of the distal phalanx, except in immunocompromised patients. Contaminated wounds should receive 3 to 5 days of cephalexin (Keflex) 500 mg tid.

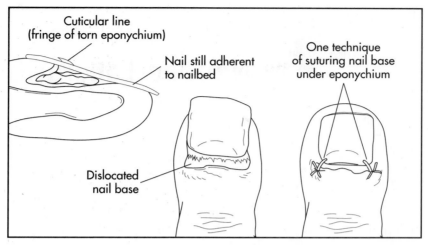

Figure 143-1 Dislocated nail root.

What Not To Do:

✗ Do not ignore the nail root dislocation and simply provide a finger-tip dressing. This is likely to lead to continued bleeding or to a later infection because tissue planes have not been replaced in their natural anatomic position.

✗ Do not debride any portion of the nailbed, sterile matrix, or germinal matrix.

 DISCUSSION

Because the nail is not as firmly attached at the base or lunula as it is to the distal nailbed, impact injuries can avulse only the base (nail root), leaving it lying on top of the eponychium. It may be surprising that this injury is often missed, but at first glance, a dislocated nail can appear to be in place, and without careful inspection, a patient can return from radiology with negative x-rays and be treated as if he only had an abrasion or contusion. The attachment of the cuticle from the nail fold of the eponychium to the base of the nail forms a constant landmark on the nail. If any nail is showing proximal to this landmark, it indicates that the nail is not in its normal position beneath the eponychium.

Nailbed Laceration

Presentation

The patient has either cut into her nailbed with a sharp edge or crushed her finger. With shearing forces, the nail may be avulsed from the nailbed to varying degrees, and there may be an underlying bony deformity.

What To Do:

✔ Provide appropriate tetanus prophylaxis (see Chapter 151).

✔ **Obtain x-rays of any crush injury.**

✔ **Perform a digital block** (see Appendix B) **for anesthesia.**

✔ **With a simple laceration through the nail, remove the nail surrounding the laceration to allow for suturing the laceration closed** as follows:

- Use a straight hemostat to separate the nail from the nailbed (Figure 144-1).
- Use fine scissors to cut away the surrounding nail.
- **Cleanse the wound with saline and suture with a fine absorbable suture (6-0 or 7-0 Vicryl or Dexon)** (Figure 144-2).
- **Apply a nonadherent dressing (e.g., Adaptic gauze) and antibiotic antiseptic ointment, and plan a dressing change within 24 hours to prevent painful adherence to the nailbed.**

✔ **When a crush injury results in open hemorrhage from under the fingernail, the nail must be completely elevated to allow proper inspection of the damage to the nailbed.** A bloodless field helps visualization. (A ½-inch Penrose drain makes a good finger tourniquet.) **Angulated fractures need to be reduced, and nailbed lacerations should be sutured with a fine absorbable suture (6-0 or 7-0 Vicryl or Dexon).** An intact nail can be cleaned and reinserted for protection or a nailbed dressing (see Chapter 136) can be applied. Cover with an appropriate finger-tip dressing (see Appendix C).

What Not To Do:

✗ Do not use nonabsorbable sutures to repair the nailbed. The patient will be put through unnecessary suffering to remove the sutures.

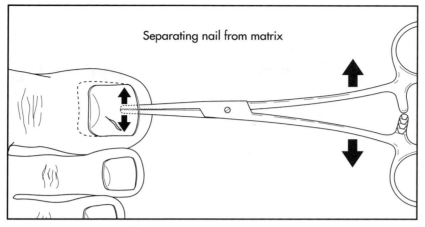

Figure 144-1 Separate nail from nailbed using straight hemostat.

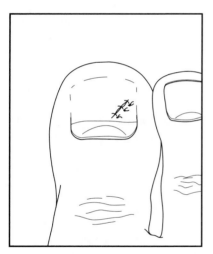

Figure 144-2 The nailbed can be repaired after it has been fully exposed.

✘ Do not attempt to suture a nailbed laceration through the nail. It can be done, but it precludes the meticulous approximation necessary for smooth nail regrowth.

 DISCUSSION

Significant nailbed injuries can be hidden by hemorrhage and a partially avulsed, overlying nail. These injuries must be repaired to help prevent future deformity of the nail. Surgical consultation should be obtained when nailbed lacerations involve the germinal matrix under the base of the nail.

Needle (Foreign Body) in Foot

Presentation

Although a needle could be embedded under any skin surface, most commonly a patient will have stepped on one while running or sliding barefoot on a carpeted floor. Generally, but not invariably, the patient will complain of a foreign body sensation with weight bearing. A very small puncture wound will be found at the point of entry, and on occasion, a portion of the needle will be palpable.

What To Do:

✔ Tape a partially opened paper clip as a skin marker to the plantar surface of the foot, with the tip of the opened paper clip over the entrance wound. Instruct the patient not to allow anyone to remove the paper clip until after the needle is removed (Figure 145-1, *A*).

✔ **Send the patient for PA and lateral radiographs of the foot with the skin marker in place** (Figure 145-1, *B*).

✔ Evaluate the x-rays. If the needle appears to be very deep, perhaps call in a consultant who can remove the needle under fluoroscopy. **If the needle is relatively superficial, inform the patient that removing a needle is not as easy as it appears.** Let him know that a simple technique will be used to locate and remove the needle, but that sometimes the needle is hidden within the tissue of the foot ("like a needle in a haystack"). If the needle cannot be located within 10 to 15 minutes, to avoid further damage to his foot, a consultant will be called in to arrange for removal under fluoroscopy.

✔ **Establish a bloodless field by elevating the leg above the level of the heart, tightly wrapping an Ace bandage around the foot and lower leg, and then inflating and clamping off a thigh cuff at approximately 50 to 75 mmHg above the patient's systolic pressure.** This will become uncomfortable within 10 to 15 minutes and thereby serve as an automatic timer for the procedure.

✔ **Remove the Ace wrap, clean, and then paint the area with Betadine solution, and locally infiltrate the appropriate area with buffered 1% lidocaine** (Xylocaine). (It will be somewhat more comfortable if the needle stick is accomplished from the medial or lateral aspect of the foot rather than directly into the plantar surface.)

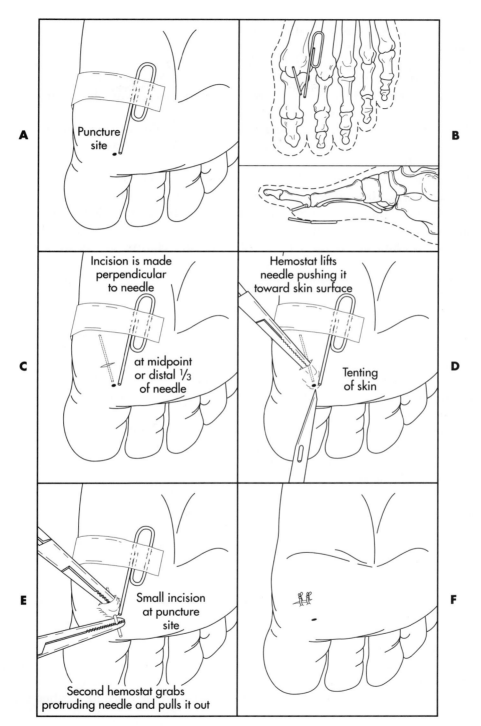

Figure 145–1 Procedure for removing a needle from the foot.

✔ **The x-rays should reveal an approximate location of the needle relative to the paper clip skin marker.**

✔ With the patient lying prone and the plantar surface of his foot facing upward, **make an incision that crosses perpendicular to the needle's apparent position at its midpoint or one third of the way toward the most superficial end of the needle.** Do not cut deep to the plantar fascia (Figure 145-1, *C*).

✔ **As the needle is cut across, there will be an audible clicking sound. Spread the incision apart, visualize the needle, and grasp it firmly with a hemostat or small Kelly clamp.**

✔ **Now, push the needle out in the direction from which it entered.** Even the eye or back end of a broken needle is sharp enough to be pushed to the skin surface. **If the needle tents up the skin and will not push through, nick the overlying skin surface with a scalpel blade until the needle exits** (Figure 145-1, *D*). **Grab this end with another clamp, let go with the first clamp, and remove the needle** (Figure 145-1, *E*).

✔ Let the thigh cuff down and suture the incision closed. Apply an appropriate dressing (Fig. 145-1, *F*).

✔ Provide tetanus prophylaxis as indicated (see Chapter 151).

What Not To Do:

✘ Do not ignore the patient who thinks he stepped on a needle but in whom a puncture wound cannot be found. Obtain an x-ray anyway, because the puncture wound is probably hidden.

✘ Do not give the patient the impression that the removal will be quick and easy.

✘ Do not make the incision near the tip of the needle or directly over and parallel to the needle. The needle will not be exactly where it is thought to be, and the incision will miss exposing the needle.

✘ Do not persist in extensively undermining or extending the incision if the needle is not located within 10 minutes of beginning the procedure. This is unlikely to be productive and may do the patient harm.

✘ Do not routinely place the patient on prophylactic antibiotics.

 DISCUSSION

Many a young doctor has been found sweating away at the foot of an emergency department stretcher, unable to locate a needle foreign body. The secret for improving the chances of success is in realizing that the x-ray only gives you an approximate location of the needle and that the incision must be made in a direction and location best suited for locating the needle, not removing it.

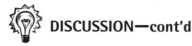 **DISCUSSION—cont'd**

There are three additional principles to keep in mind. First, the position of the needle on radiographs needs to be correlated with the anatomy of the skin surface rather than the bony anatomy of the foot. Second is the simple geometric principle that the surest way to intersect a line (the needle) is to bisect it in the plane perpendicular to its midpoint. Third, the only structures of importance in the forefoot or heel that lie plantar to the bones are the flexor tendons, and they lie close to the bones.

Let the patient know how difficult it sometimes is to locate the needle and remove it; this can create a win-win situation: the physician looks good if it is found and still looks experienced and well-informed if it is not found.

If the patient is taken to fluoroscopy, the physician or radiologist can place a hemostat around the needle under direct vision. It can then be pushed out using the same technique described above.

Linear foreign bodies such as needles can be removed from the sole of the foot without extensive dissection, complex apparatus, or repeated x-ray studies. Although blind dissection is generally not a good technique because of the risk of injury, in this particular situation, relative safety can be provided by gentle limited dissection with iris scissors of insufficient strength to sever tendons and by setting firm limits on time and depth of exploration.

SUGGESTED READINGS

Gilsdorf JR: A needle in the sole of the foot, *Surg Gynecol Obstet* 163: 573-574, 1986.

146 Paronychia

Presentation

The patient will present with finger or toe pain that is either chronic and recurrent in nature or has developed rapidly over the past several hours, accompanied by redness and swelling of the nail fold. There are three distinct varieties:

- Chronic paronychia (Figure 146-1, *A*) is most commonly seen with the "ingrown toenail" with chronic inflammation, thickening and purulence of the eponychial fold, and loss of the cuticle. There may or may not be granulation tissue. This also occurs with individuals whose hands are frequently exposed to moisture and minor trauma.
- Acute paronychia almost always involves fingers and is much more painful. It is caused by the introduction of pyogenic bacteria by minor trauma and results in acute inflammation and abscess formation within the thin subcutaneous layer between the skin of the eponychial fold and the germinal layer of the eponychial cul-de-sac (Figure 146-1, *B*). In its earliest form, there may only be cellulitis with no collection of pus.
- The third variety of paronychia is a subungual abscess, which occurs in the same location as a subungual hematoma, between the nail plate and the nailbed (Figure 146-1, *C*).

What To Do:

✔ **Perform a unilateral or bilateral digital block** (see Appendix B) and establish a bloodless field with a rubber tourniquet if a significant surgical procedure is anticipated.

✔ **With a chronic paronychia:**

- **Consider conservative treatment or temporizing the condition by sliding a cotton wedge or waxed dental floss under the corner of an ingrown nail to lift the nail edge from its embedded position (anesthesia is usually not required). Then place the patient on antibiotics like cefadroxil (Duricef) 1 g qd and warm soaks at least qid.** When candidiasis is suspected, the area should be kept dry and treated with local applications of nystatin or other topical antifungal medications. A long course of systemic medication may be required. Follow-up with a podiatrist is important for ingrown toenails. **Instruct the patient to cut toenails straight across to prevent recurrences.**
- A more aggressive approach, and one more likely to be successful, is to sharply excise the affected portion of the nail, nailbed, and matrix down to the periosteum of the dis-

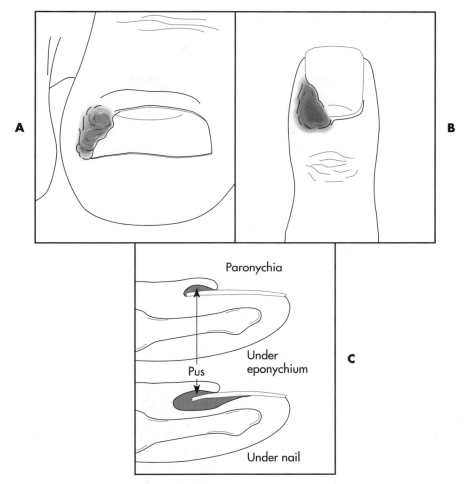

Figure 146-1 A, Chronic paronychia in an "ingrown toenail." **B,** Acute paronychia of finger. **C,** Subungual extension of pus.

tal phalanx (Figure 146-2, *A*). The patient is instructed to soak the toe in warm water for 20 minutes bid and arrange for multiple follow-up visits.

✔ **With acute paronychia:**
- **When there is minimal swelling and there appears to be only cellulitis, gently use an 18-gauge needle to separate the cuticle of the lateral nail fold from the nail to rule out or drain any collection of pus (anesthesia is usually not required).** Instruct the patient to soak the finger in warm water for 10 minutes qid and consider prescribing antibiotics for 3 or 4 days.
- **Where there is redness and swelling of the nail fold, take a #15 scalpel blade, separate the cuticle from the nail, open the eponychial cul-de-sac, and drain**

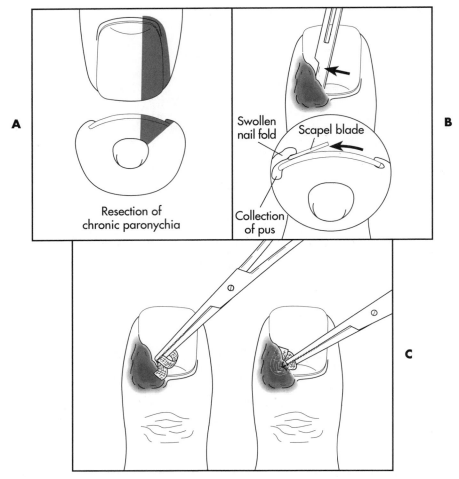

A

Resection of
chronic paronychia

B

Swollen
nail fold

Scapel blade

Collection
of pus

C

Figure 146-2 A, Extensive excision of chronic paronychia. **B,** Draining acute paronychia without invasion of skin. **C,** A gauze wick helps ensure continued drainage.

any abscess (Figure 146-2, *B*). Keep the blade flat against the dorsal surface of the nail. There is no need to make an incision and therefore a digital block should also not be necessary. A tiny wick (1 cm of ¼-inch gauze) may be slid into the opening to ensure continued drainage (Figure 146-2, *C*). Debride any periungual pustules. Most importantly, instruct the patient to perform warm soaks every 2 hours initially and then at least qid for 1 to 2 days. When drainage is complete, antibiotics are not routinely required, but where significant cellulitis is present, a short course of antibiotics may be indicated. Clindamycin (Cleocin) 150 mg qid or amoxicillin plus clavulanate (Augmentin) 250 mg tid has a wide spectrum of activity against most pathogens isolated from paronychia. The patient should be informed that if the paronychia quickly recurs, excision of a portion of the nail might be required.

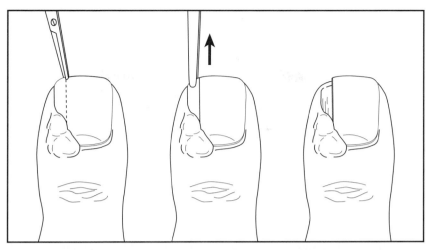

Figure 146-3 Removing a portion of the nail helps to prevent recurrence.

- **A more aggressive approach is to excise a portion of the nail. Unlike the more extensive procedure used with chronic paronychia, only a portion of the nail need be removed** (Figure 146-3). After establishing a digital block and a bloodless field, insert a fine straight hemostat between the nail and the nailbed and push and spread until you enter the eponychial cul-de-sac. Often it is at this point that pus is discovered. Then using a pair of fine scissors, cut away the quarter to third of the nail bordering the paronychia. Separate the cuticle using the hemostat and pull this unwanted fragment away. A nonadherent dressing is required over the exposed nailbed, as well as an early dressing change (within 24 hours).
- ✔ **With a subungual abscess:**
  - **Consider conservative treatment not requiring a digital block. Merely perform a trephination using the same "hot paper clip" technique used for a subungual hematoma** (see Chapter 150). The patient must perform frequent warm soaks over the next 36 hours to prevent recurrence.
  - **The more effective but more aggressive technique requires removal of the proximal third of the nail.** After performing a digital block, a straight hemostat is required to separate the cuticle of the eponychium from the underlying nail. Using the hemostat, the proximal portion of the nail is pulled out from under the eponychium and excised. On occasion, an incision will have to be made along the eponychium to allow the proximal nail to be excised. The removal of the proximal portion of the nail allows for the complete drainage of the abscess without any risk of recurrence. A nonadherent dressing is also required in this instance. Extensive damage to the germinal matrix by the infection may preclude healthy nail regrowth.
  - **When there is a distal collection of pus, a simple excision of an overlying wedge of nail using scissors should provide complete drainage.**

401

What Not To Do:

✘ Do not order cultures or x-rays on uncomplicated cases.

✘ Do not make an actual skin incision. The cuticle needs only to be separated from the nail in order to release any collection of pus.

✘ Do not remove an entire fingernail or toenail to drain simple paronychia.

✘ Do not attempt to drain an herpetic whitlow.

✘ Do not confuse a felon (tense tender finger pad) with paronychia. Felons will require more extensive surgical treatment.

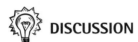 **DISCUSSION**

Whenever conservative therapy is instituted, the patient should be advised of the advantages and disadvantages of that approach. If the patient is not willing or reliable enough to perform the required aftercare or cannot accept the potential treatment failure, then it would seem prudent to begin with the more aggressive treatment modes.

No single antibiotic will provide complete coverage for the array of bacterial and fungal pathogens cultured from paronychias. Theoretically, clindamycin or amoxicillin plus clavulanate should be the most appropriate antibiotics, but because the vast majority of paronychias are easily cured with simple drainage, systemic antibiotics are usually not indicated. In immunocompromised patients and those with peripheral vascular disease, cultures and antibiotics are indeed warranted.

Remain alert to the possible complications of neglected paronychia such as osteomyelitis, septic tenosynovitis of the flexor tendon, or a closed space infection of the distal finger pad (felon). Recurrent infections may be due to a herpes simplex infection (herpetic whitlow) or fungus (onychomycosis). Tumors like squamous cell carcinoma or melanoma, cysts, syphilitic chancres, warts, or foreign body granulomas can occasionally mimic paronychia. Failure to cure paronychia within 4 or 5 days should prompt specialized culture techniques, biopsy, or referral.

147 Puncture Wounds

Presentation

Most commonly, the patient will have stepped or jumped onto a nail. There may be pain and swelling, but often the patient is only asking for a tetanus shot. He can usually be found in the emergency department with his foot soaking in a basin of Betadine solution. The wound entrance usually appears as a linear or stellate tear in the cornified epithelium on the plantar surface of the foot.

What To Do:

✔ Obtain a detailed history to ascertain the force involved in creating the puncture and the relative cleanliness of the penetrating object. Note the type of footwear (tennis or rubber-soled shoes) and the potential for foreign body retention. Also ask about tetanus immunization status and underlying health problems that may potentially diminish host defenses.

✔ Have the patient lie prone, backwards on the gurney, so that raising the head of the bed flexes his knee and brings the sole of the foot into clear view. Clean the surrounding skin and carefully inspect the wound. Provide good lighting and take your time. Examine the foot for signs of deep injury, such as swelling and pain with passive motion of the toes. Although the occurrence is unlikely, test for loss of sensory or motor function.

✔ **If the puncture was created by a slender object like a sewing needle or thumb tack, which was positively removed intact, no further treatment is necessary. If there is any question that a piece may have broken off in the tissues, obtain x-rays** (see Chapter 145). Most metal and glass foreign bodies are visualized on plain films, while plastic, aluminum, and wood are more radiolucent and may require ultrasound, CT scan, or MRI for visualization. Retained foreign bodies increase the potential for infection and should be suspected in patients who present with infection or are not responding to treatment of infection.

403

✔ **With deep, highly contaminated wounds, orthopedic or podiatric consultation should be sought** to consider a wide debridement in the operating room. This is done to prevent the catastrophic complication of osteomyelitis.

✔ **Most puncture wounds only require simple debridement and irrigation.**

✔ **Saucerize (shave) the puncture wound using a #10 scalpel blade to remove the surrounding cornified epithelium and any debris that has collected beneath its surface.** Alternatively, the jagged epidermal skin edges overlying the puncture tract may be painlessly trimmed (Figure 147-1).

✔ **If debris is found, gently slide a large-gauge blunt needle or an over-the-needle (Angiocath) catheter down the wound track and slowly irrigate with a physiologic saline solution, moving the catheter in and out until debris no longer flows from the wound.** At times, a small amount of local anesthesia will be necessary to accomplish this.

✔ **Provide tetanus prophylaxis** (see Chapter 151).

✔ Cover the wound with a Band-Aid and instruct the patient on the warning signs of infection. Arrange for follow-up at 48 hours. **Spend some time on documentation and patient education. Talk about delayed osteomyelitis and the importance of medical attention if there is continued aching or discomfort 2 to 3 weeks postinjury.** Explain that even with proper care, foreign material may be embedded deep in the wound, and infection could occur. Explain that in most cases, prophylactic antibiotics do not prevent these infections, and that the best practice is close observation and aggressive therapy if infection occurs.

✔ **Patients presenting after 24 hours will often have an established wound infection. In addition to the debridement procedures described above, these patients usually will respond to oral antistaphylococcal antibiotics like cephalexin (Keflex).** Suspect retained foreign bodies and consider imaging studies. Provide patients with crutches for nonweight-bearing and encourage them to soak the infected foot.

What Not To Do:

✘ Do not be falsely reassured by having the patient soak in Betadine. This does not provide any significant protection from infection and is not a substitute for debridement and irrigation.

✘ Do not attempt a jet lavage within a puncture wound. This will only lead to subcutaneous infiltration of irrigant and the spread of foreign material and bacteria.

✘ Do not obtain x-rays for simple nail punctures, except for the unusual case where large radio-opaque particulate debris is suspected to be deeply embedded within the wound, or the physical examination suggests bony injury.

✘ Do not routinely prescribe prophylactic antibiotics. Reserve them for established wound infections.

✘ Do not begin soaks at home unless there are early signs of infection developing.

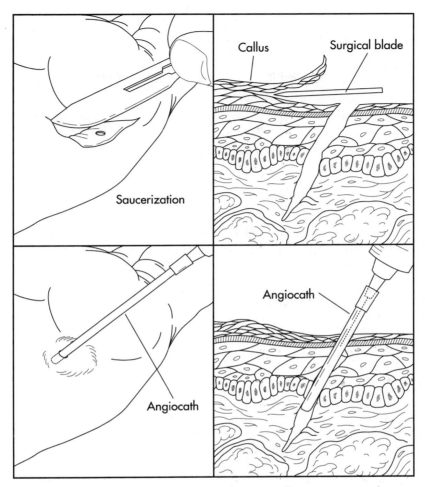

Figure 147-1 Simple debridement and irrigation for puncture wounds.

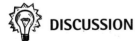 **DISCUSSION**

Small, clean, superficial puncture wounds uniformly do well. The pathophysiology and management of a puncture wound, therefore, depend on the material that punctured the foot, the location of the wound, the depth of penetration, the time to presentation, the footwear penetrated, and the underlying health status of the victim. Punctures in the metatarsophalangeal joint area may also be of higher risk for serious wound complications because of the greater likelihood of penetration of joint, tendon, or bone. Early presenters tend to be children or adults seeking tetanus prophylaxis. These patients tend to have a low incidence of infection.

Continued

DISCUSSION—cont'd

Patients who present late usually have increasing pain, swelling, or drainage as evidence of an early or established infection. Retained, unsuspected foreign bodies, often pieces of a tennis shoe or sock, are a source of serious infection.

When the foot is punctured, the cornified epithelium acts as a spatula, cleaning off any loose material from the penetrating object as it slides by. This debris often collects just beneath this cornified layer, which then acts like a trap door holding it in. Left in place, this debris may lead to early abscess formation, cellulitis, and lymphangitis. Saucerization allows for the removal of debris and the unroofing of superficial small foreign bodies or abscesses found beneath the thickly cornified skin surfaces.

Osteomyelitis caused by *Pseudomonas aeruginosa* remains the most devastating of puncture wound complications. The exact incidence of osteomyelitis remains uncertain and is estimated to be from 0.4% to 0.6%. The metatarsal heads are most at risk for osteomyelitis. A nail through the sole of a tennis shoe can inoculate *Pseudomonas* organisms. Any patient considered to have penetration of the bone, joint space, or plantar fascia, particularly over the metatarsal heads, should be referred to an orthopedic surgeon or podiatrist for appropriate follow-up evaluation.

SUGGESTED READINGS

Chisholm CD, Schlesser JF: Plantar puncture wounds: controversies and treatment recommendations, *Ann Emerg Med* 18:1352-1357, 1989.

Fitzgerald RH, Cowan JDE: Puncture wounds of the foot, *Orthop Clin North Am* 6(4):965-972, 1975.

Patzakis MJ, Wilkins J, Brien WW, et al: Wound site as a predictor of complications following deep nail punctures to the foot, *West J Med* 150:545-547, 1989.

Pennycook A, Makower R, O'Donnell AM: Puncture wounds of the foot: can infective complications be avoided? *J Roy Soc Med* 87:581-583, 1994.

Schwab RA, Powers RD: Conservative therapy of plantar puncture wounds, *J Emerg Med* 13:291-295, 1995.

Verdile VP, Freed HA, Gerard J: Puncture wounds to the foot, *J Emerg Med* 7:193-199, 1987.

148

Ring Removal

Presentation

A ring has become tight on the patient's finger after an injury (usually a sprain of the PIP joint) or after some other cause of swelling, such as a local reaction to a bee sting. Sometimes, tight-fitting rings obstruct lymphatic drainage, causing swelling and further constriction. The patient usually wants the ring removed even if it requires cutting it off, but occasionally a patient has a very personal attachment to the ring and objects to its cutting or removal.

What To Do:

✔ Limit further swelling by applying ice and elevating the extremity.

✔ When a fracture is suspected, order appropriate x-rays either before or after removing the ring.

✔ With substantial injuries, a digital or metacarpal block might be necessary to allow for the comfortable removal of the ring.

✔ **Usually, lubrication with soap and water, along with proximal traction on the skin beneath the ring, is enough to help the ring twist off the finger** (Figure 148-1).

✔ **When the ring is too tight to twist off this way, exsanguinate the finger by applying a tightly wrapped spiral of Penrose drain or flat rubber phlebotomy tourniquet tape around the exposed portion of the finger, elevate the hand above the head, wait 15 minutes, and then inflate a blood pressure cuff to 50 to 75 mmHg above the patient's systolic pressure as a tourniquet around the upper arm above the exsanguinated finger** (Figure 148-2). Wrap the cuff with cotton cast padding to keep the Velcro connection from separating and clamp the tubing to prevent a slow air leak. Remove the tight rubber wrapping from the finger and, leaving the tourniquet in place, again attempt to twist the ring off using soap and water for lubrication. If necessary, this procedure may be repeated several times until the swelling is adequately reduced.

✔ **If the ring is still too tight or if there is too much pain to allow for the above techniques, a ring cutter can be used to cut through a narrow ring band. Bend the ring apart with pliers or hemostats placed on either side of this break to allow removal** (Figure 148-3).

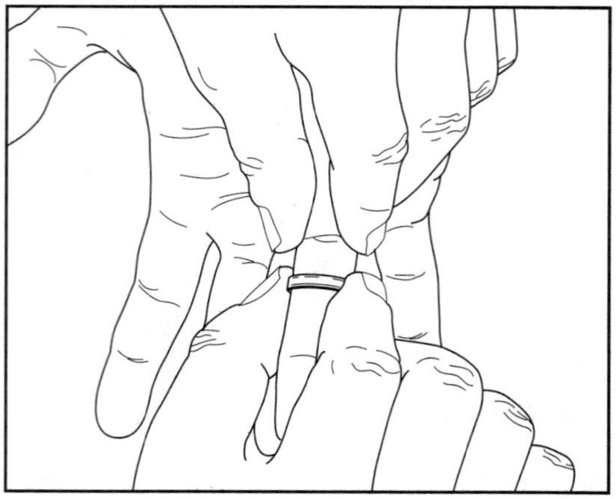

Figure 148-1 Pull skin taut and twist ring off.

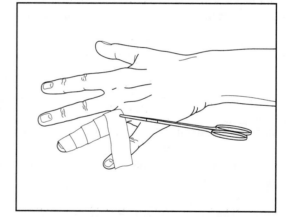

Figure 148-2 Tourniquet technique.

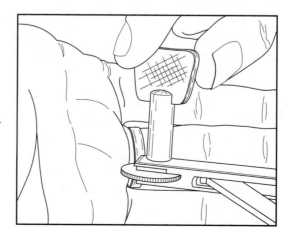

Figure 148-3 Ring-cutter technique.

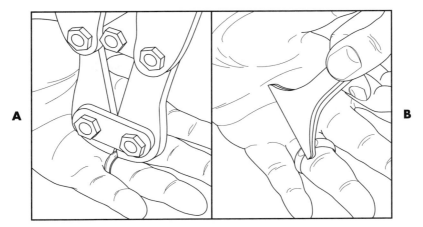

Figure 148-4 Orthopedic pin-cutter technique.

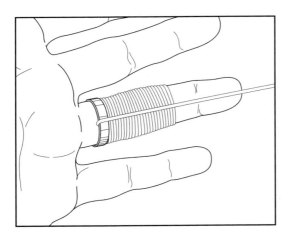

Figure 148-5 String technique.

✔ **If the band is wide or made of hard metal, it will be much easier to cut out a 5-mm wedge from the ring using an orthopedic pin-cutter** (Figure 148-4, *A*). **Then take a cast spreader, place it in the slot left by the removal of the wedge, and spread the ring open** (Figure 148-4, *B*). Alternatively, two cuts may be made on opposite sides of the ring, allowing it to be removed in halves.

✔ **Another useful device for removing constricting metal bands is the Dremel Moto-tool** with its sharp-edged grinder attachment. Protect the underlying skin with a heat-resistant shield. If a dental drill is available, it can also cut steel.

✔ **Another technique that tends to be rather time-consuming and only moderately effective (but one that can be readily attempted in the field) is the coiled-string technique.** Slip the end of a string (kite string is good) under the ring and wind a tight single-layer coil down the finger, compressing the swelling as you go. Pull up on the end of the string under the ring, then slide and wiggle the ring down over the coil (Figure 148-5).

409

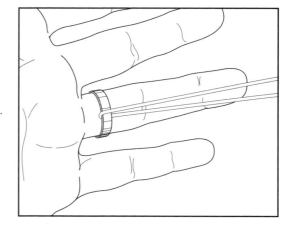

Figure 148-6 String loop technique.

✔ **Another technique is to pull a length of string under the ring using a hemostat and then tie it into a large loop that can be placed around the physician's wrist. This will allow traction to be applied and the string slid around and around the circumference of the ring as it is pulled, using lubricant as above. A small lubricated Penrose drain may be substituted for string.**

✔ Teach patients how to avoid the vicious cycle of a tourniquet effect by promptly removing rings from injured fingers.

What Not To Do:

✘ When a patient is expected to have transient swelling of the hand or finger without evidence of vascular compromise, and she requests that the ring not be removed, do not insist that the ring must be cut off. If the patient is at all responsible, she can be warned of the signs of vascular compromise (pallor, cyanosis, or pain) and instructed to keep her hand elevated and apply cool compresses. She should then be made to understand that she is to return for further care if the circulation does become compromised because of the possible risk of losing her finger. Be understanding and document the patient's request and the directions given to her.

 DISCUSSION

The constricting effects of a circumferential foreign body can lead to obstruction of lymphatic drainage, which in turn leads to more swelling and further constriction, until venous and eventually arterial circulation is compromised. If it is believed that these consequences are inevitable, be direct with the patient about having the ring removed.

DISCUSSION—cont'd

Hair-thread tourniquets can become tightly wrapped around an infant's finger, toe, or penis, causing swelling, ischemia, or discoloration distal to the band. Removing this constricting band of one or more fibers can be quite difficult. It usually requires local anesthesia, dissection, and severing of the deeply embedded fibers with a large-gauge needle and magnifying loupes. Provide for a wound check in 24 hours.

SUGGESTED READINGS

Greenspan L: Tourniquet syndrome caused by metallic bands: a new tool for removal, *Ann Emerg Med* 11:375-378, 1982.

149

Subungual Ecchymosis

Presentation

The patient had a crushing injury over the fingernail—getting it caught between two heavy objects, for example, or striking it with a hammer. The pain is initially intense but rapidly subsides over the first half hour. By the time he is examined, only mild pain and sensitivity may remain. There is a light brown or light blue-brown discoloration beneath the nail.

What To Do:

✔ Obtain an x-ray to rule out a possible fracture of the distal phalangeal tuft.
✔ **Apply a protective finger-tip splint, if necessary, for comfort.**
✔ **Explain that you are not drilling a hole in the patient's nail, because there is not a subungual hematoma to evacuate.** Inform the patient that, in time, he may lose the fingernail, but that a new nail will replace it.

What Not To Do:

✘ Do not perform a trephination of the nail.

DISCUSSION

Unlike the painful space-occupying subungual hematoma, the subungual ecchymosis only represents a thin extravasation of blood beneath the nail or a mild separation of the nail from the nailbed. Doing a trephination will not relieve any pressure or pain and may indeed cause excruciating pain, as well as open this space to possible infection. The patient's familiarity with nail trephination (above) may give him the erroneous expectation that he should have his nail drilled.

150 Subungual Hematoma

Presentation

After a blow or crushing injury to the fingernail, the patient experiences severe and sometimes excruciating pain that persists for hours and may even be associated with a vasovagal response. The fingernail has an underlying deep blue-black discoloration, which may be localized to the proximal portion of the nail or extend beneath its entire surface.

What To Do:

✔ X-ray the finger to rule out an underlying fracture of the distal phalanx.

✔ Paint the nail with 10% povidone-iodine (Betadine) solution.

✔ **Perform a trephination at the base of the nail, using a red-hot paper clip, electric cauterizing lance, or drill.** When performed quickly, patients do not feel the heat before the relief of pressure. **Tap rapidly with the cautery or drill a few times in the same spot at the base of the hematoma until the hole is through the nail. When resistance from the nail gives way, stop further downward pressure to avoid damaging the nailbed** (Figure 150-1).

✔ Persistent bleeding from this opening can be controlled by having the patient hold a folded 4 × 4 gauze pad firmly over the trephination while holding his hands over his head.

✔ **Apply an antibacterial ointment such as Betadine and cover the trephination with a Band-Aid.**

✔ To prevent infection, instruct the patient to keep his finger dry for 2 days and not to soak it or go swimming for 1 week.

✔ If there is an underlying fracture, the patient should be instructed to keep his finger completely dry for the next 10 days and return immediately at the first sign of infection.

✔ A protective aluminum finger-tip splint may also be comforting, especially if the bone is fractured.

✔ Inform the patient that he will eventually lose his fingernail, and a new nail will grow out after 2 to 6 months.

413

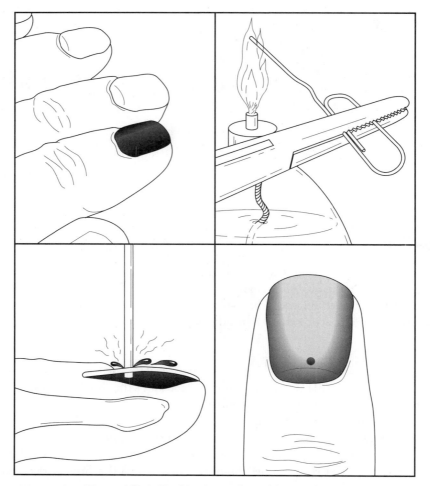

Figure 150–1 Trephination with a red–hot paper clip.

What Not To Do:

✗ Do not perform a trephination on a subungual ecchymosis (see Chapter 149).

✗ Do not perform a trephination when there is an underlying fracture (this theoretically converts a closed fracture to an open one) unless there is sufficient pain to justify it. The patient should also understand the potential risk of developing osteomyelitis, as well as the need for keeping the finger dry.

✗ Do not perform a digital block. Anesthesia should not be necessary.

✗ Do not perform a trephination on a patient who is no longer experiencing any significant pain at rest. A mild analgesic and protective splint will usually suffice.

✗ Do not make such a small opening that free drainage does not occur. The electrocautery tip may have to be bent to the side or widened to make a wide enough hole.

✘ Do not hold a hot paper clip or cautery wire on the surface of the nail without applying enough slight pressure to melt through the nail. Just holding the hot tip adjacent to the nail can heat up the hematoma and increase the pain without making a hole to relieve it.

✘ Do not send a patient home to soak his finger after a trephination. This will break down the protective fibrin clot and introduce bacteria into this previously sterile space.

✘ Do not routinely prescribe antibiotics. Even when opening a subungual hematoma with an underlying fracture of the distal phalanx, antibiotics have not been shown to be of any value in preventing infection.

✘ Do not remove the nail even with a large subungual hematoma. It is not necessary to inspect for nailbed lacerations or repair them with a closed injury.

 ## DISCUSSION

The subungual hematoma is a space-occupying mass that produces pain secondary to increased pressure against the very sensitive nailbed and matrix. Given time, the tissues surrounding this collection of blood will stretch and deform until the pressure within this mass equilibrates. Within 24 to 48 hours the pain therefore subsides and although the patient may continue to complain of pain with activity, performing a trephination at this time may not improve his discomfort to any significant extent and will expose the patient to the risk of infection. If a trephination is not performed, explain this to the patient who is requesting trephination too late.

There is some risk of missing a nailbed laceration under the hematoma but, for a small laceration, splinting by its own nail may be superior to suturing. When there are associated lacerations, open hemorrhage, or broken nails, perform a digital block and lift up the nail to inspect the nailbed and repair any lacerations. Keep in mind that not all dark patches under the nail are subungual hematomas, Consider the diagnosis of melanoma, Kaposi's sarcoma, and other tumors when the history of trauma and the physical examination are not consistent with a simple subungual hematoma.

SUGGESTED READINGS

Seaberg DC, Angelos WJ, Paris PM: Treatment of subungual hematomas with nail trephination: a prospective study, *Am J Emerg Med* 9:209-210, 1991.

151

Tetanus Prophylaxis

Presentation

The patient may have stepped on a nail or sustained any sort of laceration or puncture wound when the question of tetanus prophylaxis arises.

What To Do:

✔ Always provide appropriate wound care with adequate cleansing, debridement, irrigation, and antibiotics where indicated.

✔ **If the patient has not had tetanus immunization in the past 5 years, give adult tetanus and diphtheria toxoid (Td) 0.5 ml IM. Give pediatric diphtheria and tetanus toxoid (DT) 0.5 ml to children under 7 years of age if their history of previous immunization is unknown or includes less than three doses of DT.**

✔ **If there is any doubt that the patient has had his original series of three tetanus immunizations, add tetanus immune globulin (Hyper-Tet) 250 mg IM,** and make arrangements for him to complete the full series with additional immunizations at 4 to 8 weeks and 6 to 12 months (for children under 7 years of age, 2 to 8 weeks after the first dose, 4 to 8 weeks after the second, and 6 to 12 months after the third dose).

✔ **If there is a history of true hypersensitivity to tetanus toxoid, provide passive immunity with tetanus immune globulin, but instruct the patient that he does not have protection against future exposure.**

✔ Provide the patient with written documentation of the immunizations given.

What Not To Do:

✘ Do not assume adequate immunization. The groups most at risk in the United States today are immigrants, elderly women, and rural southern blacks. Veterans usually have been immunized. Many patients incorrectly assume they were immunized during a surgical procedure. Having had tetanus does not confer immunity.

✘ Do not give tetanus immunizations indiscriminately. Besides being wasteful, too-frequent immunizations are more likely to cause reactions, probably of the antigen–antibody type. (Surprisingly, the routine of administering toxoid and immune globulin simultaneously in two deltoid muscles does not seem to cause mutual inactivation or serum sickness.)

✘ Do not believe every story of allergy to tetanus toxoid (which is actually quite rare). Is the patient actually describing a local reaction, the predictable serum sickness of horse serum, or a reaction to older, less pure preparations of toxoid? The only absolute contraindication is a history of immediate hypersensitivity—urticaria, bronchospasm, or shock. Tetanus toxoid is safe for use in pregnancy.

✘ Do not give pediatric tetanus and diphtheria toxoid (DT) to an adult. DT contains 8 times as much diphtheria toxoid as Td.

 ## DISCUSSION

There continue to be 50 to 100 cases of tetanus in the United States each year. The CDC recommends everyone over 7 years of age receive Td every 10 years, but somehow physicians and patients alike forget tetanus prophylaxis except after a wound. Because tetanus has followed negligible injuries and spontaneous infections, the concept of the "tetanus-prone wound" is not really helpful. The CDC recommends including a small dose of diphtheria toxoid (Td) but, because this is more apt to cause local reactions, perhaps reverting to plain tetanus toxoid in patients who have complained of such reactions.

Pediatric diphtheria-pertussis-tetanus (DPT) vaccine is given at 2, 4, and 6 months, with a fourth dose at 12 to 18 months (6 months after the last dose), and a fifth dose at 4 to 6 years. Thereafter, tetanus toxoid with a reduced dose of diphtheria (Td) is given every 10 years, and boosters are given within 5 years for "tetanus-prone" wounds, which the CDC guidelines define as wounds contaminated with dirt, feces, or saliva; puncture wounds; tears; and wounds from bullets, crushing, burns, and frostbite.

SUGGESTED READINGS

Alagappan K, Rennie W, Kwiatkowski T, et al: Antibody protection to diphtheria in geriatric patients: need for ED compliance with immunization guidelines, *Ann Emerg Med* 30:455-458, 1997.

Alagappan K, Rennie W, Kwiatkowski T, et al: Seroprevalence of tetanus antibodies among adults older than 65 years, *Ann Emerg Med* 28:18-21, 1996.

Alagappan K, Rennie W, Narang V, et al: Immunologic response to tetanus toxoid in geriatric patients, *Ann Emerg Med* 30:459-462, 1997.

Gergen PJ, McQuillan GM, Kiely M, et al: A population-based serologic survey of immunity to tetanus in the United States, *N Engl J Med* 332:761-766, 1995.

Giangrasso J, Smith RK: Misuse of tetanus immunoprophylaxis in wound care, *Ann Emerg Med* 14:573-579, 1985.

Macko MB, Powell CE: Comparison of the morbidity of tetanus toxoid boosters with tetanus-diphtheria toxoid boosters, *Ann Emerg Med* 14:33-35, 1985.

152

Traumatic Tattoos and Abrasions

Presentation

The patient will usually have fallen onto a coarse surface, such as a blacktop or macadam road. Most frequently, the skin of the face, forehead, chin, hands, and knees is abraded. When pigmented foreign particles are impregnated within the dermis, tattooing will occur. An explosive form of tattooing can also be seen with the use of firecrackers, firearms, and homemade bombs.

What To Do:

✔ Cleanse the wound with nondestructive agents (e.g., normal saline, SurClens) and provide tetanus prophylaxis.

✔ With explosive tattooing, particles are generally deeply embedded and will require plastic surgery consultation. Any particles embedded in the dermis may become permanent tattoos. Abrasions that are both large (more than several square centimeters) and uniformly deep into the dermis or below (so that no skin appendages, such as hair follicles, providing a reservoir of regenerating basal epithelium, remain) may also require consultation and/or skin grafts.

✔ **With abrasions and abrasive tattooing, the area can usually be adequately anesthetized by applying 2% viscous Xylocaine or gauze soaked with TAC (tetracaine 0.5%, adrenaline 1:2000, and cocaine 11.8%) directly onto the wound for approximately 5 minutes. If this is not successful, locally infiltrate with buffered 1% lidocaine using a 25-gauge 1½- to 3-inch spinal needle for large areas.**

✔ For wounds containing tar or grease, application of bacitracin ointment prior to cleaning will help dissolve and loosen these contaminants.

✔ **The wound should now be cleaned with a surgical scrub brush, saline, and surgical soap. When impregnated material remains, use a sterile stiff toothbrush to clean the wound or use the side of a #10 or #15 scalpel blade to scrape away any debris** (Figure 152-1). While working, continuously cleanse the wound surface with gauze soaked in normal saline to reveal any additional foreign particles. Large granules may be removed with the tip of a #11 scalpel blade.

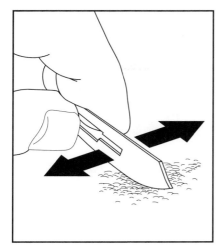

Figure 152-1 Dermabrasion with #10 scalpel blade.

✔ Wounds should be left open and povidone-iodine or bacitracin ointment applied. The patient should be instructed to gently wash the area two to three times per day and continue applying the ointment until the wound becomes dry and comfortable under a new coat of epithelium, which may require a few weeks.

✔ When the wound has been adequately cleansed, one alternative is to use a closed dressing with Adaptic gauze, ointment, and a scheduled dressing change within 2 to 3 days.

What Not To Do:

✘ Do not ignore embedded particles. If they cannot be completely removed, inform the patient about the probability of permanent tattooing and arrange a plastic surgery consultation.

 DISCUSSION

The technique of tattooing involves painting pigment on the skin and then injecting it through the epidermis into the dermis with a needle. As the epidermis heals, the pigment particles are ingested by macrophages and permanently bound into the dermis. Immediate care of traumatic tattoos is important because once the particles are embedded and healing is complete, it becomes difficult to remove them without scarring. It is advisable for a patient to protect a dermabraded area from sunlight for approximately 1 year to minimize excessive melanin pigmentation of the site.

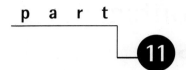

part 11

Dermatologic Emergencies

153

Allergic Contact Dermatitis

Presentation

The patient complains of a very pruritic eczematous rash at sites of skin exposure to allergens. Lesions may consist of small papules, vesicles, or bullae, at times confluent, and inflammation may exist with erythema, edema, oozing, or crusting. This dermatitis may remain localized at contact sites, or, in severe cases, can spread to involve distant body areas. Sites with thin skin (e.g., eyelids, lateral neck, dorsum of hands, genitals) show greater susceptibility, whereas areas with a thick stratum corneum (palms and soles) have more resistance. Because this is a delayed hypersensitivity reaction, the pruritus and rash may not become evident for 24 to 48 hours or longer after exposure to the allergenic substance. Although a substance new to the patient in the past few weeks is more likely to be the precipitating agent, patients do react to personal products that they have been using for years.

What To Do:

✔ Attempt to determine the offending agent. Skin lesion distribution often provides a clue to the offending allergen. Question patients about potential exposure to topical medications like neomycin and benzocaine, or other potential allergens such as sunscreens, moisturizing lotions, perfumes, nail polish, artificial nails, cosmetics, shampoos, hair dyes, household cleaners, laundry products, jewelry, footwear, clothing, and plants like rhus or toxicodendron (see Chapter 170). Metals in jewelry (e.g., nickel, chromium, cobalt) and chemicals in clothing and footwear (e.g., resins, crease resistant finishes, leather dyes, rubber accelerators) can be sources of cutaneous allergens. Vulvitis and balanitis may occur in patients who have an allergy to latex in condoms or ingredients in douches, contraceptive jellies, feminine hygiene products, or toilet paper.

✔ **Have the patient remove the offending allergen from the environment to avoid reexposure and thoroughly wash the skin with a hypoallergenic soap like Neutrogena.**

✔ **For acute reactions with considerable edema and erythema—especially those with inflamed, oozing, or crusted lesions—frequent cool or cold compresses with 1:20 aluminum acetate (Burow's) solution (Domeboro powder packets**

2 per pint of water) have cooling, soothing, and antiseptic effects. Cool baths can also help (Aveeno Colloidal Oatmeal 1 cup or 1 cup each of cornstarch and baking soda in half a bathtub of water).

✔ **For severe reactions, if there are no contraindications (tuberculosis, peptic ulcer, diabetes, herpes, or severe hypertension) prescribe systemic corticosteroids like triamcinolone 40 mg IM or prednisone 50 mg qd × 10 days.** If steroids are given less than 2 weeks, they do not suppress normal adrenocortical secretion, and if the allergen has been removed, the dosage need not be tapered to minimize rebound. Longer courses should be tapered, however.

✔ **Systemic oral antihistamine therapy, such as hydroxyzine (Atarax, Vistaril) 25 to 50 mg q6h prn helps control pruritus.**

✔ **For mild and localized reactions, corticosteroid creams or gels like desoximetasone (Topicort) 0.25% or fluocinonide (Lidex) 0.05% applied tid or qid have antiinflammatory and antipruritic effects.** More severe local reactions can be treated with the very potent topical cream clobetasol (Temovate) 0.05%. Topical steroids may be potentiated with occlusive dressings. **Avoid long-term use of these fluorinated corticosteroids on the face, where they can cause atrophy.**

✔ Impetigo due to superimposed bacterial infection should be treated with systemic antibiotics like dicloxacillin (Dynapen), cephalexin (Keflex), or erythromycin (ERYC) 250 mg qid × 10 days or azithromycin (Zithromax) 500 mg, then 250 mg qd × 4 days.

What Not To Do:

✘ Do not allow patients to apply fluorinated corticosteroids for more than 10 days to the face or genital area, where they can produce premature aging of the skin with thinning and striae.

✘ Do not prescribe systemic steroids for secondary infections such as impetigo, cellulitis, or erysipelas. Also, do not start steroids if there is a history of tuberculosis, diabetes, herpes, or severe hypertension.

DISCUSSION

Allergic contact dermatitis is a delayed cutaneous hypersensitivity or cell-mediated immune reaction. Approximately 50 chemicals cause 80% of the reactions seen in clinical practice. A contact allergic reaction normally appears 12 to 72 hours after exposure in a previously sensitized individual.

Until patch testing can identify the specific offending agent, the patient should be instructed in avoidance of the most likely source of allergen that is inferred by the history and the distribution of the rash. A patient with a facial dermatitis should be advised to avoid all cosmetics, facial creams, and lotions until the exact allergen has been identified.

423

Continued

DISCUSSION—cont'd

Photo-allergic dermatitis, primarily involving sun-exposed skin areas, requires contact with a photosensitizing agent plus exposure to long-wavelength ultraviolet (UVA) radiation, and the dermatitis is limited to exposed skin.

Contact with blister fluid does not spread the allergen, but transfer of allergen remaining under the fingernails or reexposure to allergen persisting on fomites like clothing can continue to spread the dermatitis.

Local corticosteroid therapy is not necessary when systemic therapy is used. When using a topical steroid on the face, however, a less potent agent such as hydrocortisone or desonide is recommended.

SUGGESTED READINGS

Leung DYM, Diaz LA, DeLeo V, et al: Allergic and immunologic skin disorders, *JAMA* 278:1914-1923, 1997.

Williams SR, Clark RF, Dunford JV: Contact dermatitis associated with capsaicin: Hunan hand syndrome, *Ann Emerg Med* 25:713-715, 1995.

c h a p t e r

Contusion (Bruise)

Presentation

The patient has fallen, has been thrown against an object, or has been struck at a site where now there is point tenderness, swelling, ecchymosis, hematoma, or pain with use. On physical examination, there is no loss of function of muscles and tendons (beyond mild splinting because of pain), no instability of bones and ligaments, and no crepitus or tenderness produced by remote stress (such as weight-bearing on the leg or manual flexing of a rib) (Figure 154-1).

What To Do:

✔ Take a thorough history to ascertain the mechanism of injury and perform a complete examination to document structural integrity and intact function.

✔ **Reserve x-rays for possible foreign bodies and bony injury.** Fractures are uncommon after a direct blow but are suggested by pain with remote percussion, stressing of bone (i.e., applying torsion), or an underlying deformity or crepitus. The yield is very low when x-rays are ordered on the basis of pain and swelling alone.

✔ Explain to the patient that swelling will peak in 1 day, then resolve gradually, and that swelling, stiffness, and pain may be reduced by good treatment during the first 1 to 2 days.

✔ **Prescribe R.I.C.E.:**
- Rest the affected part
- Immobilization (the ultimate in rest, best achieved with a splint)
- Cold (usually an ice bag, wrapped in a towel, applied to the injury for 10 to 20 minutes per hour for the first 24 hours)
- Elevation of the affected part (ideally, above the level of the heart)

✔ Provide appropriate analgesia.

✔ **Explain to the patient the late migration and color change of ecchymoses, so that green or purple discoloration appearing farther down the limb 1 week after the injury does not frighten her into thinking she has another injury or complication.**

✔ Large intramuscular hematomas (especially of the anterior thigh) may require drainage or orthopedic consultation.

✔ Arrange for reevaluation and follow-up if there is any continued or increasing discomfort.

425

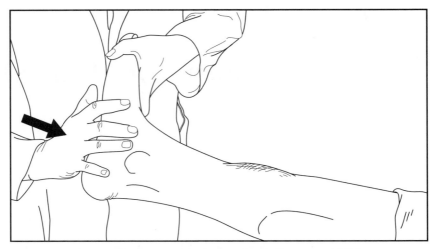

Figure 154-1 Foot percussion provides indirect stress of tibia.

What Not To Do:

✗ Do not apply an elastic bandage to the middle of a limb, where it may act as a venous tourniquet. Include all of the distal limb in the wrapping if a compression dressing is necessary.

✗ Do not confuse patients with instructions for application of heat and exercises to prevent stiffness and atrophy. Concentrate on the here-and-now therapy of the acute injury; namely, rest, immobilization, elevation, and cold: all designed to decrease acute edema. Leave other instructions to follow-up and physical therapy consultants. Patients who confuse today's correct therapy with next week's can complicate their problem.

✗ Do not take for granted that all patients understand rest, immobilization, elevation, and cold. Walking on a fresh foot injury or soaking it for long periods in ice water or Epsom salts is not usually therapeutic.

 DISCUSSION

The acute therapy of contusions concentrates on reduction of the acute edema; all other components of treatment are postponed for 3 to 4 days until the inflammation and edema are reduced. Patients need to know this time course and must understand that the more the swelling can be reduced, the sooner the injuries can heal, function can return, and the pain will decrease. Edema of hands and feet is especially slow to resolve because these structures usually hang in a dependent position and require much modification of activity to rest and elevate.

155

Cutaneous Abscess or Pustule

Presentation

A patient with an abscess may or may not have a history of minor trauma (such as an embedded foreign body) but has localized pain, swelling, and redness of the skin. The area is warm, firm, and usually fluctuant to palpation. Sometimes there is surrounding cellulitis or lymphangitis and, in the more serious case, fever. There may be a spot where the abscess is close to the skin, the skin is thinned, and pus may break through to drain spontaneously ("pointing"). A pustule will appear only as a cloudy tender vesicle surrounded by some redness and induration, and occasionally will be the source of an ascending lymphangitis.

What To Do:

✔ **A pustule should not require any anesthesia for drainage. Simply snip open the cutaneous roof with fine scissors or an inverted #11 scalpel blade, grasp an edge with pickups, and excise the entire overlying surface.** Cleanse the open surface with normal saline and cover it with povidone-iodine ointment and a dressing.

✔ **When the location of an abscess cavity is uncertain, attempt to aspirate it with a #18-gauge needle after prepping the area with povidone-iodine.** If an abscess cavity cannot be located, send the patient out on antibiotics and intermittent, warm, moist compresses. Have him seen again in 24 hours.

✔ **When the abscess is pointing or has been located by needle aspiration, prepare the overlying skin for incision and drainage with povidone-iodine solution. Anesthetize the area with a regional field block,** accomplished by injecting a ring of subcutaneous 1% lidocaine solution approximately 1 cm away from the erythematous border of the abscess. In addition, inject lidocaine into the roof of the abscess along the line of the projected incision (Figure 155-1, *A*).

✔ **Incise with a #11 or #15 scalpel blade at the most dependent and thin-roofed area of fluctuance.** The incision should be large and directed along the relaxed skin-tension lines to reduce future scarring (Figure 155-1, *B*).

✔ **In larger abscesses insert a hemostat into the cavity to break up any loculated collections of pus** (Figure 155-1, *C*). **The cavity may then be irrigated with nor-**

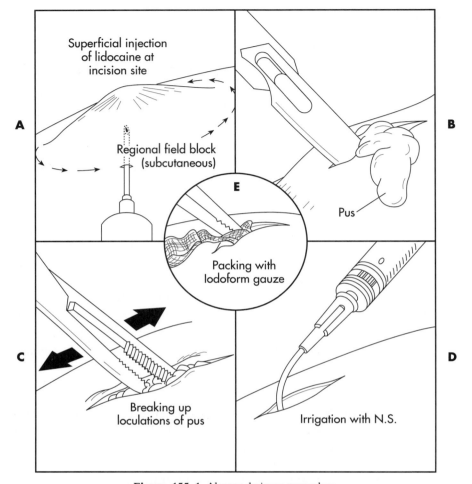

Figure 155-1 Abscess drainage procedure.

mal saline and loosely packed with Iodoform or plain gauze (Figure 155-1, *D* and *E*). Leave a small wick of this gauze protruding through the incision to allow for continued drainage and easy removal after 48 hours. To prevent recurrence, patients who have infected epidermoid cysts containing foul-smelling, cheesy material should be referred for complete excision of the cyst after the infection and inflammation have resolved.

✔ **Instruct the patient to use intermittent warm water soaks or compresses for a few days when there is no packing used or after the packing is removed.**

✔ With multiple infected hair follicles as seen with folliculitis (many pustules pierced by hairs) and with furuncles and carbuncles (abscesses often occurring on the neck with singular or multiple pustular openings), the patient may benefit from the use of antibiotics, in addition to incision, drainage, and treatment with warm compresses.

✔ Provide a dressing to collect continued drainage.

What Not To Do:

✗ Do not incise an abscess that lies in close proximity to a major vessel, such as in the axilla, groin, or antecubital space, without first confirming its location and nature by needle aspiration.

✗ Do not treat deep infections of the hands as simple cutaneous abscesses. When significant pain and swelling exist, or there is pain on range-of-motion of a finger, seek surgical consultation.

DISCUSSION

Either trauma or obstruction of glands in the skin can lead to cutaneous abscesses. Incision and drainage is the definitive therapy for most of these lesions and, therefore, routine cultures and antibiotics are generally not indicated. Systemic antibiotics should, however, be given to the immunologically suppressed patient; the toxic, febrile patient; or where there is a large area of cellulitis or lymphangitis, in which cases an antibiotic can be selected on the basis of a Gram's stain or presumptively based on body location. Staphylococci and group A beta-hemolytic streptococci are the most common isolates from abscesses of the head, neck, extremities, and trunk, with anaerobes predominating in abscesses of the buttocks and perirectal area.

It is sometimes not possible to achieve total regional anesthesia for incision and drainage of an abscess, perhaps because local tissue acidosis neutralizes local anesthetics. In such cases, additional analgesia may be obtained by premedication with narcotics or brief inhalation of nitrous oxide.

SUGGESTED READINGS

Llera JL, Levy RC: Treatment of cutaneous abscess: a double-blind clinical study, *Ann Emerg Med* 14:15-19, 1985.

156

Cutaneous Larva Migrans (Creeping Eruption)

Presentation

The patient has an intensely pruritic, erythematous, serpiginous raised lesion on the sole of the foot, hand, or buttock. She may remember recently walking barefoot or sitting in the sand or soil in an area frequented by dogs or cats (Figure 156-1).

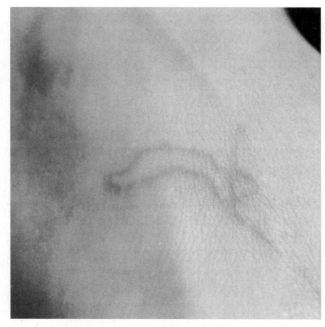

Figure 156-1 Cutaneous larva migrans. *(From Schleicher SM: Diagnosis at a glance,* Emerg Med *April: 57-58, 1997.)*

What To Do:

✔ **Prescribe ivermectin (Mectizan) 150 mcg/kg one oral dose.** Alternatively, prescribe albendazole (Albenza) 200 mg PO bid × 3 days or topical thiabendazole lotion tid × 7 to 10 days.

✔ **Prescribe hydroxyzine (Atarax, Vistaril) 25 to 50 mg qid** or diphenhydramine (Benadryl) 25 to 50 mg qid prn to reduce itching.

What Not To Do:

✘ Do not refer patients for cryotherapy. This was an historic treatment but has been shown to be ineffective.

DISCUSSION

These lesions result from infestation by the skin-penetrating filiform larvae of hookworms that hatch from eggs that are passed in dog and cat feces. The incidence of this rash is greatest in warm, moist, sandy areas, such as tropical beaches. Migration of the larvae a few millimeters a day results in the characteristic snake-like burrow in the epidermis. Man is not the normal host for these parasites, so the infection does not penetrate the dermis, and the larvae die, even without treatment, within 2 to 8 weeks.

157

Diaper Rash

Presentation

An infant has worn a wet diaper too long and has developed an uncomfortable rash, which may range from simple redness to macerated and superinfected skin. Hallmarks of *Candida (Monilia)* infection are often present, including intensely red, raw areas, satellite lesions, and white exudate (Figure 157-1).

What To Do:

✔ **For a mild rash, recommend frequent diaper changes (the most important intervention) and have the parents avoid excessive cleansing, especially with baby wipes,** which may actually add to the irritation. **Have parents apply a topical antifungal such as 2% miconazole (Micatin) cream, 1% clotrimazole (Lotrimin) cream, or 1% naftifine (Naftin) cream after each diaper change until the rash has been healed for 2 days.** They may also apply 1% hydrocortisone cream or ointment bid, as well as an occlusive agent such as Triple Paste, Diaperene, Desitin, or Balmex.

✔ **For a persistent rash, also instruct the parents that the child go "bare" and wear no plastic-covered diapers as much as possible, but especially at nap time until the rash has healed.** This may increase the laundry load, but it allows the skin to dry, avoid physical trauma, and restore its natural defenses.

✔ **For a severe *Candida* diaper rash, prescribe oral treatment with nystatin to clear the gastrointestinal tract. Use nystatin oral suspension (60-ml bottle, 100,000 units/ml) 4 to 6 ml PO qid, 2 ml for infants.**

✔ For secondary bacterial infection (e.g., crusting, vesicles, bullae) prescribe mupirocin (Bactroban) 2% ointment tid for 10 days.

✔ Make sure the family has a pediatrician for further follow-up.

What Not To Do:

✘ Do not use combination antifungal-steroid creams such as Lotrisone and Mycolog because they contain potent fluorinated steroids that may cause skin atrophy or striae.

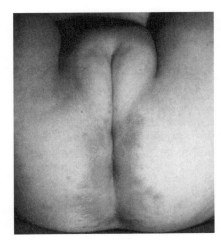

Figure 157–1 Incipient erosions are present in a patient with *Candida* diaper dermatitis. *(From Fallon Freidlander S: Cutaneous fungal infections in children, Resident & Staff Physician 44(2):46, 1998.)*

✘ Do not recommend talcum powder or "talcum-free" powders for use when diapers are changed. They add little in terms of medication or absorbency and are occasionally aspirated by infants as their diapers are being changed.

 DISCUSSION

Irritant contact diaper dermatitis is a very common disorder during infancy and predisposes the baby to developing a secondary infection with *Candida* organisms. Excessive moisture accompanied by chafing, elevated ammonia and pH levels within the diaper, as well as proteolytic enzymes present in the stool, all irritate and damage the baby's skin. Superinfection with *Candida* organisms is probably common enough to treat presumptively in every case of a diaper rash present for longer than 72 hours and severe enough to be brought for medical treatment.

158

Erysipelas, Cellulitis, Lymphangitis

Presentation

The cardinal signs of infection (pain, redness, warmth, and swelling) are present. *Erysipelas* is very superficial and bright red with indurated, edematous, sharply demarcated borders, giving the skin a pitted appearance like an orange peel (peau d'orange). *Cellulitis* is deeper, involving the subcutaneous connective tissue, and has an indistinct advancing border. *Lymphangitis* has minimal induration and an unmistakable erythematous linear pattern ascending along lymphatic channels.

These superficial skin infections are often preceded by minor trauma, such as an abrasion or the presence of a foreign body, and are most common in patients who have predisposing factors such as diabetes, drug addiction, alcoholism, immunosuppression, arterial or venous insufficiency, and lymphatic drainage obstruction. They may be associated with an abscess or dermatologic abnormality, such as tinea pedis, or they may have no clear-cut origin. With any of these skin infections the patient may have tender lymphadenopathy proximal to the site of infection and may or may not have signs of systemic toxicity (fever, rigors, and listlessness).

What To Do:

✔ Look for a possible source of infection and remove it. Debride and cleanse any wound, remove any foreign body, or drain any abscess.

✔ When the patient is very sick with high fever or severe pain, or there is discoloration of the entire limb, obtain medical consultation and prepare for hospitalization. Obtain a CBC and blood cultures, and obtain x-rays to look for gas-forming organisms. Hospitalization should also be strongly considered for deep facial cellulitis, a deep infection of the hand, or an immunocompromised patient.

✔ **If there is low-grade fever, or none at all, treat the patient on an outpatient basis. Prescribe dicloxacillin (Dynapen) 500 mg qid × 10 days, cephalexin (Keflex) 500 mg tid × 10 days, cefadroxil (Duricef) 1 g qd × 10 days, or azithromycin (Zithromax) 500 mg, then 250 mg qd × 4 days. Instruct the patient to keep the infected part at rest and elevated, and to use intermittent, warm, moist compresses.**

✔ **Follow-up within 24 to 48 hours to ensure that the therapy has been adequate.**
Infections still worsening after 48 hours of outpatient treatment may require hospital
admission for better immobilization, elevation, and IV antibiotics.

What Not To Do:

✗ Do not try to aspirate the border of a lesion for bacterial culture. It is not helpful and produces unnecessary pain and expense.

DISCUSSION

The most common etiologic agents are group A beta-hemolytic streptococci or *Staphylococcus aureus*. Erysipelas and lymphangitis are often a result of group A streptococci alone, although *S. aureus* may produce a similar picture.

It may be easier to evaluate on follow-up whether a cellulitis is improving or not if the initial margin of redness, swelling, tenderness, or warmth was marked on the skin with a ballpoint pen. Because response to treatment is often equivocal at 24 hours, reevaluation is usually best scheduled at 48 hours.

Necrotizing fasciitis is a serious deep-seated infection of the subcutaneous tissue that results in the progressive destruction of fascia and fat. It is most commonly seen in the elderly, especially those with atherosclerosis and diabetes. Early on, there may be marked systemic toxicity out of proportion to the degree of local involvement. The first cutaneous clue to group A streptococcal necrotizing fasciitis is diffuse swelling of an arm or leg, followed by the appearance of bullae filled with clear fluid, which rapidly takes on a maroon or violaceous color. Without immediate and aggressive debridement and IV antibiotics, necrotizing fasciitis can evolve into gangrene or myonecrosis.

SUGGESTED READINGS

Bisno AL, Stevens DL: Streptococcal infections of skin and soft tissues, *N Engl J Med* 334:240-245, 1996.
Powers RD: Soft tissue infections in the emergency department: the case for the use of "simple" antibiotics, *South Med J* 84:1313-1315, 1991.

159

Fire Ant Stings

Presentation

Usually the patient has experienced multiple burning stings and is seeking help because of local swelling, itching, and pain. After the initial wheal and flare at the sting site, there is formation of a small (2 mm) sterile pustule, which is virtually pathognomonic for a fire ant sting (Figure 159-1). At times there are large local reactions, and it is not unusual for an entire extremity to be affected. Systemic reactions are analogous to those caused by Hymenoptera stings (see Chapter 163).

What To Do:

✗ Examine the patient for any signs of an immediate, systemic, allergic reaction (anaphylaxis) such as decreased blood pressure, generalized urticaria or erythema, or wheezing. Reassure the patient who has come in after 12 to 24 hours that anaphylaxis is no longer a problem.

✔ **Relieve itching and burning with cold compresses.**

✔ **Treat minor reactions with topical steroids like Aristocort A 0.1% or 0.5% cream or Topicort emollient cream 0.25% or gel 0.05%. Dispense 15 g to apply tid or qid.**

✔ **For pruritus prescribe an antihistamine like hydroxyzine (Atarax, Vistaril) 25 to 50 mg qid.**

✔ **When swelling is severe and there are no signs of infection or other contraindications to systemic corticosteroids, prescribe a brief course of prednisone 40 to 60 mg qd × 4 to 5 days or give one dose of triamcinolone (Aristocort Forte) 40 mg IM.**

✔ Have the patient return or seek follow-up immediately at any sign of infection.

✔ If there are signs of infection, with surrounding swelling, tenderness, heat, and erythema, treat aggressively with cephalexin (Keflex) 500 mg tid or cephadroxil (Duricef) 500 mg bid × 10 days, or azithromycin (Zithromax) 500 mg, then 250 mg qd × 4 days.

What Not To Do:

✗ Do not open pustules. They are initially sterile, and opening them only increases the chance that they will become infected.

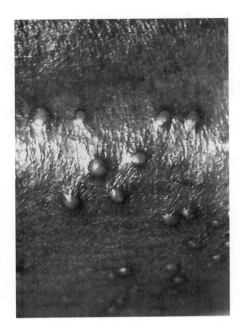

Figure 159-1 Fire ant stings. *(Courtesy Richard R. Lockey, Division of Allergy and Immunology, University of South Florida College of Medicine, Tampa, 1999.)*

✗ Do not belittle the patient's complaint or make him feel guilty about his visit if it turns out to be a simple problem.

✗ Do not send a patient out less than 1 hour after the initial sting. Observe for possible anaphylaxis.

✗ Do not apply heat, even if an infection is suspected. The swelling and discomfort will worsen.

 DISCUSSION

Imported red fire ants now infest 13 of the southeastern United States and Puerto Rico and are spreading into New Mexico and Arizona. In heavily infested areas, approximately 30% of the population is stung by fire ants each year, with consequences ranging from local reactions to life-threatening anaphylaxis. Secondary infection, which can be severe, is an additional threat even when the immediate reaction is relatively minor. The fire ant gets its name from the fierce burning discomfort caused by its sting, not from its color, which ranges from dark red to brown or black. Most stings occur during the late spring and early summer, when the ants are most active and their venom is most potent.

chapter

160 Friction Blister

Presentation

After wearing a pair of new or ill-fitting shoes, the patient complains of an uncomfortable open or intact blister on the heel or sole of the foot. Secondary infection may cause pustules, cellulitis, or lymphangitis.

What To Do:

✔ **For torn or open blisters or blisters that have become infected, remove the overlying cornified epithelium with fine scissors and forceps. Clean the area thoroughly with hydrogen peroxide or povidone-iodine solution. Cover the wound with antibiotic ointment and a simple strip bandage. Have the patient wash the area and repeat the dressings until complete healing has taken place.**

✔ When cellulitis or lymphangitis is present, provide appropriate antibiotics like erythromycin (EES) or cephalexin (Keflex) 500 mg tid for 5 to 10 days.

✔ **For untorn or closed blisters that are not infected, the skin may be left intact and covered with a protective dressing or, for additional comfort, the blister can be decompressed. Cleanse the area with povidone-iodine and then, using a 25-gauge needle, aspirate the blister fluid until the blister has completely collapsed. To prevent contamination and infection, either provide continuous antibacterial ointment (bacitracin) and strip bandage protection or cover the punctured blister with a polyurethane film like OpSite or a hydrogel dressing like Spenco 2nd Skin or Vigilon or seal the needle puncture with cyanoacrylate (Dermabond).** Additional padding may also be protective and comforting.

✔ **Instruct the patient on friction blister prevention.** A properly fitting shoe is essential, and even comfortable shoes need to be broken in gradually. Good socks and padded insoles can also help prevent friction blisters. US Military Academy cadets who applied an antiperspirant solution containing 20% aluminum chloride to their feet for at least 3 consecutive days reduced their risk of developing foot blisters during a 21 km hike by approximately half.

What Not To Do:

✖ Do not use neomycin-containing ointments because of the potential for allergic reactions.

 DISCUSSION

Active people often develop friction blisters on their feet. Although such blisters rarely cause significant medical problems, they can be quite painful and hinder athletic performance. Treatment goals include maintaining comfort, promoting healing, and preventing infection.

161

Frostbite and Frostnip

Presentation

Frostnip occurs when skin surfaces such as the tip of the nose and ears are exposed to an environment cold enough to freeze the epidermis. These prominent exposed surfaces become blanched and develop paresthesias and numbness. As they are rewarmed, they become erythematous and at times painful.

Superficial frostbite can be either a partial- or a full-thickness freezing of the dermis. The frozen surfaces appear white and feel soft and doughy. With rewarming these areas will become erythematous and edematous with severe pain. Blistering will occur within 24 to 48 hours with deeper partial-thickness frostbite.

What To Do:

✔ **When there is no longer any danger of reexposure and refreezing, rapidly warm the affected part with heated blankets (warm hands in the case of frostnip) or in a warm bath (38 to 40° C).**

✔ **A strong analgesic such as meperidine (Demerol) or morphine may be required to control pain.**

✔ When blistering occurs, bullae should not be ruptured. If the blisters are open, though, they should be debrided and gently cleansed with povidone-iodine and normal saline. Silvadene cream may be applied, followed by a sterile absorbent dressing.

✔ Patients should be provided with follow-up care and warned that healing of the deeper injuries may be slow and produce skin that remains sensitive for weeks. In addition, there may be permanent damage to fingernails, long-term paresthesia, and permanent cold sensitivity.

What Not To Do:

✘ Do not warm the injured skin surface while in the field if there is a chance that refreezing will occur. Reexposing even mildly frostbitten tissue to the cold without complete rewarming can result in additional damage.

✘ Do not rub the injured skin surface in an attempt to warm it by friction: this can also create further tissue destruction.

✖ Do not allow the patient to smoke. Smoking causes vasoconstriction and may further decrease blood flow to the frostbitten extremity.

✖ Do not confuse frostnip and superficial frostbite with deep frostbite. Severe frostbite, when the deep tissue or extremity is frozen with a woody feeling and lifeless appearance, requires inpatient management and could be associated with life-threatening hypothermia.

 DISCUSSION

Frostbite is more common in persons exposed to cold at high altitudes. The areas of the body most likely to suffer are those farthest from the trunk or large muscles: ear lobes, nose, cheeks, hands, and feet. Touching cold metal with bare hands can cause immediate frostbite, as can the spilling of gasoline or other volatile liquids on the skin at very low temperatures. Of course, prevention is the best "treatment" for frostbite. Heavily insulated, waterproof clothing gives the best protection against frostbite.

162

Herpes Zoster (Shingles)

Presentation

Patients complain of pain, tenderness, dysesthesias, paresthesia, hypersensitivity, or an itch that covers a specific dermatome and then after several days develops into a characteristic unilateral rash. The discomfort may be difficult to describe, often alternating between an itch, a burning, or even a deep, aching pain. Prior to the onset of the rash, zoster can be confused with pleuritic or cardiac pain, cholecystitis, or ureteral colic. The pain may precede the eruption by as much as a few weeks and occasionally pain alone is the only manifestation.

Approximately 3 to 5 days from the onset of symptoms, an eruption of erythematous macules and papules usually appear, first posteriorly then spreading anteriorly along the course of the involved nerve segment. In most instances grouped vesicles on an erythematous base will appear within the next 24 hours. Herpes zoster occurs in thoracic dermatomes in 50% to 60% of patients. Cranial, cervical, and lumbar dermatomes each account for about 10% of cases (Figure 162-1, *A* to *D*).

What To Do:

✔ **If it has been 3 days or less since the onset of the rash, prescribe famciclovir (Famvir) 500 mg or valacyclovir (Valtrex) 1000 mg tid × 7 days.**

✔ **Prescribe analgesics appropriate for the level of pain the patient is experiencing. NSAIDs may help, but narcotics are often required (e.g., Percocet q4h).** When prescribing narcotics for the elderly, remember to warn them that they are likely to suffer constipation as a side effect (see Chapter 70). If the pain is severe, consider referring the patient for an epidural nerve block, which has been successful in relieving the acute pain and may decrease the incidence of postherpetic neuralgia.

✔ **Cool compresses with Burow's solution will be comforting** (e.g., Domeboro powder, 2 packets in 1 pint of water).

✔ Dressing the lesions with gauze and splinting them with an elastic wrap may also help bring relief. Superficial infection may be prevented by a topical antibiotic ointment.

✔ **Secondary infection should be treated with systemic antibiotics like cephalexin 500 mg tid or azithromycin 500 mg, then 250 mg qd × 4 days.**

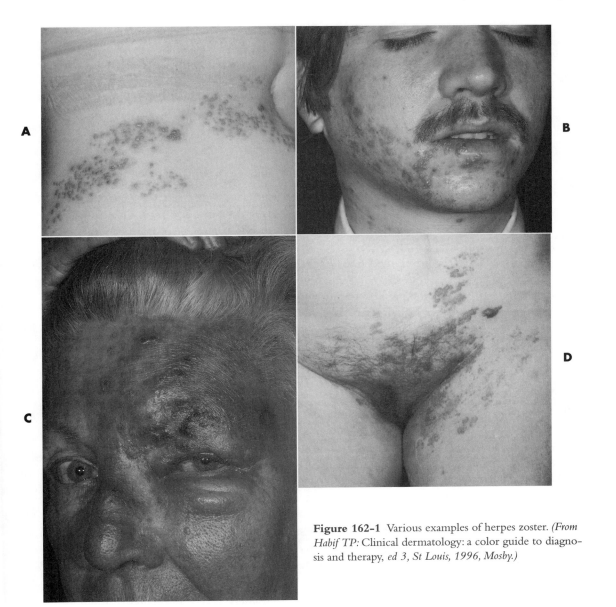

Figure 162-1 Various examples of herpes zoster. *(From Habif TP: Clinical dermatology: a color guide to diagnosis and therapy, ed 3, St Louis, 1996, Mosby.)*

443

✔ **Ocular lesions should be evaluated by an ophthalmologist and treated with topical ophthalmic corticosteroids.** Although topical steroids are contraindicated in herpes simplex keratitis because they allow deeper corneal injury, this does not appear to be a problem with herpes zoster ophthalmicus. **If the rash extends to the tip of the nose, the eye will probably be involved,** because it is served by the same ophthalmic branch of the trigeminal nerve. Look for a punctate keratopathy on fluorescein staining, although patients may have only pain, lacrimation, conjunctivitis, or scleritis. Herpes zoster ophthalmicus can result in corneal scarring, uveitis, glaucoma, corneal perforation, or blindness. Patients with AIDS are at risk for developing acute retinal necrosis.

✔ **Until all lesions are crusted, instruct patients to stay away from immunocompromised individuals and pregnant women who have not had chickenpox.** Explain that they can transmit varicella to a susceptible individual.

What Not To Do:

✘ Do not prescribe systemic steroids to prevent postherpetic neuralgia, especially for patients at high risk (i.e., with latent tuberculosis, immunocompromise, peptic ulcer, diabetes mellitus, hypertension, and congestive heart failure). There is also no indication for prescribing steroids in patients under 60 years of age, when the risk of postherpetic neuralgia is minimal.

✘ Do not initiate a comprehensive diagnostic work up looking for an occult malignancy simply on the basis of zoster. The incidence of cancer among patients with zoster is no greater than that of the general population. Patients with cancers and particularly lymphomas are, however, at increased risk of zoster.

DISCUSSION

Herpes zoster can usually be readily diagnosed by its clinical appearance. One well-known diagnostic caveat is that the pain and rash do not cross the midline; however, it is not impossible for the disease to be bilateral and involve more than one dermatome, and multidermatomal zoster may be the presenting finding for HIV. Bell's palsy (see Chapter 1) following zoster dermatitis of the geniculate ganglion is well known and can be part of the Ramsey Hunt syndrome.

When the diagnosis is in doubt, the Tzanck test can help. Select an intact early vesicular lesion, unroof it, and using the belly of a #15 scalpel blade, scrape the floor of the vesicle to obtain as much exudate as possible. Gently transfer this material to a clean glass slide and allow it to air dry. A Wright or Giemsa stain will reveal multinucleated giant cells.

Herpes zoster affects 10% to 20% of the US population. It results from reactivation of latent herpes varicella/zoster (chickenpox) virus residing in dorsal root or cranial nerve ganglion cells. The virus migrates peripherally along axons into the skin. Two thirds of the patients are over 40 years of age. In immunocompetent patients, zoster is usually a self-limiting, localized disease and usually heals within 3 to 4 weeks, so most patients can be reassured that their disease will abate without permanent problems. The incidence in immunocompromised patients is up to 10 times higher than in immunocompetent hosts, and usually their treatment must be more aggressive.

DISCUSSION—cont'd

Postherpetic neuralgia in patients over 60 years of age can be an extremely painful, recurrent misery. Before the availability of antiviral agents, the best prophylaxis was systemic corticosteroids, but these have not been shown to improve outcome when added to a week of antiviral treatment. Now, famciclovir and valacyclovir (when taken within the first 3 days of onset) appear to reduce duration of postherpetic neuralgia, as well as time to resolution of the acute lesions.

SUGGESTED READINGS

Grant DM, Mauskopf JA, Bell L, et al: Comparison of valacyclovir and acyclovir for the treatment of herpes zoster in immunocompetent patients over 50 years of age, *Pharmacotherapy* 17:333-341, 1997.

Tyring S, Barbarash RA, Nahlik JE, et al: Famciclovir for the treatment of acute herpes zoster: effects on acute disease and postherpetic neuralgia, *Ann Intern Med* 123:89-96, 1995.

Whitley RJ, Weiss H, Gnann JW, et al: Acyclovir with and without prednisone for the treatment of herpes zoster, *Ann Intern Med* 125:376-383, 1996.

Wood MJ, Johnson RW, McKendrick MW, et al: A randomized trial of acyclovir for 7 days or 21 days with and without prednisolone for treatment of acute herpes zoster, *N Engl J Med* 330:896-900, 1994.

163

Hymenoptera (Bee, Wasp, Hornet) Envenomation

Presentation

Sometimes a patient comes to a hospital emergency department (ED) immediately after a painful sting because he is alarmed at the intensity of the pain or worried about developing a serious life-threatening reaction. Sometimes he seeks help the next day because of swelling, redness, and itching. Parents may not be aware that their child was stung by a bee and may be concerned only about the local swelling. Symptoms of a severe reaction may include generalized pruritus, shortness of breath, chest constriction, stomach pain, dizziness, nausea, hoarseness, thickened speech, weakness, confusion, and feelings of impending doom.

Erythema develops soon after the sting with varying degrees of localized edema. Often there is a central punctate discoloration at the site of the sting, or rarely, a stinger may be protruding (only honeybees leave a stinger). A delayed hypersensitivity reaction will produce varying degrees of edema, which can be quite dramatic when present on the face (Figure 163-1), and may involve all of an arm or leg. Tenderness and occasionally ascending lymphangitis can occur.

What To Do:

✔ Scrape away the stinger with the back edge of a scalpel blade or a long fingernail (Figure 163-2). **Within the first few minutes of being stung, it is most important to remove the stinger quickly, even if it is grasped and pulled off, rather than delaying to find a hard edge to scrape with.**

✔ **Examine the patient for any signs of an immediate, systemic, allergic reaction (anaphylaxis), such as decreased blood pressure, generalized urticaria or erythema, wheezing, tongue swelling,** pharyngeal edema, or laryngeal spasm. Treat any of these findings aggressively with airway support, IV fluids, corticosteroids, antihistamines, and epinephrine. On discharge from the hospital, prescribe a sting kit to carry at all times (e.g., Ana-Kit, Epi-Pen) and refer the patient to an allergist for possible desensitization.

✔ **Apply a cold pack to an acute sting to give pain relief and reduce swelling.** Try ibuprofen or acetaminophen for analgesia.

✔ Observe the patient with an acute sting for approximately 1 hour to watch for the rare late anaphylaxis.

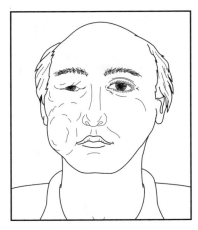

Figure 163-1 Localized reaction to bee sting.

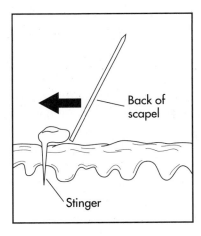

Back of scapel

Stinger

Figure 163-2 Removal of a stinger.

✔ Reassure the patient who has come in after 12 to 24 hours that anaphylaxis is no longer a problem.

✔ **Prescribe hydroxyzine (Vistaril) 50 mg qid for itching. A minor reaction will also benefit from a topical steroid cream like hydrocortisone or triamcinolone. For a severe local reaction with no contraindications, prescribe a systemic corticosteroid like prednisone 50 mg qd for 3 to 4 days.**

✔ **If an ascending lymphangitis or possible cellulitis is present, treat the patient with an appropriate antibiotic** like cephadroxil (Duricef) 1 g qd, cephalexin (Keflex) 500 mg tid, dicloxacillin (Dynapen) 500 mg qid for 5 to 10 days, or azithromycin (Zithromax) 500 mg, then 250 qd for 4 days.

✔ **Provide tetanus prophylaxis** (see Chapter 151) **as for a clean minor wound.**

✔ **If an extremity is involved, have the patient keep it elevated** and instruct him that the swelling may worsen if the hand or foot is held in a dependent position. This swelling may continue for several days. Severe hand swelling may be prevented or reduced by

447

placing the patient's hand in a splint and compression dressing. Promptly remove any rings (see Chapter 148) in cases of hand stings.

✔ To help prevent future stings, instruct patients to avoid wearing brightly colored clothing and using fragrances when outside, and to avoid recreational activities when bees or wasps are nearby.

What Not To Do:

✘ Do not belittle the patient's complaint or make him feel guilty about his visit if the injury turns out to be minor.

✘ Do not send the patient with an acute sting home less than 1 hour after the sting.

✘ Do not apply heat, even if an infection is suspected—the swelling and discomfort will worsen.

✘ Do not prescribe the Ana-Kit, Epi-Pen, or other anaphylaxis treatment for patients who have only had a localized reaction.

 DISCUSSION

Bee stings are very painful and frightening. There are many misconceptions about the danger of bee stings, and many patients have been instructed unnecessarily to report to an ED or clinic immediately after being stung. Many of these people have only suffered localized hypersensitivity reactions in the past and are not at a significantly greater risk than the general public for developing anaphylaxis, which is defined as an immediate, generalized reaction. Besides some relief of pain for the acute sting, there is little more than reassurance to offer these patients.

Anaphylactic reactions generally occur within a few minutes to 1 hour after the sting. Most victims have no previous history. Patients with a history of systemic reactions should carry a kit containing injectable epinephrine and chewable antihistamines to be used at the first sign of a generalized reaction. Venom-specific immunotherapy for hymenopteran allergy can markedly reduce approximately 30% to 60% of the risk of repeat systemic reaction. Patients who have had extensive local but not general reactions tend to react the same way to subsequent stings despite venom immunotherapy.

Although it is most prudent to treat an ascending lymphangitis with an antibiotic, it should be realized that after a bee sting the resultant local cellulitis and lymphangitis are usually chemically-mediated, inflammatory reactions.

SUGGESTED READINGS

Jerrard DA: Emergency department management of insect stings, *Am J Emerg Med* 14:429-433, 1996.
Visscher PK, Vetter RS, Camazine S: Removing bee stings, *Lancet* 348:301-302, 1996.

164

Impetigo

Presentation

Parents will usually bring their children in because they are developing unsightly skin lesions, which may be pruritic and are found most often on the face (Figure 164-1) or other exposed areas. Streptococcal lesions consist of irregular or somewhat circular, red, oozing erosions, often covered with a yellow-brown honey-like crust. These may be surrounded by smaller erythematous macular or vesiculopustular areas. Staphylococcal lesions present as bullae, which are quickly replaced by a thin, shiny crust over an erythematous base.

What To Do:

✔ **For a few lesions involving a relatively small area, prescribe mupirocin 2% (Bactroban) ointment or cream to be applied to the rash tid for 10 days.** Have parents soften and cleanse crusts with warm soapy compresses before applying the antibiotic ointment.

✔ **For severe or resistant cases, add a 10-day course of erythromycin ethyl succinate (EES) 400 mg qid (30 mg/kg/day) or penicillin VK 250 mg qid (25 mg/kg/day),** or one IM injection of benzathine penicillin 600,000 units IM for children 6 years of age and younger, 1.2 million units IM for children over 7 years of age. **For suspected staphylococcal infections, use dicloxacillin (Dynapen) 250 mg qid (12.5 mg/kg/day) in place of penicillin.** Alternative regimens include cephalexin (Keflex) 250 mg qid (25 mg/kg/day), cefadroxil (Duricef) 250 to 500 mg bid (30 mg/kg/day), amoxicillin/clavulanate (Augmentin) 250 mg tid (2 mg/kg/day), all for 10 days, or azithromycin (Zithromax) 500 mg, then 250 mg qd (10 mg/kg, then 5 mg/kg/day) for 4 days.

✔ To prevent the spread of this infection, have the patient and his family wash their hands frequently, change towels and bed linens every day, and keep infected school children home until the acute phase has cleared.

What Not To Do:

✗ Do not routinely culture these lesions. This is only indicated for unusual lesions or for lesions that fail to respond to routine therapy.

✗ Do not use bacitracin or similar antibacterial ointments on these lesions. They are ineffective and may cause an unnecessary contact dermatitis.

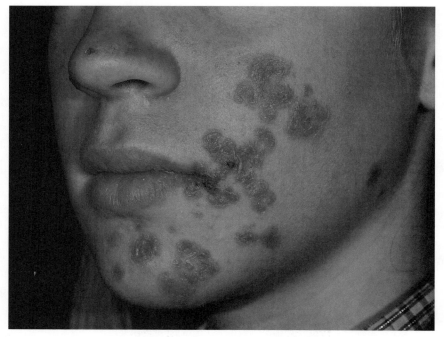

Figure 164-1 Impetigo on the face. *(From Habif TP: Clinical dermatology: a color guide to diagnosis and therapy, ed 3, St Louis, 1996, Mosby.)*

 DISCUSSION

Impetigo is usually self-limiting, and it is believed that antibiotic treatment does not alter the subsequent incidence of secondary glomerulonephritis. Impetigo is very contagious among infants and young children and may be associated with poor hygiene or predisposing skin eruptions such as chickenpox, scabies, and atopic and contact dermatitis. When lesions occur singly, they may be mistaken for herpes simplex.

SUGGESTED READINGS

Bass JW, Chan DS, Creamer KM, et al: Comparison of oral cephalexin, topical mupirocin and topical bacitracin for treatment of impetigo, *Ped Infect Dis J* 16:708-710, 1997.

165

Partial-Thickness (Second-Degree) Burns and Tar Burns

Presentation

Partial-thickness burns can occur in a variety of ways. Spilled or splattered hot water and grease are among the most common causes, along with hot objects, explosive fumes, and burning (volatile) liquids. The patient will complain of excruciating pain, and the burn will appear erythematous with vesicle formation. Some of these vesicles or bullae may have ruptured before the patient's arrival, while others may not develop for 24 hours. Tar burns are special in that tar adheres aggressively to the burned skin.

What To Do:

✔ **To stop the pain, immediately cover the burned area with sterile towels that have first been soaked in iced normal saline or an iced 1% povidone-iodine solution.** Continue irrigating the burn with the iced solution for the next 20 to 30 minutes or until the patient can remain comfortable without the cold compresses.

✔ **Provide the patient with any necessary tetanus prophylaxis** (see Chapter 151) **and pain medication (e.g., Percodan, Demerol).**

✔ Examine the patient for any associated injuries and check the airway and pulmonary status of any patient with significant facial burns.

✔ **When the pain has subsided, gently cleanse the burn with povidone-iodine scrub and rinse this off with normal saline.**

✔ **If the vesicles are not perforated, have a relatively thick wall, and are on a hairless surface such as the palm of the hand, they should be left intact.** With small burns such as these, patients can be sent home to continue cold compresses for comfort. Otherwise, **these vesicles should be protected from future rupture with a bulky sterile dressing.**

✔ **Vesicles that are already open, large, thin-walled, and prone to rupture; or vesicles occurring on hairy surfaces that are prone to infection should be com-**

pletely debrided. Using fine scissors and forceps, strip away any loose epithelium from the burn. **(With tar burns, debridement should be accomplished in the same manner, removing the tar along with the loose epithelium. Tar adhering to normal epithelium can be left in place,** acting as a sterile dressing in itself.) Rinse off any remaining debris with normal saline and **cover all the open areas with an oil emulsion gauze (e.g., Adaptic), followed by silver sulfadiazine (Silvadene) cream and a bulky absorbent sterile dressing.** The first dressing change should be scheduled in 2 days.

✔ **Small burns and facial burns can often be treated with an open technique of using Silvadene cream only.** Patients are instructed to gently wash the burn four times each day, followed by reapplication of the Silvadene cream.

✔ Small clean burns can alternatively be covered with synthetic dressings. Biobrane collagen Silastic is designed to be placed tightly against the wound with a compressive gauze dressing wrapped over it. Within 2 days, as long as the wound is clean and has no seroma formation, the collagen side of the dressing adheres to the surface of the burn and effectively seals it. The dressing acts as a skin substitute and allows the underlying skin to heal and reepithelialize more comfortably. **Biobrane may be left in place for 1 month. Other synthetic dressings can be applied in the same manner and may be more available, including Duoderm and OpSite.**

✔ Patients can be reassured that superficial, partial-thickness burns will generally heal in 7 to 21 days with full function and, unless there are complications (such as infection), patients do not have to worry about scarring.

What Not To Do:

✗ Do not use ice-containing compresses that might increase tissue damage. Compresses soaked in iced saline should be avoided on large burns (greater than 15% total body surface) because they may lead to problems with hypothermia. When pain cannot be controlled with compresses, use strong parenteral analgesics such as morphine sulfate.

✗ Do not confuse partial-thickness burns with full-thickness burns. Full-thickness burns have no sensory function or skin appendages, such as hair follicles, remaining, do not form vesicles, and may have evidence of thrombosed vessels. If areas of full-thickness burn are present or suspected, seek surgical consultation because these areas will not grow new skin and may later require skin grafting.

✗ Do not discharge patients with suspected respiratory burns or extensive burns of the hands or genitalia. These patients require special inpatient observation and management.

✗ Do not use caustic solvents in an attempt to remove tar from burns. It is unnecessary, painful, and will cause further tissue destruction.

✗ Do not use synthetic dressings on old or contaminated burns, which have a high risk for infection.

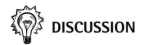

DISCUSSION

Simple partial-thickness burns will do well with nothing more than cleansing, debridement, and a sterile dressing. All other therapy, therefore, should be directed at making the patient more comfortable. Silvadene cream is not always necessary, but it is soothing and may reduce the risk of infection. Bacitracin ointment may also be used on small burns. When it is possible to leave vesicles intact, the patient will have a shorter period of disability and will require fewer dressing changes and follow-up visits. If the wound must be debrided, the closed-dressing technique may be more convenient and less of a mess than the open technique of washings and cream applications.

Some physicians believe it is important to remove all traces of tar from a burn. Removal can be accomplished relatively easily by using a petroleum-based antibiotic ointment such as bacitracin, which will dissolve the tar. This can be mixed with an equal amount of Unibase (ingredients: water, cetyl alcohol, stearyl alcohol, white petrolatum, glycerin, sodium citrate, sodium laurel sulfate, propyl paraben). Others have found the citrus and petroleum distillate industrial cleanser Medi-Sol (Orange-Sol Inc., Chandler, AZ) effective, as well as nontoxic and nonirritating. Other effective solvents include polysorbate and Tween 80.

SUGGESTED READINGS

Levy DB, Barone JA, York JM, et al: Unibase and triple antibiotic ointment for hardened tar removal, *Ann Emerg Med* 15:765-766, 1986.

Stratta RJ, Saffle JR, Kravitz M, et al: Management of tar and asphalt injuries, *Am J Surg* 146:766-769, 1983.

Pediculosis (Lice, Crabs)

Presentation

Patients arrive with emotions ranging from annoyance to sheer disgust at the discovery of an infestation with lice or crabs and request acute medical care. There may be extreme pruritus and the patient may bring in a sample of the creature to show you. The adult forms of head lice (pediculosis) can be very difficult to find but their oval, light gray eggs (nits) can be readily found firmly attached to the hairs above the ears and toward the occiput. Secondary impetigo and furunculosis can occur. The adult forms of pubic lice (*Phthirus* organisms or crab lice) are more easily found, but their light yellow-gray color still makes them difficult to see. Small black dots present in infested areas represent either ingested blood in adult lice or their excreta. Identification of lice, larvae, or nits with a magnifying glass makes the diagnosis (Figure 166-1).

What To Do:

✔ **Instruct the patient and other close contacts on the use of nonprescription louse treatments. The most effective is 1% permethrin (Nix),** which should be applied undiluted to the hair until the affected area is entirely wet. After 10 minutes, shampoo and rinse with warm water. It is not necessary to remove nits. Less than 1% of patients require a second treatment in 7 days. A second choice is pyrethrins and piperonyl butoxide (RID), which is applied in the same fashion. This product does not kill all of the unhatched eggs and has no residual activity, so a second treatment is required 7 to 10 days later to kill newly hatched lice. Use Eserine ophthalmic ointment to kill adult lice on eyelashes.

✔ **As lice have become resistant to OTC treatments, some clinicians have had to escalate to prescription strength 5% permethrin cream (Elimite)** applied to clean dry hair and left on overnight (8 to 14 hours) under a shower cap. **For head lice resistant to all other treatments, give a single oral dose of ivermectin (Mectizan) 200 mcg/kg repeated once after 10 days.**

✔ Instruct families to disinfect sheets and clothing by machine washing in hot water, machine drying on the hot cycle for 20 minutes, ironing, dry cleaning, or storage in plastic bags for 2 weeks. Combs and brushes should be soaked in 2% Lysol or heated in water to about 65° C for 10 minutes.

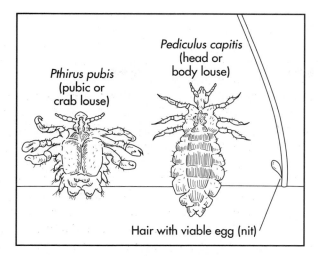

Figure 166-1 Pediculosis.

✔ Nit removal can help identify if there is a later recurrence and may reduce the risk of recurrence. Application of a 1:1 solution of white vinegar and water may help to loosen nits before removal with a fine-toothed comb.

✔ **When pubic or body lice are sexually transmitted, treat sex partners.**

What Not To Do:

✗ Do not recommend comprehensive cleaning of the whole house. Adult lice cannot survive for more than 1 day if they cannot find a meal of blood.

✗ Do not have the family use commercial sprays (R&C Spray or Li-Ban Spray) to control lice on inanimate objects. Their use is no more effective than vacuuming.

✗ Do not let patients use lindane (Kwell) shampoo on mucous membranes, around the eyes, or on acutely inflamed areas, and do not prescribe it for pregnant women and infants. It is absorbed and can be toxic to the central nervous system.

 DISCUSSION

Head and pubic lice are obligatory blood-sucking ectoparasites whose eggs are firmly attached to the hair shafts near the skin, and incubate for about 1 week before hatching. Nits located more than one-half inch from the scalp are no longer viable. The itching is believed to be due to allergic sensitization.

A common alternate treatment for lice is lindane (Kwell) shampoo, which is only available by prescription. One ounce is worked into the affected area for 4 minutes and then thor-

Continued

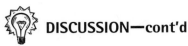 **DISCUSSION—cont'd**

oughly rinsed out. Because of the very toxic nature of lindane, its use should be reserved for those cases that fail to respond to the initial therapies above. Resistance to lindane appears to be growing more common in the United States. Lindane lotion is used for scabies (see Chapter 171).

Ivermectin (Mectizan) is an antiparasitic drug now available in the United States for oral use to treat strongyloidiasis and onchocerciasis. It is also highly effective for scabies.

SUGGESTED READINGS

Drugs for head lice, *The Medical Letter* 39:6-7, 1997.

Fischer TF: Lindane toxicity in a 24-year-old woman, *Ann Emerg Med* 24:972-974, 1994.

Meinking TL, Taplin D, Kalter DC, et al: Comparative efficacy of treatments for pediculosis capitis infestations, *Arch Dermatol* 122:267-271, 1986.

Pencil Point Puncture

Presentation

The patient will tell you that he was stabbed or stuck with a sharp pencil point. He may be overtly or unconsciously worried about lead poisoning. A small puncture wound lined with graphite tattooing will be present. The pencil tip may or may not be present, visible, or palpable. If the puncture wound is palpated, an underlying pencil point may give the patient a foreign body sensation.

What To Do:

✔ **Reassure the patient or parent that there is no danger of lead poisoning.** Pencil "leads" are made of clay and graphite, which is carbon and nontoxic.

✔ **Palpate and inspect for a foreign body.** If uncertain, obtain an x-ray, xerogram, or ultrasound to rule out the presence of a foreign body.

✔ Scrub the wound.

✔ Administer tetanus prophylaxis, if necessary (see Chapter 151).

✔ **In order to reduce the amount of tattooing, the wound may be anesthetized and scraped (dermabraded) with the tip of a scalpel blade** (Figure 167-1).

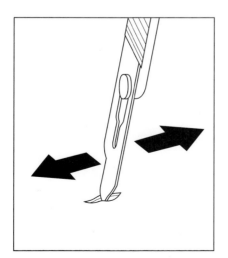

Figure 167-1 Dermabrade to reduce tattooing.

✔ **Warn the patient or family about signs of infection, and inform them that there may be a permanent black tattoo that can be removed later if the resulting mark is cosmetically unacceptable.**

What Not To Do:

✗ Do not excise the entire wound on the initial visit.

 DISCUSSION

It is unwise to excise the entire wound because the resultant scar might be more unsightly than the tattoo. If a superficial pencil tip foreign body exists, then see Chapter 174 for an easy removal technique. Deep punctures or foreign bodies may require exploratory surgery in the operating room.

168   Pityriasis Rosea

Presentation

Patients with this benign disorder often seek acute medical help because of the worrisome sudden spread of a rash that began with one local skin lesion. This "herald patch" may develop anywhere on the body and appears as a round 2 to 6 cm mildly erythematous scaling plaque. There is no change for a period of several days to 2 weeks; then the rash appears, composed of small (1 to 2 cm), pale, salmon-colored, oval macules or plaques with a coarse surface surrounded by a rim of fine scales. The distribution is truncal, with the long axis of the oval lesions running in the planes of cleavage of the skin (parallel to the ribs) giving it a "Christmas tree" appearance (Figure 168-1). The condition may be asymptomatic or accompanied by varying degrees of pruritus and occasionally mild malaise. The lesions will gradually extend in size and may become confluent with one another. The rash persists for 6 to 8 weeks then completely disappears. Recurrences are uncommon.

What To Do:

✔ **Reassure the patient about the benign nature of this disease.** Be sympathetic and let her know that it is understandable how frightening it can seem.

✔ **Draw blood for serologic testing for syphilis** (e.g., RPR, VDRL). Secondary syphilis can mimic pityriasis rosea. Make a note to track down the results of the test.

✔ **Provide relief from pruritus by prescribing hydroxyzine (Atarax) 50 mg q6h or an emollient such as Lubriderm.** Tepid cornstarch baths (1 cup in ½ tub of water) may also be comforting.

✔ Low- to mid-potency topical steroids can be used when pruritus is significant.

✔ **Inform the patient that she should anticipate a 6- to 14-week course of the disease,** but to seek follow-up care if the rash does not resolve within 12 weeks.

What Not To Do:

✘ Do not routinely use topical or systemic steroids. These are only effective in the most severe inflammatory varieties of this syndrome.

✘ Do not send off a serologic test for syphilis without assuring the results will be seen and acted on.

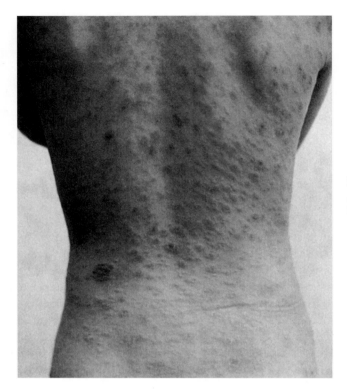

Figure 168-1 Pityriasis rosea. *(From Leung AKS, Wong BE, Chan PYH: Pediatrics Review,* Resident & Staff Physician *43(5):109, 1997.)*

 DISCUSSION

Pityriasis rosea is seen most commonly in adolescents and young adults during the spring and fall seasons. It is probably a viral syndrome. The "herald patch" may not be seen in 20% to 30% of the cases, and there are many variations from the classic presentation described. Infrequently oral lesions will accompany the skin rash and resolve along with it: these include punctate hemorrhages, erosions, ulcerations, erythematous macules, annular lesions, and plaques. Other diagnostic considerations besides syphilis include tinea corporis, seborrheic dermatitis, acute psoriasis, and tinea versicolor.

169

Pyogenic Granuloma (Proud Flesh)

Presentation

Often there is a history of a laceration or minor trauma to the skin or mucous membrane several days to a few weeks before. The lips, oral mucosa, and fingers are most commonly involved. The wound has not healed and now bleeds with every slight trauma. Objective findings usually include a crusted, sometimes purulent collection of erythematous, well-demarcated granulation tissue arising from a moist, sometimes hemorrhagic wound. There are usually no signs of a deep tissue infection (Figure 169-1).

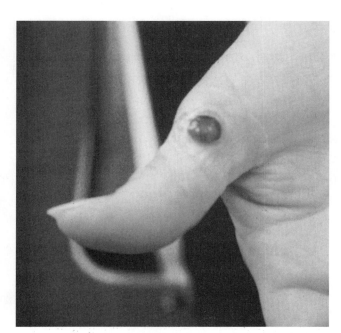

Figure 169-1 Pyogenic granuloma. *(From Schleicher SM: Diagnosis at a glance, Emerg Med Sept 1997, p 91-92.)*

What To Do:

✔ **Cleanse the area with hydrogen peroxide and povidone-iodine solution.**
✔ **Cauterize the granulation tissue with a silver nitrate stick until it is completely discolored.**
✔ Dress the wound after applying povidone-iodine ointment and have the patient repeat ointment and dressings 2 to 3 times per day until healed.
✔ **Warn the patient about the potential signs of developing infection.**

What Not To Do:

✘ Do not cauterize any lesion that by history and appearance might be neoplastic in nature. Pyogenic granuloma is occasionally confused with melanoma, basal cell carcinoma, and squamous cell carcinoma. Suspicious lesions should be referred for complete excision and pathologic examination.
✘ Do not cauterize a large or extensive lesion. These should also be completely excised.

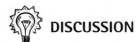 **DISCUSSION**

It is not uncommon for a secondary cellulitis to develop after cauterizing the pyogenic granuloma. It is therefore reasonable to place a patient on a short course (3 to 4 days) of a high dose antibiotic (dicloxacillin or cephalexin 500 mg tid or cefadroxil l g qd) when the wound is located on a distal extremity.

The term *pyogenic granuloma* is a misnomer. These lesions are actually capillary hemangiomas.

170

Rhus (Toxicodendron) Contact Dermatitis (Poison Ivy, Oak, or Sumac)

Presentation

The patient is troubled with an intensely pruritic rash made up of tense vesiculo-papular lesions on a mildly erythematous base. Typically some of these are found in groups of linear streaks with weeping, crusting, confluence, and sometimes large bullae (Figure 170-1). If involvement is severe, there may be marked edema, particularly on the face, periorbital areas, and genital areas. The thick, protective stratum corneum of the palms and the soles generally protect these areas. The patient is often not aware of having been in contact with poison ivy, oak, or sumac but may recall working in a field or garden from 24 to 48 hours before the onset of symptoms. In general, the shorter the reaction time, the greater is the degree of the individual's sensitivity.

What To Do:

✔ **Have the patient apply cool or cold compresses of Burow's solution** (Domeboro Powder Pkts 2 packets in 1 pint of refrigerated water) for 20 minutes every 3 to 4 hours (more often if comforting).

✔ **Small areas can be treated with potent topical steroids such as fluocinonide (Lidex) or desoximetasone (Topicort) 0.05% cream or gel 3 to 4 times per day after using cool compresses, which can be enhanced at night with an occlusive plastic (Saran) wrap dressing.** A severe local reaction can be treated with clobetasol (Temovate) 0.05% cream, a very powerful topical steroid. It may require 2 days of application before itching subsides significantly.

✔ **Diphenhydramine (available over the counter as Benadryl) or hydroxyzine (Vistaril) 25 to 50 mg PO q6h will help mild itching between application of compresses.**

✔ Tepid tub baths with Aveeno colloidal oatmeal (one cup in ½ tub) or cornstarch and baking soda (1 cup of each in ½ tub) will provide soothing relief.

463

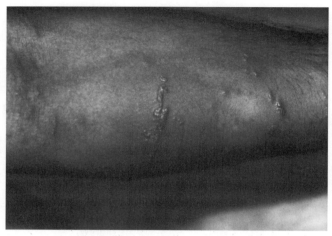

Figure 170-1 Poison ivy dermatitis. *(Photo taken by David Effron, MD, F.A.C.E.P. In Rosen P et al: Emergency medicine: concepts and clinical practice, St Louis, 1998, Mosby, p 2790 and 2794.)*

✔ **When there is involvement of the face, in severe reactions, or in situations where the patient's livelihood is threatened, early and aggressive treatment with systemic corticosteroids should be initiated. Prednisone (60 to 80 mg a day tapered over 2 weeks) will be necessary to prevent a late flare-up or rebound reaction. One 40 mg dose of IM triamcinolone acetonide (Kenalog) will be equally effective.** For pediatric patients, use prednisolone syrup, 15 mg/5 ml (Prelone) 1 mg/kg/day, tapered over 2 to 3 weeks.

✔ **Inform patients about preventing future exposures by using IvyBlock,** an OTC lotion containing bentoquatam 5% that binds with plant allergens, preventing them from penetrating the skin. This is of no use for patients who already have a rash. Avoidance of the offending agent is the key to prevention, so instruct patients to cover up in the future with long pants, a long-sleeved shirt, gloves, and boots.

✔ **Treat secondary infections with antibiotics like dicloxacillin, erythromycin, or cefalexin 250 mg qid for 10 days or azithromycin 500 mg, then 250 mg qd × 4 days.**

✔ Although hyperpigmentation can occur in dark-skinned individuals, patients can usually be reassured that even severe lesions will not leave any visible skin markings when healing is complete.

What Not To Do:

✘ Do not have the patient use heavy-duty skin cleansers, alcohol, or other strong solvents to remove any remaining antigen. This would be ineffective and may do harm.

✘ Do not try to substitute prepackaged steroid regimens (Medrol Dosepak, Aristopak). The course is not long enough and may lead to a flare up.

✗ Do not allow patients to apply fluorinated corticosteroids such as Lidex or Valisone for more than 3 weeks to the face or intertriginous areas, where they can produce thinning of skin and telangiectasias. A 10- to 14-day course should not be a problem. Any significant involvement of the face should be treated with systemic corticosteroids.

✗ Do not institute systemic steroids in the presence of secondary infections such as impetigo, cellulitis, or erysipelas. Also, do not start steroids if there is a history of tuberculosis, peptic ulcer, diabetes, herpes, or severe hypertension.

✗ Do not recommend OTC topical steroid preparations that are not potent enough to be effective.

✗ Do not prescribe topical steroids if systemic steroids are being given.

✗ Do not recommend the use of topical antihistamines or topical benzocaine because of the added risk of causing a second contact dermatitis.

 DISCUSSION

Poison oak and poison ivy are forms of allergic contact dermatitis that result from the exposure of sensitized individuals to the allergen urushiol in the sap of these plants. These allergens induce sensitization in more than 70% of the population, may be carried by pets, and are frequently transferred from hands to other areas of the body that may unfortunately include the genital area. In a dry environment, the allergen can remain under fingernails for several days and on clothes for longer than 1 week.

The gradual appearance of the eruption over a period of several days is a reflection of the amount of antigen deposited on the skin and the reactivity of the site, not an indication of any further spread of the allergen. The vesicle fluid is a transudate, does not contain antigen, and will not spread the eruption elsewhere on the body or to other people. The allergic skin reaction usually runs a course of about 2 weeks, sometimes longer, and is not shortened by any of the above treatments. The aim of therapy is to reduce the severity of symptoms, not to shorten the course. Those skin areas with the greatest degree of initial reaction tend to be affected the longest.

Urushiol is degraded by soap and water. Washing skin immediately after exposure can abort the rash. Washing clothes in a standard washing machine will inactivate the antigen remaining on the patient's clothing. Shoes may require separate cleansing and can be the source of late spread.

171 Scabies (Itch Mite)

Presentation

Patients may rush to the emergency department or call for medical help shortly after having gone to bed, unable to sleep because of severe itching. Papules and vesicles (marking deposition of eggs) along thread-like tracks (mite burrows) are chiefly found in the interdigital web spaces, as well as on the volar aspects of the wrists, axillae, olecranon area, nipples, umbilicus, lower abdomen, genitalia, and gluteal cleft (Figures 171-1 and 171-2). Scabies lesions can occur anywhere on the body, including the face and scalp. Infants and young children may also have palm and sole involvement with vesicular and pustular lesions. Secondary bacterial infection is often present.

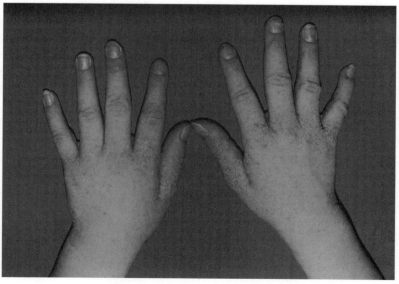

Figure 171-1 Itch mite lesions. *(Photo taken by David Effron, MD, F.A.C.E.P. In Rosen P et al: Emergency medicine concepts and clinical practice, St Louis, 1998, Mosby, p 2790 and 2794.)*

What To Do:

✔ Attempt identification of the mite by placing mineral oil over 5 or 6 nonexcoriated papules or vesicles at the proximal end of a track and scraping them with a #15 scalpel blade onto a microscope slide. Examine under low magnification for the mite, its oval eggs, or fecal concretions. If the clinical picture is convincing, especially if there is someone else at home (a source) who is itching, treatment should be instituted without the help of microscopic examination, or even in the face of negative scrapings.

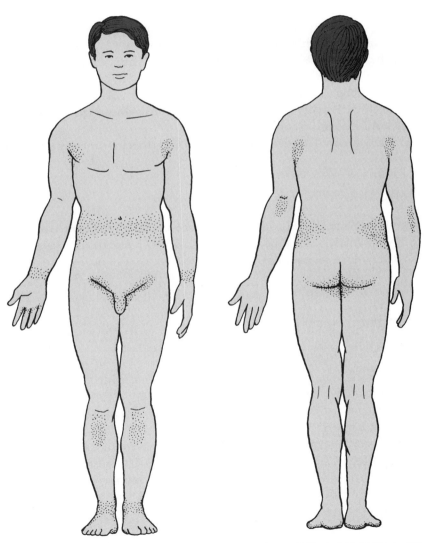

Figure 172-2 Characteristic distribution of scabies lesions. *(From Goldstein BG, Goldstein AO: Practical dermatology, ed 2, St Louis, 1997, Mosby.)*

✔ **Prescribe prescription-strength permethrin (Elimite) 5% insecticidal cream 60 g for the patient to massage from his neck to the soles of his feet and have him leave it on for 8 to 14 hours before washing it off.** An alternative therapy is crotamiton (Eurax) 10%, which is applied but initially not washed off, repeated at 24 hours, then washed off at 48 hours. Less safe but a third the cost and still effective if used correctly is lindane (Kwell) lotion 1%, which is left on for 24 hours. **Mites tend to persist in subungual areas, so have the patient trim fingernails, scrub beneath them, and then apply one of the above scabicides under the nails. If available, an alternative is ivermectin (Mectizan) 200 mcg/kg in one oral dose.**

✔ Tell the patient that the itching will not go away at once and that this does not mean the treatment was ineffective. Dead mites and eggs continue to itch as they are absorbed by the body. **An antipruritic agent such as hydroxyzine (Atarax, Vistaril) 25 to 50 mg q6h can be prescribed for comfort. Adding a short course of oral prednisone may be most effective when pruritus is severe.**

✔ Clothing, bedding, and towels should be washed with hot water or dry cleaned to prevent reinfection. **Family members, frequent household guests, and sexual contacts should also be treated.**

✔ Reexamine patients 1 to 2 weeks after initiating therapy to ensure that there is not a recurrence.

What Not To Do:

✗ Do not use lindane (Kwell) on infants, young children, pregnant women, or in widespread "Norwegian" scabies, because enough of this pesticide may be absorbed percutaneously to produce seizures or CNS toxicity.

 DISCUSSION

Scabies is caused by infestation with the mite *Sarcoptes scabiei*. The female mite, which is just visible to the human eye, excavates a burrow in the stratum corneum and travels about 2 mm a day for about 1 to 2 months before dying. During this time she lays eggs that reach maturity in about 3 weeks.

Scabies is transmitted principally through close personal contact, but may be transmitted through clothing, linens, or towels. Severe pruritus is probably caused by an acquired sensitivity to the organism and is first noted 2 to 4 weeks after primary infestation.

Less than 25% of cases show the characteristic 2 to 3 mm serpiginous tracks. Immunocompromised patients are prone to crusted "Norwegian" scabies rather than the classic inflammatory papules and vesicles. This form may involve the palms and soles and may not itch.

172

Sea Bather's Eruption (Sea Lice)

Presentation

Patients seek help because of an intense pruritic eruption of red welts like mosquito bites, appearing in areas that had been covered by their swimwear, within a few hours after bathing in the Caribbean or off the coasts of Mexico, Florida, or Long Island. Symptoms usually resolve spontaneously in a few days; however, some individuals (especially children) experience a more severe delayed hypersensitivity reaction occurring 10 days after exposure. This rash extends to exposed areas of the body not previously affected, and victims may also experience severe itching, fatigue, fever, chills, nausea, and headache. Outbreaks occur between March and August, with a peak incidence in May.

What To Do:

✔ Inform the patient about the nature of this rash and that it will usually last for 3 to 5 days.

✔ **Prescribe a topical steroid in combination with a topical anesthetic to be applied tid-qid. Pramosone cream or lotion 2.5% is supplied in 1- and 2-ounce tubes and bottles of 2, 4, and 8 fluid ounces.**

✔ **Prescribe an oral antihistamine such as hydroxyzine (Atarax, Vistaril) 25 to 50 mg qid for itching.**

✔ **If systemic symptoms are present or if the rash is extensive and severe, prescribe 3 to 4 days of a systemic steroid like prednisone 40 to 60 mg qd.**

✔ Wash swimwear in detergent and fresh water and dry before wearing again. Without washing and drying, unreleased nematodes can fire, producing lesions without additional exposure to ocean water.

✔ Instruct the patients about future prevention by either avoiding ocean bathing during known outbreaks, or by immediately removing their swimwear after sea bathing and then showering. Showering with fresh water while still wearing swimwear may cause a discharge of nematocysts and worsening of symptoms.

469

What Not To Do:

✗ Do not prescribe systemic steroids to patients who have contraindications. This is a self-limiting condition.

 DISCUSSION

Sea bather's eruption typically occurs 4 to 24 hours after exposure, although some persons may develop a "prickling" sensation or urticarial lesions while still in the water. The larvae of a jellyfish, *Linuche unguiculata,* is implicated as the cause. Water flows through bathing suits and traps larvae, which discharge nematocysts when they contact skin. Lesions also occur on uncovered skin surfaces subjected to friction, like axillae and inner thighs. Surfers develop lesions on the chest and abdomen that were in contact with surfboards. Sea lice do not infest humans.

Cercarial dermatitis or "swimmer's itch" is a different condition that occurs sporadically in fresh water as well as ocean water, in exposed skin rather than under bathing suits, and is thought to be caused by an avian schistosome, *Microbilharzia variglandis.*

SUGGESTED READINGS

Tomchik RS, Russell MT, Szmant AM, et al: Clinical perspectives on seabather's eruption, also known as "sea lice," *JAMA* 269:1669–1672, 1993.

Sliver, Superficial

Presentation

The patient has caught himself on a sharp splinter (usually wooden) and either cannot grasp it, has broken it trying to remove it, or has found that it is too large and painful to remove. The history may be somewhat obscure. On examination, a puncture wound should be found with a tightly embedded sliver that may or may not be palpable over its entire length (Figure 173-1). There may only be a puncture wound without a clearly visible or palpable foreign body.

What To Do:

✔ Obtain a careful history. Find out if the patient has any foreign body sensation. Be suspicious of all puncture wounds (especially on the foot) that have been caused by a wooden object.

✔ **If it is unclear whether a wooden foreign body is beneath the skin, order a high-resolution ultrasound study employing a linear array transducer that focuses in the near field-of-view. CT scanning can be used to detect deep wooden foreign bodies when ultrasound has failed.**

✔ **If the sliver is visible or easily palpated, locally infiltrate with 1% lidocaine (Xylocaine) with epinephrine and clean the skin with povidone-iodine solution. With proper lighting, and using a #15 scalpel blade, cut down over the entire length of the sliver, completely exposing it. The sliver can now be easily lifted out and completely removed. Cleanse the track with normal saline or 1% povidone-iodine on a gauze sponge.** Debride contaminated tissue if necessary (Figure 173-2).

✔ If the sliver is not visible or easily palpable but it seems to be relatively superficial and buried within subcutaneous tissue, try excising the surrounding tissue, although this should rarely be required. First, when possible, create a bloodless field by using a tourniquet or self-retaining retractors in combination with lidocaine with epinephrine. Make a narrow oval incision on the skin surface surrounding the puncture site. Undermine the outer wound edges and then excise the central skin plug along with the subcutaneous tissue containing the foreign body. Make certain that the entire wooden fragment has been recovered.

✔ **Close the wound with sutures or wound closure strips.** Avoid sutures, especially absorbable buried sutures, when possible because of the increased risk of infection.

✔ Give tetanus prophylaxis, if necessary (see Chapter 151).

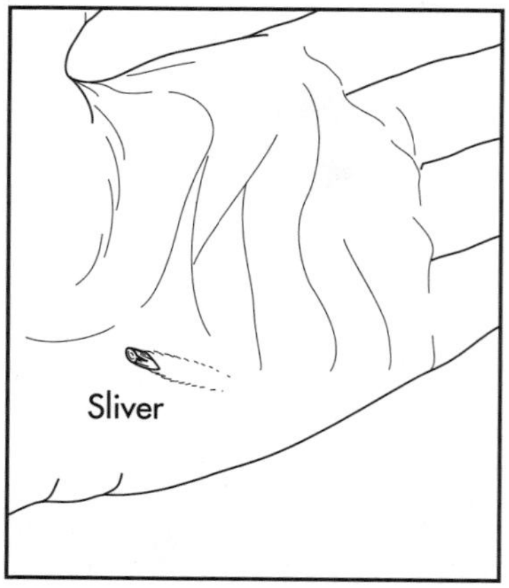

Figure 173-1 Sliver visible.

Sliver

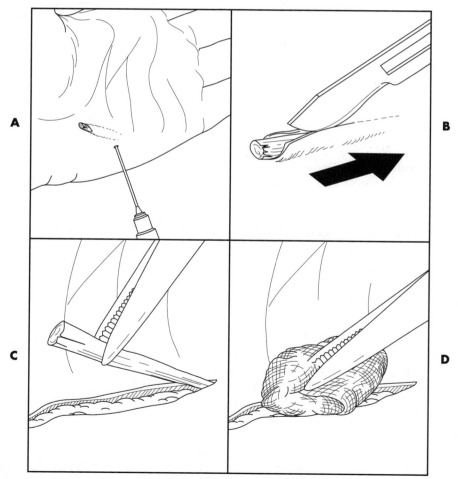

Figure 173-2 A, Injection with anesthetic. **B,** Incision down to sliver. **C,** Lift out with forceps.
D, Clean track with wet gauze fluff.

✔ Warn the patient about the signs of infection and schedule a 48-hour wound check. Prophylactic antibiotics are generally not required.

What Not To Do:

✗ Do not order plain radiographs. Wooden foreign bodies are radiolucent. After 1 day absorbing water from adjacent tissue, they tend to be isodense on xerography and tomography. In addition, cactus and sea urchin spines, thorns, plastic, and aluminum all tend to be difficult to visualize on plain radiographs.

✗ Do not try to pull the sliver out by one end. It is likely to break and leave a fragment behind.

✗ Do not try to locate a foreign body in a bloody field.

✗ Do not make an incision across a neurovascular bundle, tendon, or other important structure.

✗ Do not attempt to remove a deep, poorly localized foreign body. Those cases should be referred to a surgeon for removal in the OR, perhaps with fluoroscopic or ultrasound guidance.

✗ Do not rely entirely on ultrasound to rule out the possibility of a retained foreign body.

✗ Do not be lulled into a false sense of security because the patient thinks the entire sliver has already been removed. This is often not the case.

DISCUSSION

The most common error in the management of soft tissue foreign bodies is failure to detect their presence. An organic foreign body is almost certain to create an inflammatory response and become infected if any part of it is left beneath the skin. It is for this reason, along with the fact that wooden slivers tend to be friable and may break apart during removal, that complete exposure is generally necessary before the sliver can be taken out. Of course, very small and superficial slivers can be removed by loosening them and picking them out with a #18-gauge needle, avoiding the more elaborate technique previously described. When only the outer skin layers are involved, reassuring the patient and gently manipulating the wound can usually obviate the need for anesthesia.

If the foreign body is thought to be relatively superficial but cannot be located, explain to the patient that by exploring and excising any further more harm may be caused, and therefore the splinter will be watched until it forms a "pus pocket," thus making it more easily removed at a later time. If this procedure is followed, it should always be coordinated with a follow-up surgeon. The patient should be placed on an antibiotic and provided with follow-up care within 48 hours.

When making an incision over a foreign body, always take the underlying anatomic structures into consideration. Never make an incision if there is any chance that a neurovascular bundle, tendon, or other important structure may be severed.

When a patient returns after being treated for a puncture wound, and there is evidence of nonhealing or recurrent exacerbations of inflammation, infection, or drainage, assume that the wound still contains a foreign body, begin antibiotics, and refer him for surgical consultation.

174

Subcutaneous Foreign Body

Presentation

Small, moderate-velocity metal fragments can be released when a hammer strikes a second piece of metal, such as a chisel. The patient has noticed a stinging sensation and a small puncture wound or bleeding site and is worried that there might be something inside. A BB shot will produce a more obvious but very similar problem. Another mechanism for producing radio-opaque foreign bodies includes punctures with glass shards, especially by stepping on glass fragments or receiving them in a motor vehicle accident. Physical findings will show a puncture wound and may show an underlying, sometimes palpable, foreign body.

What To Do:

✔ Be suspicious of a retained foreign body in all wounds produced by a high-velocity missile or sharp fragile object. The most common error in the management of soft tissue foreign bodies is failure to detect their presence.

✔ **X-ray the wound to document the presence and location of the suspected foreign body.** Explain how difficult it often is to remove a small metal fleck and that often these are left in without any problem (like shrapnel injuries).

✔ Inform the patient that a simple technique will be attempted, but that in order to avoid more damage, the search will not extend beyond 15 to 20 minutes.

✔ **If the foreign body is in an extremity, then it is preferable, and sometimes essential, to establish a bloodless field.**

✔ **Anesthetize the area with a small infiltration of 1% lidocaine (Xylocaine) with epinephrine (avoid tissue swelling).**

✔ **Take a blunt stiff metal probe (not a needle) and gently slide it down the apparent track of the puncture wound. Move the probe back and forth, fanning it in all directions, until a clicking contact between the probe and the foreign body can be felt and heard.** This should be repeated several times until it is certain that contact is being made with the foreign body (Figure 174-1).

✔ **After contact is made, fix the probe in place** by resting the hand holding the probe against a firm surface and then, with the other hand, **cut down along the probe with**

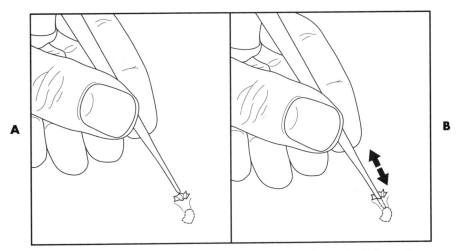

Figure 174-1 A, Puncture wound. **B,** Fan probe until foreign body is struck.

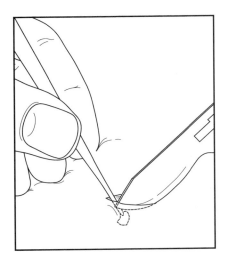

Figure 174-2 Cut down probe to foreign body.

a #15 scalpel blade until the foreign body is reached. Do not remove the probe (Figure 174-2).

✔ **Reach into the incision with a pair of forceps and remove the foreign body (located at the end of the probe)** (Figure 174-3).

✔ Close the wound with strip closures or sutures.

✔ If the track is relatively long and the foreign body is very superficial and easily palpable beneath the skin, then it may be advantageous to eliminate the probe and just cut down directly over the foreign body.

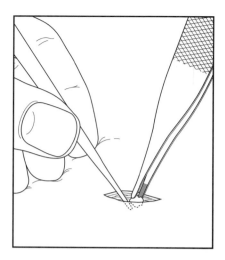

Figure 174-3 Foreign body removed with forceps while probe remains in contact with it.

✔ If the entrance wound is large, a hemostat may be inserted using a spreading technique to search for and then remove the foreign body.

✔ Provide tetanus prophylaxis (see Chapter 151).

✔ Warn the patient about signs of developing infection.

✔ If the foreign body cannot be located in 15 to 20 minutes, inform the patient that in the case of a small metal fleck the wound will probably heal without any problem. It may migrate to the skin surface over a period of months or years, at which time it can be more easily removed. Should the wound become infected, it can be successfully treated with an antibiotic, and the foreign body can be more easily removed if a small abscess forms. Patients with glass, sea shell fragments, gravel, or other potentially harmful objects embedded subcutaneously should have them removed as soon as possible and will require surgical consultation or referral if they cannot be located and removed. Always inform the patient and document when a retained foreign body is suspected.

✔ **Ultrasonography is the most reliable method for detecting radiolucent, superficial foreign bodies and may be used for guidance in their retrieval.** The 7.5 MHz probe should be used for small objects suspected to be superficial in nature, whereas the 5.0 MHz probe should be used for larger, deeper objects. The linear scan is best for initially locating the foreign body, while the sector scan may be easier to use as a guide in retrieval. Note that a negative ultrasound does not reliably rule out the possibility of a retained subcutaneous foreign body.

✔ Always provide the patient with a physician who can perform the necessary follow-up care.

✔ Schedule a wound check within 48 hours or warn the patient about signs of infection.

What Not To Do:

✗ Do not disregard a patient's suspicion that a foreign body may be present, especially when glass or wood may have been involved.

✘ Do not cut down on the metal probe if there is any possibility of cutting across a neurovascular bundle, tendon, or other important structure.

✘ Do not attempt to cut down to the foreign body unless it is very superficial and there is a probe in place and in contact with the foreign body.

✘ Do not blindly grab something in a wound with a hemostat. An important anatomic structure may be damaged.

 ## DISCUSSION

Any patient who complains of a foreign body sensation should be assumed to have one, even in the face of negative x-rays.

Almost all glass is visible on plain x-rays, but small fragments, between 0.5 and 2.0 mm, may not be visible, even when left and right oblique projections are added to the standard PA and lateral views.

X-rays are usually of little value in accurately locating metallic flecks. Even when skin markers are used, because of variances in the angle of the x-ray beam to the film, relative to the skin marker and foreign body, the apparent location of the foreign body is often significantly different from the real location. An incision made over the apparent location therefore usually produces no foreign body. Needle localization under fluoroscopy may be required for those objects that must be removed, if the simple probe technique described fails to deliver the foreign body.

If removal of a metallic object is attempted and a strong eye magnet is available, it can be substituted for the probe described earlier. First, enlarge the entrance wound and then, after contact with the magnet, the object can be dissected out or even pulled out with the magnet.

Moderate-velocity, metallic foreign bodies rarely travel deeply into the subcutaneous tissue, but a potentially serious injury must be considered when these objects strike the eye. A specialized orbital CT scan may be obtained in these cases. An MRI is better at detecting nonmetallic foreign bodies within the orbit or globe of the eye.

SUGGESTED READINGS

Chisholm CD, Wood CO, Chua G, et al: Radiographic detection of gravel in soft tissue, *Ann Emerg Med* 29:725-730, 1997.

Courter BJ: Radiographic screening for glass foreign bodies—what does a "negative" foreign body series really mean? *Ann Emerg Med* 19:997-1000, 1990.

Ginsburg MJ, Ellis GL, Flom LL: Detection of soft-tissue foreign bodies by plain radiography, xerography, computed tomography and ultrasonography, *Ann Emerg Med* 19:701-703, 1990.

Manthey DE, Storrow AB, Milburn JM, et al: Ultrasound versus radiography in the detection of soft tissue foreign bodies, *Ann Emerg Med* 28:7-9, 1996.

Montano JB, Steele MT, Watson WA: Foreign body retention in glass-caused wounds, *Ann Emerg Med* 21:1360-1363, 1992.

Schlager D, Sanders AB, Wiggins D, et al: Ultrasound for the detection of foreign bodies, *Ann Emerg Med* 20:189-191, 1991.

Turner J, Wilde CH, Hughes KC, et al: Ultrasound-guided retrieval of small foreign objects in subcutaneous tissue, *Ann Emerg Med* 29:731-734, 1997.

175 Sunburn

Presentation

Patients generally seek help only if their sunburn is severe. There will be a history of extended exposure to sunlight or to an artificial source of ultraviolet radiation, such as a sunlamp. The burns will be accompanied by intense pain, and the patient will not be able to tolerate anything touching the skin. There may be systemic complaints of "sun poisoning" that include nausea, vomiting, chills, and fever. The affected areas are erythematous and are accompanied by mild edema. The more severe the burn, the earlier it will appear and the more likely it will progress to edema and blistering.

What To Do:

✔ Inquire as to whether or not the patient is using a photosensitizing drug (e.g., tetracyclines, thiazides, sulfonamides, phenothiazines, sulfonylurea hypoglycemic agents, griseofulvin) and have the patient discontinue its use and avoid the sun for at least 3 weeks.

✔ **Have the patient apply cool compresses of skim milk and water or Burow's solution** (Domeboro Powder Packets, two pkts in 1 pint of water) as often as desired to relieve pain. This is the most comforting therapy.

✔ **NSAIDs such as ibuprofen (Motrin) 800 mg tid or naproxen (Naprosyn) 500 mg bid will help reduce pain and inflammation. When pain is severe, prescribe narcotics like hydrocodone or oxycodone.**

✔ Suggest an emollient such as Lubriderm or cold cream for topical treatment. The patient may also be helped by a topical steroid spray such as dexamethasone (Decaspray), although some investigators have not found topical steroids to be of any significant value. Most recommend not using them unless there is a coexistent contact dermatitis.

✔ **With a more severe burn, especially with the systemic symptoms of "sun poisoning," prescribe a short course of systemic steroids (50 to 100 mg of prednisone qd × 3 days) to reduce inflammation, swelling, pain, and itching.** Add a mild sedative like hydroxyzine (Vistaril) 50 mg qid.

✔ **Instruct the patient to avoid the sun for a minimum of 3 weeks.**

What Not To Do:

✘ Do not allow the patient to use OTC sunburn medications that contain local anesthetics (benzocaine, dibucaine, or lidocaine). They are usually ineffective or only provide very transient relief. In addition, there is the potential hazard of sensitizing the patient to these ingredients.

✘ Do not trouble the patient with unnecessary burn dressings. These wounds have a very low probability of becoming infected. Treatment should be directed at making the patient as comfortable as possible.

✘ Do not overlook toxic shock syndrome in the hypotensive patient with fever, diarrhea, vomiting, altered mental status, or abnormal liver functions. The rash looks like a sunburn.

 DISCUSSION

With sunburn, the onset of symptoms is usually delayed for 2 to 8 hours. Maximum discomfort usually occurs after 14 to 20 hours, and symptoms last between 24 and 72 hours.

Patients should be instructed on the future use of sunscreens containing paraaminobenzoic acid (PABA) (e.g., Pabanol and PreSun). The majority of ultraviolet carcinogenic skin damage occurs by 18 years of age, making it especially important that children use protective sunscreen with a sun protective factor (SPF) of at least 15, to decrease the incidence of skin cancer later in life. Common glass and most clothing (except wet light cotton) are also good sunscreens. Prophylactic use of aspirin before sun exposure has also been recommended.

176 Tick Removal

Presentation

The patient arrives with a tick attached to the skin, often the scalp, often frightened or disgusted and concerned about developing Lyme disease, Rocky Mountain spotted fever (RMSF), or "tick fever."

What To Do:

✔ **Promptly remove the tick. Grasp the tick as close to the skin as possible with a pair of narrow-tipped forceps and slowly pull up until the tick mouth parts separate from the skin** (Figure 176-1). Be careful not to squeeze the tick's body. Alternatively, the tick's jaws may be pried away from the skin using a 20-gauge needle tip as a wedge.

✔ **After removal of the tick, disinfect the attachment site and wash your hands with soap and water.** Dispose of the tick in a container of alcohol or flush it down the toilet after it has been properly identified.

✔ **If the mouth parts appear to remain embedded, anesthetize the area with an infiltration of 1% Xylocaine and use a #10 scalpel blade to scrape (dermabrade) these fragments away.**

✔ Instruct the patient or family to record the patient's temperature daily for the next 2 weeks and to notify a physician or return at the first sign of a fever.

✔ If any rash, fever, cranial or peripheral neuropathies, or systemic symptoms such as headache, myalgia, malaise, sweats, chills, or joint pains occur during the initial visit or subsequently, evaluate for possible tick-borne illness and initiate treatment.

✔ **If this was a 5-mm *Ixodes* or deer tick** (Figure 176-2), **which was attached for more than 24 to 48 hours, consider prescribing antibiotics to prevent Lyme disease** (doxycycline 100 mg bid × 10 days, amoxicillin 500 mg tid × 10 days, or azithromycin 500 mg, then 250 mg qd × 4 days). Instruct the family to watch for a pink patch at the site, which could be the beginning of erythema chronicum migrans. Transmission of the infecting organism, *Borrelia burgdorferi,* occurs in about 10% of bites by infected ticks. If the risk of Lyme disease in the area is greater than 1%, these prophylactic antibiotics may be appropriate.

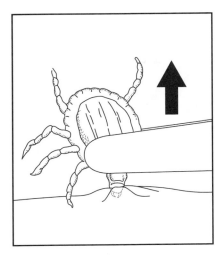

Figure 176-1 Remove tick with narrow-tipped forceps.

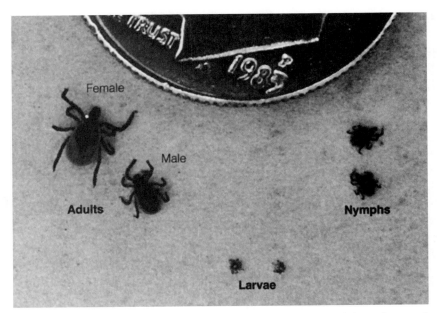

Figure 176-2 Three phases in the life cycle of *Ixodes*. (*From Marzouk JB: Tick-borne diseases: where to expect and how to detect such bite-caused syndromes,* Consultant *June 1985, p 21.*)

✔ **If this was a 1–cm *Dermacentor* or *Amblyomma* tick** (Figure 176-3), **reassure the patient and family that the likelihood of developing RMSF is very small** (1%), and that if it should occur, prompt treatment will be quite effective upon development of fever. It is counterproductive to give prophylactic antibiotics in an attempt to prevent RMSF.

481

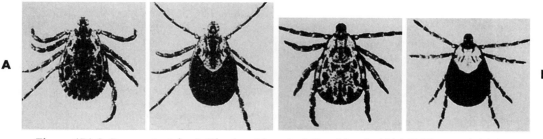

Figure 176-3 *Dermacentor* ticks. **A,** The dog tick, male *(left)* and female *(right).* **B,** The wood tick, male *(left)* and female *(right). (Courtesy Dr. RA Cooley, US Public Health Service, Hamilton, Montana.)*

What Not To Do:

✗ Do not use heat, occlusion, or caustics to remove a tick. A multitude of techniques have been promoted, but they may only increase the chance of infection.

✗ Do not contaminate fingers with potentially infected tick products.

✗ Do not mutilate the skin attempting to remove the tick's "head." Usually what is seen left behind is cementum secreted by the tick, which is easily scraped off.

✗ Do not prescribe prophylactic antibiotics for RMSF.

✗ Do not prescribe prophylactic antibiotics for Lyme disease if its prevalence is low or if the tick was attached less than 24 to 48 hours.

✗ Do not initiate serologic testing in the asymptomatic patient. It is costly and unnecessary.

 DISCUSSION

Ixodes scapularis (previously *Ixodes dammini*) (Figure 176-4), the tiny deer tick of the Eastern United States, and *Ixodes pacificus* of the Western United States can carry babesiosis, human granulocytic ehrlichiosis, and Lyme disease. Lyme disease is usually transmitted by ticks in the nymph stage, when they are tiny and likely to be missed. Unfortunately, nymphs are most active from May through August, just when people are most likely to be outdoors.

Dermacentor variabilis, the dog tick, is the major vector of RMSF, which is also carried by *D. andersoni,* the western wood tick, and *Amblyomma americanum,* the Lone Star tick. *A. americanum* has particularly long mouth parts, and its larvae are also capable of infesting human hosts. Other diseases carried by ticks include tick paralysis (usually cured by removing the tick), Colorado tick fever, relapsing fever, Q fever, and tularemia (Figure 176-5).

People in high-risk areas can minimize exposure by avoiding heavily wooded areas, wearing long-sleeved shirts and long trousers, tucking pants cuffs into boots or socks, wearing light-colored clothes that will not hide ticks, and checking diligently for ticks on clothing and skin each day. Applying repellents containing permethrin to clothing and DEET to skin also reduces risk but follow the manufacturer's instructions, especially when applying DEET to children. Special graspers for removing ticks are available and can be handy in the field.

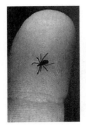

Figure 176-4 Life-size deer tick. *(From Gorman C: Deer tick turn deadly,* Time *July 24, 1995, p 56.)*

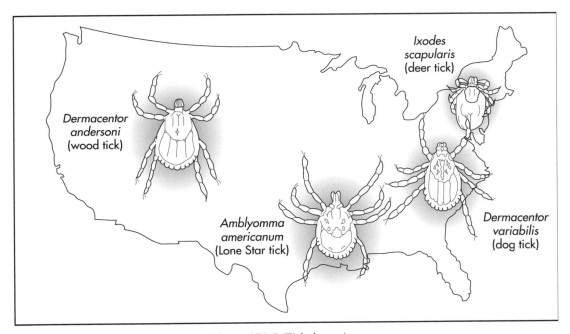

Ixodes
scapularis
(deer tick)

Dermacentor
andersoni
(wood tick)

Amblyomma
americanum
(Lone Star tick)

Dermacentor
variabilis
(dog tick)

Figure 176-5 Ticks by region.

SUGGESTED READINGS

Kirkland KB, Wilkinson WE, Sexton DJ: Therapeutic delay and mortality in cases of Rocky Mountain spotted fever, *Clin Infect Dis* 20:1118-1121, 1995.

Magid D, Schwartz B, Craft J, Schwartz JS: Prevention of Lyme disease after tick bites, *N Engl J Med* 327:534-541, 1992. (letters NEJM 1993;328:1418-1420.)

Nadelman RB, Nowakowski J, Forseter G, et al: The clinical spectrum of early Lyme borreliosis in patients with culture-confirmed erythema migrans, *Am J Med* 100:502-508, 1996.

Needham GR: Evaluation of five popular methods for tick removal, *Pediatrics* 75:997-1002, 1985.

chapter

177

Tinea (Athlete's Foot, Jock Itch, Ringworm)

Presentation

Patients usually seek medical care for "athlete's foot," "jock itch," or "ringworm" (Figure 177-1) when pruritus is severe or when secondary infection causes pain and swelling. *Tinea pedis* is usually seen as interdigital scaling, maceration, and fissuring between toes. At times, tense, pruritic, inflamed vesicular lesions spread to dorsal or plantar surfaces. *Tinea cruris* is usually a moist, mildly erythematous eruption, symmetrically affecting both groin and upper inner thigh but sparing the scrotum and penis. *Tinea corporis* appears most often on the hairless skin of children as dry erythematous patchy lesions with sharp annular and arciform borders that are elevated, scaling, or vesicular, while the center of the ring shows progressive clearing.

What To Do:

✔ When microscopic examination of skin scrapings in potassium hydroxide is readily available, definite identification of the lesion can be made by looking for the presence of hyphae or spores. Using a #10 scalpel blade, scrape flakes or scales from the active border of the lesion onto a glass slide. Sweep the particles towards the center of the slide and add a drop of 10% to 20% KOH and a cover slip. Warm with a flame and then view under low (100×) magnification with the microscope light condenser lowered. Branching fungal filaments (hyphae and myceliae) identify superficial dermatophytes. Budding cells and pseudohyphae ("spaghetti and meatballs") suggest yeast, particularly *Candida* organisms. Fungal cultures are rarely necessary for acute, uncomplicated lesions. Treatment can be started presumptively when microscopic examination is not easily accomplished, but always consider the "herald patch" of pityriasis rosea (see Chapter 168), seborrheic dermatitis, psoriasis, impetigo (see Chapter 164), and neurodermatitis in the differential diagnosis.

✔ **Clotrimazole (Lotrimin) and miconazole (Micatin) are available over the counter. Naftifine (Naftin), terbinafine (Lamisil), oxiconazole (Oxistat), and ciclopirox (Loprox) require a prescription. Either as a lotion or a cream, if applied to the rash bid, they will cause involution of most superficial lesions within 2 to 3 weeks.** Advise the patient to apply the topical medication 2 cm past the border of the skin lesion. **More severe lesions can be treated with fluconazole (Diflucan)**

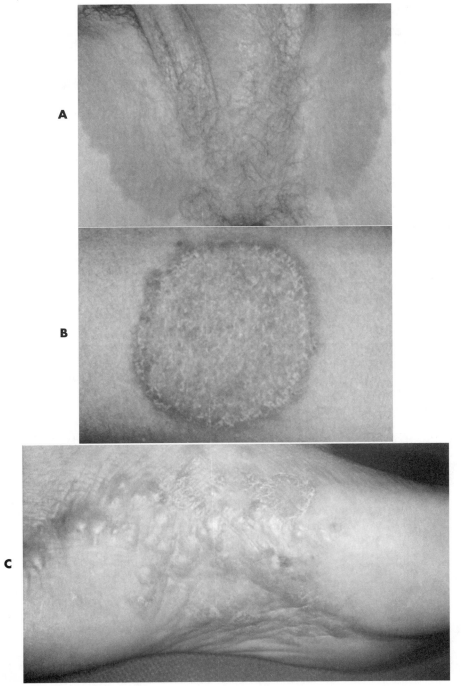

Figure 177-1 **A,** Jock itch. **B,** Ringworm. **C,** Athlete's foot. *(From Litz JZ:* Emerg Med *30(4):68-93, 1998.)*

150 mg once a week for 1 to 4 weeks (see the PDR® for adverse side effects and interactions).

✔ **With signs of secondary infection, begin treatment first with wet compresses of Burow's solution** (2 pkts of Domeboro powder in 1 pint water) for one half hour every 3 to 4 hours. With signs of deep infection (cellulitis, lymphangitis) begin systemic antibiotics in addition, like cefadroxil (Duricef) 1 g qd × 5 to 7 days, cephalexin (Keflex) or dicloxacillin (Dynapen) 250 to 500 mg tid × 5 to 7 days, or azithromycin (Zithromax) 500 mg, then 250 mg qd × 4 days.

✔ **With inflammation and weeping lesions, a topical antifungal and steroid cream such as Lotrisone in addition to the compresses will be most effective.** Warn patients that this medication has a potent steroid that can lead to skin atrophy or striae if used for an extended period, especially in the groin.

✔ For tinea pedis, instruct patients to wear nonocclusive footwear like sandals that allow the foot to "breathe." Have them put on socks before underwear to avoid spreading the fungus from feet to groin. For tinea cruris, suggest loose undergarments made of absorbent materials like cotton rather than synthetics. Skin should be dried well with a towel or hair dryer. Absorbent powders and drying agents such as Zeasorb-AF and Drysol can be applied lightly.

What Not To Do:

✘ Do not attempt to treat fungal infections of the scalp (tinea capitis) with local therapy. A boggy swelling (tinea kerion) or patchy hair loss with inflammation and scaling requires systemic antifungals like griseofulvin.

✘ Do not treat with corticosteroids alone. They will reduce signs and symptoms, but allow increased fungal growth.

 DISCUSSION

Tinea infections are caused by superficial fungi known as dermatophytes, which are true saprophytes that take all their nutrients from dead keratin in the stratum corneum of the skin and the keratinized tissue of hair and nails. They cannot invade live epidermis.

Tinea pedis or athlete's foot is the most common fungal infection. It is seen most in populations that wear occlusive footwear because shoes promote warmth and sweating that encourage fungal growth. Tinea must be differentiated from allergic and irritant contact dermatitis (see Chapter 153).

Candidiasis and erythrasma may resemble tinea cruris, but candidiasis is usually more moist, red, and tender. Pustules may be seen within the indistinct border, and satellite lesions may be scattered over adjacent skin. Candidiasis also may involve the scrotum or penis, which are usually spared by tinea. *Candida* organisms may be treated topically with naftifine (Naftin), ciclopirox (Loprox), or clotrimazole (Lotrimin, Mycelex).

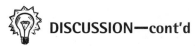

DISCUSSION—cont'd

Erythrasma is a skin infection caused by *Corynebacterium minutissimum,* a gram-positive bacteria. The rash is characteristically asymptomatic, reddish-brown, superficial, dull patches with well-defined margins and no central clearing. The peripheral edge is not usually any more raised than the center (Figure 177-2). When illuminated with an ultraviolet Wood's lamp, the infected skin glows with coral-red fluorescence. Erythrasma is treated with oral erythromycin 250 mg qid × 14 days.

All superficial dermatophytes of the skin, except those involving the scalp, beard, face, hands, feet, groin, and nails, are known as tinea corporis or ringworm of the body. Contact with pets is often the source of the infection. Systemic diseases (e.g., diabetes, leukemia, AIDS) predispose patients to tinea corporis.

Tinea versicolor (Figure 177-3) is a misnomer because it is not caused by a dermatophyte fungus but a lipophilic yeast. Pityriasis versicolor is the more correct name. It is asymptomatic, and its presentation to an acute care facility usually is incidental with some other problem. There is, however, no reason to ignore this chronic superficial skin infection, which causes cosmetically unpleasant, irregular patches of varying pigmentation that tend to be lighter than the surrounding skin in the summer and darker than the surrounding skin in the winter. Wood's light examination sometimes reveals a white or yellow fluorescence. Differential diagnosis includes pityriasis rosea, vitiligo, leprosy, and secondary syphilis. Prescribe a 2.5% selenium sulfide lotion (Selsun) to apply as a lather, leave on 10 minutes, then wash off daily for 7 days or 3 to 5 times a week for 2 to 4 weeks. Alternatively, use keto-conazole (Nizoral) cream 2%, applied daily for 2 weeks, or ketoconazole or fluconazole (Diflucan) as a single 400 mg oral dose (see the PDR® for adverse side effects and interactions). Superficial scaling should resolve in a few days and the pigmentary changes will slowly clear over a period of several months.

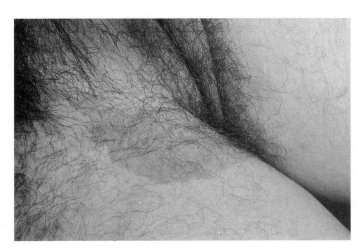

Figure 177-2 Erythrasma. *(From Habif TP: Clinical dermatology: a color guide to diagnosis and therapy, ed 3, St Louis, 1996, Mosby.)*

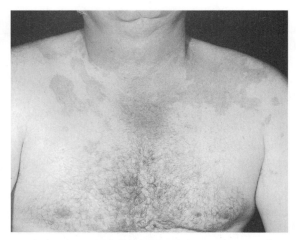

Figure 177-3 Tinea versicolor. *(From Habif TP:* Clinical dermatology: a color guide to diagnosis and therapy, *ed 3, St Louis, 1996, Mosby.)*

178 Urticaria (Hives), Acute

Presentation

The patient is generally very uncomfortable with intense itching. There may be a history of similar episodes and perhaps a known precipitating agent (bee sting, food, or drug). More often the patient will only have a rash. Sometimes this is accompanied by nonpitting edematous swelling of the lips, face, and/or hands (angioedema). In the more severe cases, patients may have wheezing, laryngeal edema, and/or frank cardiovascular collapse (anaphylaxis).

The urticarial rash consists of sharply defined, slightly raised wheals surrounded by erythema and tending to be circular or serpiginous. Each eruption is transient, lasting no more than 8 to 12 hours, but it may be replaced by new lesions in different locations. These eruptions may occur immediately after exposure to an allergen, or they may be delayed for several days. With drug allergies, the initial rash may disappear in 1 to 2 days, but new lesions may reappear for up to 1 week.

What To Do:

✔ **Attempt to elicit a precipitating cause, including drugs, foods, stress, or an underlying infection or illness** (e.g., collagen vascular disease, malignancy, or, when accompanied by arthralgias, anicteric hepatitis or infectious mononucleosis). **Question patients about their use of all drugs, especially antibiotics, aspirin (which they may not think of as a drug or is hidden in Alka-Seltzer), oral contraceptives, foods or drugs containing tartrazine (FD&C yellow dye #5), and aspartame (NutraSweet). Inquire about the foods they have eaten 6 to 12 hours before developing the rash. Pay particular attention to nuts, shellfish, eggs, chocolate, dairy products, and fish, as well as fresh fruits and vegetables.** When angioedema of the lips, tongue, pharynx, and larynx is the predominant finding, consider ACE inhibitors (e.g., Capoten, Vasotec, Lotensin, Prinivil, Zestril, others) as the precipitating cause.

✔ If the cause is identified, it should be removed or avoided. **In food or drug hypersensitivity, avoidance is critical.**

✔ **For immediate relief of severe pruritus, especially if accompanied by systemic symptoms, give 0.3 ml of epinephrine (1:1000) subcutaneously,** this may wear off quickly, and may need to be repeated q20min. Epinephrine adds a number of side effects the patient may find worse than the itching: tachycardia, shaking, dry mouth, wet palms, hypertension, and even angina and very rarely myocardial infarction.

✔ **For relief of itching, administer H1 blockers diphenhydramine (Benadryl) or hydroxyzine (Vistaril, Atarax) 50 mg PO, or IM stat, followed by a prescription for 25 to 50 mg PO qid,** or cyproheptadine hydrochloride (Periactin) 4 mg qid, or cetirizine (Zyrtec) 10 to 20 mg qd for the next 48 to 72 hours.

✔ **To reduce the rash, administer H2 blockers cimetidine (Tagamet) 300 mg IV/IM/PO, ranitidine (Zantac) 50 mg IV or 150 mg PO,** or nizatidine (Axid) 150 to 300 mg PO stat, followed by a prescription of cimetidine 400 mg bid, or ranitidine or nizatidine 150 mg bid for the next 48 to 72 hours.

✔ **To blunt the entire allergic process, give prednisone 60 mg PO stat and prescribe 20 to 50 mg qd for 4 days.** Avoid systemic corticosteroids in patients with diabetes, active peptic ulcers, or other steroid risks.

✔ In resistant cases, the tricyclic antidepressant doxepin (Sinequan) can be used in doses of 10 to 25 mg qd or bid. This drug has activity against both H1 and H2 histamine receptors and is 700 times more potent than diphenhydramine. Sedation is common.

✔ Inform the patient that the cause of hives cannot be determined in the majority of cases. Let her know that the condition is usually of minor consequence but can at times become chronic and, under unusual circumstances, is associated with other illnesses. Therefore, the patient should be provided with elective follow-up care, preferably by an allergist.

✔ Patients who experience a more severe reaction should be given a prescription for injectable epinephrine (Epi-Pen, Ana-Kit, Ana-Guard) that will be available to them at all times.

What Not To Do:

✘ Do not let the patient take aspirin. Some patients experience a precipitation or worsening of their symptoms with the use of aspirin or other NSAIDs. Morphine, codeine, reserpine, and alcohol, as well as certain food additives such as azo food dyes, tartrazine dye, and benzoates, are often allergens or potentiate allergic reactions and should probably also be avoided.

✘ Do not recommend or prescribe topical steroids, topical antihistamines, or topical anesthetic creams or sprays. They are ineffective and have no role in the management of urticaria.

✘ Do not overlook the possibility of an urticarial vasculitis when the presenting rash is more painful than itchy, and there are systemic symptoms like purpura, arthralgias, fever, abdominal pain, and nephritis. Obtain an ESR, consider the diagnosis of systemic lupus erythematosus or Sjögren's syndrome, and consult appropriately.

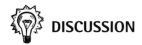 **DISCUSSION**

Urticaria present for less than 6 weeks is termed acute, greater than 6 weeks is considered chronic. Simple urticaria affects approximately 20% of the population at some time. This local reaction is due at least in part to the release of histamines and other vasoactive peptides from mast cells following an IgE-mediated antigen-antibody reaction. This results in vasodilatation and increased vascular permeability, with the leaking of protein and fluid into extravascular spaces. The heavier concentration of mast cells within the lips, face, and hands explains why these areas are more commonly affected.

The ideal treatment for urticaria is identification and elimination of its cause. Because the cause is often obscure, however, only symptomatic treatment may be possible. The spontaneous resolution of symptoms obviates the need for an extensive evaluation. Patients with ACE inhibitor–induced angioedema are usually less responsive to the measures above.

Although the treatment of anaphylactic shock is beyond the scope of this book, when there is airway compromise or hypotension, add airway control and IV fluid therapy to the medications above.

SUGGESTED READINGS

Horan RF, Schneider LC, Sheffer AL: Allergic skin disorders and mastocytosis, *JAMA* 268:2858-2868, 1992.

Kemp SF Lockey RF, Wolf BL, et al: Anaphylaxis: a review of 266 cases, *Arch Intern Med* 155:1749-1754, 1995.

Pollack CV, Romano TJ: Outpatient management of acute urticaria: the role of prednisone, *Ann Emerg Med* 547-551, 1995.

Runge JW, Martinez JC, Caravati EM, et al: Histamine antagonists in the treatment of acute allergic reactions, *Ann Emerg Med* 21:237-242, 1992.

Rusli M: Cimetidine treatment of recalcitrant acute allergic urticaria, *Ann Emerg Med* 15:1363-1365, 1986.

chapter

Zipper Caught on Penis or Chin

Presentation

Usually a child has gotten dressed too quickly and, not wearing underpants, accidentally pulled up penile skin into his zipper. The skin becomes entrapped and crushed between the teeth and the slide of the zipper, thereby painfully attaching the article of clothing to the body part involved (most often the penis or less often the area beneath the chin) (Figure 179-1).

What To Do:

✔ Paint the area with a small amount of povidone-iodine and **infiltrate the skin with 1% buffered lidocaine (plain).** This will allow the comfortable manipulation of the zipper and the article of clothing (Figure 179-2).

✔ **Cover the area with mineral oil. This lubricates the moving parts, and with some traction and manipulation often frees the skin without having to cut the zipper.**

✔ If the mineral oil alone does not work, then cut the zipper away from the article of clothing to leave yourself with a less cumbersome problem.

✔ **Cut the slide of the zipper in half with a pair of metal snips or an orthopedic pin cutter.** The patient is less likely to be frightened if this procedure is kept hidden from his view. **If unable to break the two halves of the slide apart using a metal cutter, then take two heavy-duty surgical towel clamps and place their tongs into the side grooves at both ends of the slide. Grip one clamp firmly in each hand and twist your wrists in opposite directions. This often will pop the two halves of the slide apart, releasing the entrapped skin** (Figure 179-3).

✔ Pull the exposed zipper teeth apart, cleanse the crushed skin, and apply an ointment such as povidone-iodine or bacitracin (Figure 179-4).

✔ Tetanus prophylaxis should be administered as needed (see Chapter 151).

What Not To Do:

✗ Do not cut clothing if mineral oil releases the zipper.

492

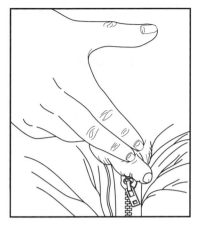

Figure 179-1 Penis caught in zipper.

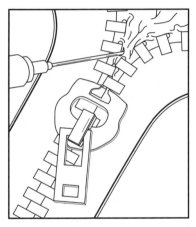

Figure 179-2 Injection of lidocaine.

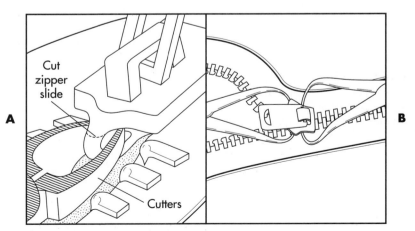

Figure 179-3 Cut zipper slide with a metal snip or an orthopedic pin cutter **(A)** or use two heavy-duty surgical towel clamps **(B)**.

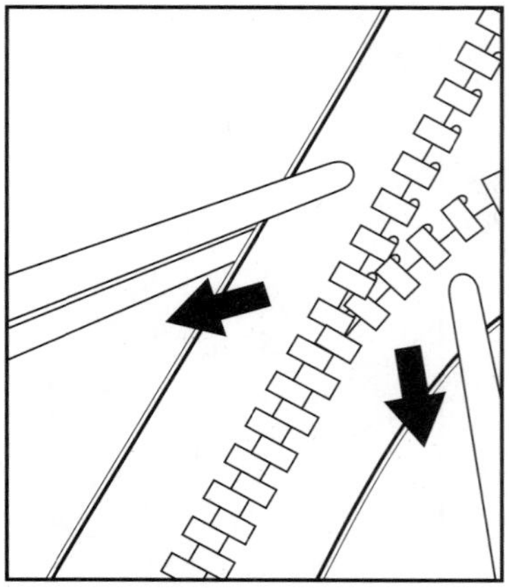

Figure 179-4 Pull exposed zipper teeth apart.

✘ Do not destroy the entire article of clothing by cutting into it. Only the zipper needs to be cut away, allowing repair of the clothing.

✘ Do not excise an area of skin or perform a circumcision; it only creates unnecessary morbidity for the patient.

DISCUSSION

Newer plastic zippers have made this problem less common than in the past, but it still occurs, and it is a very grateful patient who is released from this entrapment.

SUGGESTED READINGS

Kanegaye JT, Schonfeld N: Penile zipper entrapment: a simple and less threatening approach using mineral oil, *Pediatric Emergency Care* 9:90-91, 1993.

Nolan JF, Stillwell TJ, Sands JP: Acute management of the zipper-entrapped penis, *J Emerg Med* 8:305-307, 1990.

Appendixes

Appendix A

Complete Eye Exam

What To Do:

✔ Record visual acuity, using a Snellen (wall) or Jaeger (hand–held) chart first without and then with the patient's own corrective lenses. If glasses are not available, a pinhole will compensate for most refractory errors.

✔ While wearing gloves, inspect the lids, conjunctivae, extraocular movements, and pupillary reflexes.

✔ Use a 10× magnification slit lamp to examine the cornea and anterior chamber; look for any injection of ciliary vessels at the corneal limbus, which indicates iritis. When the slit lamp is stopped down to a pinhole, look for light reflected from protein exudate or suspended white cells in the normally clear aqueous humor of the anterior chamber (a late sign of iritis). Look for red cells (hyphema) or white cells (hypopyon) settling to the bottom of the anterior chamber after the patient has been sitting up for 15 minutes.

✔ Demonstrate the integrity of the corneal epithelium with fluorescein dye, which is taken up by exposed stroma or nonviable epithelium and glows green in ultraviolet or cobalt blue light.

✔ Note the depth of the anterior chamber with tangential lighting.

Appendix B

Digital Block

It is necessary to provide complete anesthesia before treatment of most finger-tip injuries. Many techniques for performing a digital nerve block have been described. The following technique is both effective and rapid in onset. This type of digital block provides anesthesia only distal to the distal interphalangeal joint, the site that most often demands a nerve block.

What To Do:

✔ Cleanse the finger and paint the area with povidone–iodine (Betadine) solution.

✔ Using a 27-gauge needle, slowly inject 1% lidocaine (Xylocaine buffered 10:1 with sodium bicarbonate, no epinephrine) midway between the dorsal and palmar surfaces of the finger at the midpoint of the middle phalanx.

✔ Inject straight in along the side of the periosteum; then pull back without removing the needle from the skin and fan the needle dorsally.

✔ Advance the needle dorsally and inject again. Pull the needle back a second time and, without removing it from the skin, fan the needle in a palmar direction.

✔ Advance the needle and inject the lidocaine in the vicinity of the digital neurovascular bundle (Figure B-1).

✔ With each injection, instill enough lidocaine to produce visible soft tissue swelling.

✔ Repeat this procedure on the opposite side of the finger.

✔ For anesthesia of the proximal finger as well, a similar block may be performed as far proximally as the middle of the metacarpal. There the connective tissue is looser and the needle need not be fanned into digital septa as described earlier. Be prepared to wait 3 to 10 minutes for adequate anesthesia.

✔ With fractures, burns, crush injuries, or other conditions in which the pain will be prolonged, substitute bupivacaine (Marcaine) 0.5% for the lidocaine.

497

What Not To Do:

✘ Do not use lidocaine with epinephrine. The digital arteries are end arteries that can spasm and provide prolonged anesthesia, ischemia, and potential necrosis of the finger tip.

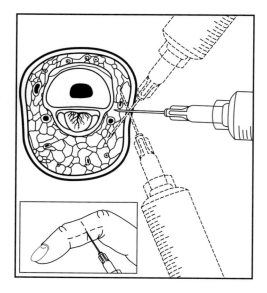

Figure B-1 Needle insertion points for a digital block.

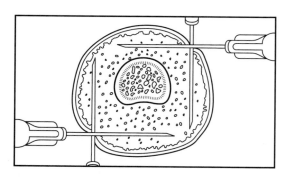

Figure B-2 Needle insertion points for a modified ring block. *(Illustration courtesy of Mary Albury-Noyes. From Gillette RD: Practical management of ingrown toenails,* Postgraduate Medicine *84(8):146, 1998.)*

 DISCUSSION

Digital nerve blocks are often described as being injected at the base of the proximal phalanx, but it is not necessary to block the whole digit when only the distal tip is injured, and the first technique described here provides anesthesia faster. Toes are difficult to separate, and it may be easier to perform a modified ring block at their base (Figure B-2). Over the dorsum of the proximal interphalangeal joint, the connective tissue is loose enough for direct injection of anesthetic with minimal discomfort, and a digital block is not required. Some studies have demonstrated digital anesthesia by injecting 2 ml of buffered lidocaine directly into the flexor tendon sheath, using a 25- or 27-gauge needle at a 45-degree angle at the distal palmar crease of the hand.

Appendix C

Finger-Tip Dressing, Simple

To provide a complete nonadherent compression dressing for an injured finger tip, first cut out an L-shaped segment from a strip of polyurethane or oil-emulsion (Adaptic) gauze. Cover the gauze with antibiotic ointment to provide occlusion and prevent adhesion to the wound surface.

What To Do:

- ✔ Place the tip of the finger over the short leg of the gauze and then fold it over the top of the finger (Figure C-1).
- ✔ Take the long leg of the gauze and wrap it around the tip of the finger.
- ✔ For absorption and compression, fluff a cotton gauze pad and apply it over the end of the finger.
- ✔ Cover with roller or tube gauze and secure with adhesive tape.

What Not To Do:

- ✘ Do not place tight circumferential wraps of tape around a finger, especially if swelling is expected. Such a wrap may act as a tourniquet and lead to vascular compromise. For the same reason, use caution applying tight layers of tube gauze: 3 or 4 layers will suffice.

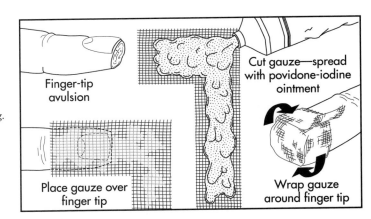

Figure C-1 Simple finger-tip dressing.

Finger-tip avulsion

Place gauze over finger tip

Cut gauze—spread with povidone-iodine ointment

Wrap gauze around finger tip

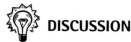 **DISCUSSION**

For small finger-tip injuries or partially healed injuries that allow the patient to apply his own simple dressing, use the two halves of an adhesive strip bandage cut lengthwise and crossed over the finger tip, encircled by a second, uncut strip bandage.

Appendix D

Oral Nerve Blocks

What To Do:

✔ An **inferior alveolar nerve block** provides rapid relief of pain in all teeth on one side of the mandible, the lower lip, and the chin (Figure D-1).

✔ Palpate the retromolar fossa with the index finger and identify the convexity of the mandibular ramus.

✔ Hold the syringe parallel to the occlusal surfaces of the teeth so that its barrel is in line between the first and second premolars on the opposite side of the mandible.

✔ Retract the soft tissue toward the cheek and find the pterygomandibular triangle.

✔ Puncture the triangle, ensuring that the needle passes through the ligaments and muscles of the medial mandibular surface.

✔ Stop advancing the needle when it reaches the bone, withdraw it a few millimeters, aspirate to be sure the tip is not in a vein, and deposit 1 to 2 ml of local anesthetic (e.g., lidocaine 1%, bupivacaine 0.5%).

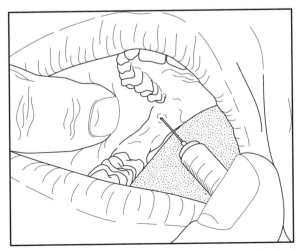

Figure D-1 Needle placement for an oral nerve block.

✔ **Supraperiosteal infiltration** provides intraoral local anesthesia for pain arising from maxillary teeth.

✔ Puncture the mucobuccal fold, holding the bevel of the needle toward the bone, aspirate the area, and then inject 1 to 2 ml of anesthetic near the apex of the affected tooth. This technique usually produces full anesthesia in 5 to 10 minutes. For best results, inject as close as possible to the tooth-bearing maxillary bone (Figure D-2).

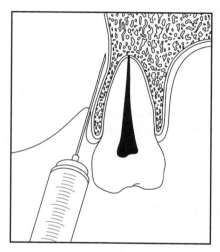

Figure D-2 Schematic illustration of supraperiosteal injection. *(From* Manual of Local Anesthesia in Dentistry. *New York, Cook-Waite Laboratories, Inc. Reprinted courtesy of Eastman Kodak Company.)*

Appendix E

Rabies Prophylaxis

Presentation

A possibly contagious animal has bitten the patient, or the animal's saliva has contaminated an abrasion or mucous membrane.

What To Do:

✔ Clean and debride the wound thoroughly. Irrigate with soap and water or 1% benzalkonium chloride, and rinse with normal saline.

✔ Know the local prevalence of rabies, or ask someone who knows (e.g., local health department).

✔ If the offending animal was an apparently healthy dog or cat, arrange to have the animal confined and observed for 10 days. During that period, an animal infected with rabies will show symptoms. If the animal has symptoms of rabies, it should be euthanized and examined using a fluorescent rabies antibody (FRA) technique. If the FRA test is positive for rabies, the patient must be treated with rabies immune globulin (RIG) and human diploid cell vaccine (HDCV) or another rabies vaccine. If the animal is not available for observation, the decision regarding whether or not to provide rabies prophylaxis depends on the local prevalence of rabies in domestic animals, rodents, and lagomorphs.

✔ An unprovoked attack is more likely than a provoked attack to indicate that the animal is rabid. Bites inflicted on a person attempting to feed or handle an apparently healthy animal should generally be regarded as provoked.

✔ If the patient has been bitten by a wild animal (e.g., bat, coyote, fox, opossum, raccoon, skunk) capable of transmitting rabies, the animal should be caught, killed, and sent to the local public health department for brain examination with immunofluorescence. If the animal did not appear to be healthy or if the bite is on the patient's face, the patient should be started on RIG and HDCV in the meantime. Treatment should be stopped only if the FRA test is negative.

✔ If the offending wild animal is not captured, no matter how normal-appearing, assume it was rabid, and provide a full course of RIG and HDCV.

503

✔ Postexposure prophylaxis should be considered when contact with a bat or a bite from a bat is possible but uncertain, such as when a bat is found near a sleeping person or a previously unattended child and the animal is unavailable for testing.

✔ Provide passive immunity with 20 IU/kg of RIG (Imogam Rabies-HT, BayRab). Infiltrate around the wound (if anatomically feasible) as much as possible and administer the remainder IM in the gluteus. Give two separate injections if the remaining volume is greater than 5 ml. This passive protection has a half-life of 21 days.

✔ Begin immunization with rabies vaccine, HDCV (Imovax), rabies vaccine adsorbed (RVA), or purified chick embryo cell culture (PCEC, RabAvert) 1 ml IM in the deltoid (or the anterolateral thigh in children) at a site distant from the immune globulin.

✔ Make arrangements for repeat doses of rabies vaccine at 3, 7, 14, and 28 days postexposure, and obtain an antibody level after the series.

What Not To Do:

✘ Do not treat the bites of rodents and lagomorphs (hamsters, rabbits, squirrels, rats, etc.) unless rabies is endemic in your area. To date, rodent and lagomorph bites have not caused human rabies in the United States.

✘ Do not omit RIG from treatment. Treatment failures have resulted from giving rabies vaccine alone.

DISCUSSION

The older, duck embryo vaccine (DEV) for rabies required 21 injections and produced more side effects and less of an antibody response than the new HDCV. Sometimes, neurologic symptoms would arise from DEV treatment, raising the agonizing question of whether the symptoms represented early signs of rabies or side effects of the treatment and thus whether treatment should be continued or discontinued. Today it is much easier to initiate immunization with HDCV or a newer rabies vaccine and follow through because side effects are minimal and antibody response is excellent. Roughly 25% of patients experience redness, tenderness, and itching around the injection site, and another 20% experience headache, myalgia, or nausea. The new rabies vaccine that is prepared in purified chick embryo cell culture appears to be as effective as HDCV but does not cause the serum-sickness-like hypersensitivity reactions noted earlier.

Patients with immunosuppressive illness or those taking immunosuppressive medications, corticosteroids, or antimalarials may have an inadequate response to vaccination and require serum antibody assays.

The incubation period of rabies varies from weeks to months, roughly in proportion to the length of the axons up which the virus must propagate to the brain, which is why prophylaxis is especially urgent in facial bites.

Pregnancy is not a contraindication to postexposure prophylaxis.

SUGGESTED READINGS

Kauffman FH, Goldmann BJ: Rabies, *Am J Emerg Med* 4:525–531, 1986.

Noah DL, Drenzek CL, Smith JS, et al: Epidemiology of human rabies in the United States, 1980 to 1996, *Ann Intern Med* 128(11):922–930, 1998.

Appendix F

Regional Poison Control Center Phone Numbers

Many of these centers also have 800 numbers for in-state use only.

Alabama		**Kentucky**	(502) 629-7275	**Oregon**	(503) 494-8968
Birmingham	(205) 939-9201	**Maryland**	(410) 528-7702	**Pennsylvania**	
Tuscaloosa	(205) 345-0600	**Massachusetts**	(617) 232-2120	Hershey	(800) 521-6110
Arizona		**Michigan**	(313) 745-5711	Philadelphia	(215) 386-2100
Phoenix	(602) 253-3334	**Minnesota**		Pittsburgh	(412) 681-6669
Tucson	(602) 626-6016	Minneapolis	(612) 347-3141	**Rhode Island**	(410) 277-5727
California		St Paul	(612) 221-2113	**Texas**	
Fresno	(209) 445-1222	**Missouri**	(314) 772-5200	Dallas	(214) 590-5000
Sacramento	(916) 734-3692	**Montana**	(303) 629-1123	Galveston	(409) 765-1420
San Diego	(619) 543-6000	**Nebraska**	(402) 390-5555	San Antonio	(800) 764-7661
San Francisco	(800) 523-2222	**New Jersey**	(800) 962-1253	**Utah**	(801) 581-2151
Santa Clara	(408) 885-6000	**New Mexico**	(505) 843-2551	**Virginia**	(804) 924-5543
Colorado	(303) 629-1123	**New York**		**West Virginia**	(304) 348-4211
District of Columbia	(202) 625-3333	Hudson Valley	(914) 366-3030	**Wyoming**	(402) 390-5555
Florida		Long Island	(516) 542-2323		
Jacksonville	(904) 549-4480	New York City	(212) 340-4494		
Tampa	(813) 253-4444	**Ohio**			
Georgia	(404) 616-9000	Cincinnati	(513) 558-5111		
Indiana	(317) 929-2323	Columbus	(614) 228-1323		

Index

508

513

517

519